# Handbook of Dermatology
## A Practical Manual

**Margaret W. Mann, MD**
Department of Dermatology
University of California, Irvine
Irvine, California, USA

**David R. Berk, MD**
Division of Dermatology
Washington University
St Louis, Missouri, USA

**Daniel L. Popkin, MD, PhD**
Department of Immunology
The Scripps Research Institute
La Jolla, California, USA

**Susan J. Bayliss, MD**
Division of Dermatology
Washington University
St Louis, Missouri, USA

**WILEY-BLACKWELL**

This edition first published 2009, © 2009 by Margaret W. Mann, David R. Berk, Daniel L. Popkin, and Susan J. Bayliss

Blackwell Publishing was acquired by John Wiley & Sons in February 2007. Blackwell's publishing program has been merged with Wiley's global Scientific, Technical and Medical business to form Wiley-Blackwell.

Registered office: John Wiley & Sons Ltd, The Atrium, Southern Gate, Chichester, West Sussex, PO19 8SQ, UK

Editorial offices:     9600 Garsington Road, Oxford, OX4 2DQ, UK
                       The Atrium, Southern Gate, Chichester, West Sussex, PO19 8SQ, UK
                       111 River Street, Hoboken, NJ 07030-5774, USA

For details of our global editorial offices, for customer services and for information about how to apply for permission to reuse the copyright material in this book please see our website at www.wiley.com/wiley-blackwell

2  2009

Library of Congress Cataloging-in-Publication Data
Handbook of dermatology : a practical manual / Margaret W. Mann ... [et al.].
    p. ; cm.
  Includes bibliographical references and index.
  ISBN 978-1-4051-8110-5 (pbk. : alk. paper)  1. Dermatology—Handbooks, manuals, etc. 2. Skin—Diseases—Handbooks, manuals, etc.  I. Mann, Margaret W.
  [DNLM: 1. Skin Diseases—diagnosis—Handbooks. 2. Skin Diseases—therapy—Handbooks. 3. Dermatologic Agents—therapeutic use—Handbooks. WR 39 H2357  2008]
  RL74.H36  2008
  616.5—dc22                                                                        2008015533

ISBN: 978-1-4051-8110-5

A catalogue record for this book is available from the British Library.

Set in 6.5/8.5 Frutiger by  Macmillan Publishing Solutions
Printed in Singapore by Fabulous Printers Pte Ltd

# Contents

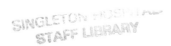

**Part 2  Surgery**

*Color plate section can be found facing page* 208

# Preface

Welcome to the first edition of *Handbook of Dermatology: A Practical Manual*, a pocket guide designed for practicing dermatologists, dermatology residents, medical students, and physicians in other fields who may be interested in dermatology. Written and edited by former residents and attending physicians in the Division of Dermatology at Washington University School of Medicine, this book is based on an in-house resident handbook which has been used by our department for the past five years. Our goal was to compile and consolidate need-to-know dermatologic information for daily use in patient care and resident and fellow education. As such, it represents the indispensable pocket-sized quick reference which we had wanted during our training and which we now use in our practices.

Currently, there are multiple in-depth dermatology textbooks and atlases, most of which are too bulky to be carried around in the clinic. Our manual concisely presents data in outline, bullet-point, and table formats such that information is manageable and easily retrievable. The compact design is lightweight, allowing information to be accessible in seconds during clinics, facilitating patient care. We have tried to balance space limitations with the need to cover a subject in sufficient detail.

Our manual has three main sections — medical dermatology, surgical dermatology, and pharmacology/treatment. Each section is designed to provide the reader with up-to-date, comprehensive yet concise information for patient care. In addition to core material, we sought to consolidate the information which we found ourselves most often looking up, which our attendings most frequently quizzed us on, and which were emphasized on the dermatology board exam. The manual consolidates the dermatologic algorithms, protocols, guidelines, staging and scoring systems which we find most essential. Each section is designed for easy reference, with tabular and graphic information throughout. The diseases covered are those which we frequently encountered in clinic, on call, during teaching conferences, and on board exams.

We hope you will find this manual helpful to you in providing care to your patients. We welcome your input as this manual continues to evolve.

Margaret W. Mann
David R. Berk
Daniel L. Popkin
Susan J. Bayliss

# Dedication

We wish to express our thanks to the many people who have inspired us to write this book and supported us in our careers. Special thanks to the following physicians who contributed to the manuscript: Drs. Paul Klekotka, Alison Klenk, and Neel Patel – who helped make the prototype possible – without you, this manual would never have happened; Drs. Milan Anadkat, Grace Bandow, Amy Cheng, Michael Heffernan, Yadira Hurley, and David Smith for their valuable contributions; Drs. Stacey Tull and Quan Vu for the beautiful drawings; Drs. Senait Dyson, Kristen Kelly, and Anne Lind for their proofreading and comments; and finally Drs. Lynn Cornelius, Arthur Eisen, and all the faculty in the Division of Dermatology at Washington University for their support and encouragement.

Margaret Mann would like to thank her parents and her ever-patient husband, Daniel, for all the love and support over the years.

David Berk wishes to thank his family, especially his wife Melissa and his parents, for their constant support and patience.

Daniel Popkin would like to thank his parents and his wife Margaret.

Susan Bayliss wishes to thank her grandsons Cai and Eli Kenemore, and her daughters Elizabeth Kenemore and Meredith Mallory for all the joy they constantly bring her.

# Abbreviations

| | |
|---|---|
| ACD | allergic contact dermatitis |
| AD | autosomal dominant |
| AFB | acid fast bacilli |
| AK | actinic keratoses |
| ANA | anti-nuclear antibody |
| ANCA | anti-neutrophilic cytoplasmic antibody |
| APS | antiphospholipid syndrome |
| AR | autosomal recessive |
| ASO | antistreptolysin O titer |
| asx | asymptomatic |
| BCC | basal cell carcinoma |
| BID | twice daily |
| BM | bone marrow |
| BMP | basic metabolic panel |
| BMZ | basement membrane zone |
| BP | bullous pemphigoid |
| BP | blood pressure |
| Bx | biopsy |
| $Ca^{++}$ | calcium |
| CAD | coronary artery disease |
| CBC | complete blood count |
| CCB | calcium channel blocker |
| CF | cystic fibrosis |
| cGVHD | chronic graft-versus-host disease |
| CH50 | total hemolytic component |
| CMP | complete metabolic panel |
| CMV | cytomegalovirus |
| CN | cranial nerve |
| CNS | central nervous system |
| CP | cicatricial pemphigoid |
| CR | creatinine |
| CRF | chronic renal failure |
| CRP | C-reactive protein |
| Cryo | cryoglobulinemia |
| CT | computed tomography |
| CTCL | cutaneous T-cell lymphoma |
| CTD | connective tissue disease |
| CVA | cerebral vascular accident |
| Cx | culture |
| CXR | chest X-ray |
| DCN | doxycycline |

| | |
|---|---|
| DEJ | dermal–epidermal junction |
| DF | dermatofibroma |
| DFA | direct fluorescent antibody |
| DFSP | dermatofibrosarcoma protuberans |
| DH | dermatitis herpetiformis |
| DHEA-S | dehydroepiandrosterone sulfate |
| DI | diabetes insipidus |
| DIF | direct immunofluorescence |
| DM | dermatomyositis |
| DM2 | diabetes mellitus type II |
| Dsg | desmoglein |
| Dz | disease |
| EBA | epidermolysis bullosa acquisita |
| EBV | Epstein–Barr virus |
| EDS | Ehlers–Danlos syndrome |
| EED | erythema elevatum diutinum |
| EKG | electrocardiogram |
| EM | electromicroscopy |
| EMG | electromyogram |
| ENA | extractable nuclear antigen |
| eos | eosinophils |
| ESR | erythrocyte sedimentation rate |
| ETOH | alcohol |
| F | fever |
| FLP | fasting lipid panel |
| FMF | Familial Mediterranean fever |
| G6PD | glucose-6-phosphate dehydrogenase |
| GA | granuloma annulare |
| GF | granuloma faciale |
| GI | gastroenterology |
| GVHD | graft-versus-host disease |
| h/o | history of |
| HA | headache |
| HBV | hepatitis B virus |
| HCV | hepatitis C virus |
| HDL | high density lipoprotein |
| Hep | hepatitis |
| HSM | hepatosplenomegaly |
| HSV | herpes simplex virus |
| HTN | hypertension |
| IBD | inflammatory bowel disease |
| IIF | indirect immunofluorescence |
| IL | intralesional |
| IM | intramuscular |

| | |
|---|---|
| IV | intravenous |
| IVIG | intravenous immunoglobulin |
| KOH | potassium hydroxide |
| LAN | lymphadenopathy |
| LCH | Langerhans Cell Histiocytosis |
| LCV | leukocytoclastic vasculitis |
| LDH | lactate dehydrogenase |
| LDL | low density lipoprotein |
| LE | lupus erythematosus |
| LFT | liver function test |
| LN | lymph nodes |
| LP | lichen planus |
| MCN | minocycline |
| MCTD | mixed connective tissue disease |
| MEN | multiple endocrine neoplasia |
| MF | mycosis fungoides |
| MM | malignant melanoma |
| MR | mental retardation |
| MRI | magnetic resonance imaging |
| MTX | metrotrexate |
| nl | normal |
| NLD | necrobiosis lipoidica diabeticorum |
| NSAIDs | non-steroidal anti-inflammatory drugs |
| NXG | necrobiosis xanthogranuloma |
| OCP | oral contraceptive pill |
| OTC | over the counter |
| PAN | polyarteritis nodosa |
| PCN | penicillin |
| PCR | polymerase chain reaction |
| PCT | porphyria cutaneous tarde |
| PET | positron emission tomography |
| PFTs | pulmonary function tests |
| PIH | post inflammatory hyperpigmentation |
| PMLE | polymorphous light eruption |
| PMNs | polymorphonuclear leukocytes |
| po | per oral |
| PPD | tuberculosis skin test |
| PT/PTT | prothrombin time/ partial thromboplastin time |
| PUVA | psoralen + ultraviolet A |
| PV | pemphigus vulgaris |
| QD | once a day |
| QHS | every night |
| QOD | every other day |
| RA | rheumatoid arthritis |

# Part 1
# General Dermatology

*Handbook of Dermatology: A Practical Manual.* By Margaret W. Mann, David R. Berk, Daniel L. Popkin, and Susan J. Bayliss. Published 2009 by Blackwell Publishing, ISBN: 978-1-4051-8110-5.

## Work-up Quick Reference

CTCL

CBC, LDH, Sezary prep, flow cytometry, CXR

Vasculitis

CBC, ESR, BMP, UA, consider drug-induced vasculitis, further testing guided by ROS and type of vasculitis suspected (CRP, SPEP, UPEP, cryo, LFT, HBV, HCV, RF, C3, C4, CH50, ANA, ANCA, ASO, CXR, guaiac, cancer screening, HIV, ENA, echo, electromyogram, nerve conduction, biopsy (nerve, respiratory tract, kidney))

Urticaria

In children, often due to Strep
Consider ASO, Rapid Strep

Urticarial vasculitis

CBC, UA, ANA, C1, C3, C4, CH50, anti-C1q, ESR

Lupus

ANA, ENA (Ro/La), CBC, BMP, ESR, C3, C4, UA, G6PD

Sarcoid

BMP, $Ca^{++}$, CXR, PFTs, G6PD, EKG, ophtho consult

Angioedema

CBC, C1 est inhib, C1,C2,C4; Hereditary: C1-nl; C2,C4 and C1 est inhib-↓ (C1est inhib levels may be nl but non-functional); Acquired: C1-↓; C2,C4 and C1 est inhib-↓

Photosensitivity

ENA (Ro/La)

Hypercoagulable

CBC, PT/PTT, Factor V Leiden,
Anti-phospholipid Ab, protein C&S, prothrombin G20210A, anti-thrombin III activity, homocysteine

TEN

Tx: IVIG 2–4 gm/kg (total dose, divided over 2–5 days) use GammaGard if possible (low IgA)
Check for IgA deficiency. See TEN protocol p. 282–283

## Direct immunofluorescence – where to biopsy?

| Diseases | Where to biopsy |
| --- | --- |
| LE, MCTD, PCT, LP, Vasculitis | Erythematous border of active lesion/involved skin (avoid old lesions, facial lesions, ulcers) |
| Pemphigus group, Pemphigoid group, Linear IgA | Erythematous perilesional skin (avoid bullae, ulcers, erosions) |
| DH | Normal-looking perilesional skin (0.5–1 cm away) |
| Lupus band | Uninvolved, non-photoexposed skin (buttock) |

*Source:* http://www.mayoclinic.org/dermatology-rst/immunofaqs.html

## False positive/negative DIFs

*False negative in BP*: (1) low yield of biopsy on distal extremity (esp. legs) (controversial), (2) predominantly IgG4 subclass of auto-antibody (poorly recognized on DIF)

*False positive in LE*: chronically sun-exposed skin of young adults

*To increase DIF yield*: transport in saline (reduces dermal background) – cannot do DIF on formalin-fixed specimen

## Biopsy for GVHD

Biopsy for GVHD vs. lymphocyte recovery vs. drug eruption
- In general, path is indistinguishable between GVHD, lymphocyte recovery, and drug eruption except high grade GVHD
- Lymphocyte recovery occurs in the first 2 weeks after transplant
- Acute GVHD occurs between 3 weeks and 100 days (or longer in persistent, recurrent, or late-onset forms)
- Chronic GVHD classically was considered to occur after 40 days but has no time limit
- Eosinophils may be found in both drug eruption and acute GVHD.

Marra DE *et al.* Tissue eosinophils and the perils of using skin biopsy specimens to distinguish between drug hypersensitivity and cutaneous graft-versus-host disease. *JAAD.* 2004; 51(4):543–545.
Zhou Y *et al.* Clinical significance of skin biopsies in the diagnosis and management of graft vs host disease in early postallogeneic bone marrow transplantation. *Arch Derm.* 2000; 136(6):717–721.

# The Dermatologic Differential Algorithm

1. Is it a rash or growth?
2. If it is a rash, is it mainly epidermal, dermal, subcutaneous, or a combination?
3. If the rash is epidermal or a combination, try to define the characteristics of the rash. Is it mainly papulosquamous? Papulopustular? Blistering?
4. After defining the characteristics, then think about causes of that type of rash (CITES MVA PITA):
   **C**ongenital, **I**nfections, **T**umor, **E**ndocrinologic, **S**olar related, **M**etabolic, **V**ascular, **A**llergic, **P**sychiatric, **I**atrogenic, **T**rauma, **A**utoimmune. When generating the differential, take the history and location of the rash into account.
5. If the rash is dermal or subcutaneous, then think of cells and substances that infiltrate and associated diseases (histiocytes, lymphocytes, mast cells, neutrophils, metastatic tumors, mucin, amyloid, immunoglobulin, etc.).

6. If the lesion is a growth, is it benign or malignant in appearance? Think of cells in the skin and their associated diseases (keratinocytes, fibroblasts, neurons, adipocytes, melanocytes, histiocytes, pericytes, endothelial cells, smooth muscle cells, follicular cells, sebocytes, eccrine cells, apocrine cells, etc.).

## Alopecia Work-Up

| Hair | Duration | % of Hair | Microscopic/Hair pull |
|------|----------|-----------|----------------------|
| Anagen | 2–6 years | 85–90 | Sheaths attached to roots |
| Catagen | 2–3 weeks | <1 | Intermediate appearance (transitional) |
| Telogen | 3 months | 10–15 | Tiny bulbs without sheaths, 'club' root |
| Exogen | Active shedding of hair shaft | | |
| Kenogen | Rest period after shedding telogen; empty follicle | | |

### Associations

1. Medications? Telogen effluvium-associated meds: anticonvulsants, anticoagulants, chemotherapy, psychiatric meds, antigout, antibiotics, beta-blockers
2. Hormones (pregnancy, menstruation, OCPs)?
3. Hair care/products?
4. Diet (iron or protein deficiency)?
5. Systemic illness/stress?

### Cicatricial or non-cicatricial?

1. **Non-cicatricial:** Is hair breaking off or coming out at the roots? Is hair loss focal or diffuse?

| Breakage | Coming out at roots |
|----------|---------------------|
| Hair shaft defects, trichorrhexis nodosa, hair care (products, traction, friction), tinea capitis, trichotillomania, anagen arrest/chemotherapy | Telogen effluvium, alopecia areata, androgenetic, syphilis, loose anagen, OCPs |

| Focal loss | Diffuse loss |
|------------|--------------|
| Hair care (traction), tinea capitis, trichotillomania, alopecia areata, syphilis, hair shaft defects | Telogen effluvium, anagen effluvium, androgenetic alopecia, hair shaft defects |

2. **Cicatricial:** Is biopsy predominantly lymphocytic, neutrophic, or mixed?

## Classification of cicatricial alopecia

| Lymphocytic | Neutrophilic | Mixed |
| --- | --- | --- |
| • LPP (including classic, frontal fibrosing, Graham-Little)<br>• Central centrifugal<br>• Alopecia mucinosa<br>• Keratosis follicularis spinulosa decalvans<br>• Chronic cutaneous LE<br>• Pseudopelade (Brocq) | • Folliculitis decalvans<br>• Dissecting cellulitis/ folliculitis | • Folliculitis/acne keloidalis<br>• Folliculitis/acne necrotica<br>• Erosive pustular dermatosis |

Adapted from Olsen EA *et al.* North American hair research Society Summary of sponsored Workshop on Cicatricial Alopecia. *J Am Acad Dermatol* 2003; 48:103–10.

## Structural hair abnormalities classified by hair fragility

| Increased fragility | No increased fragility |
| --- | --- |
| Trichorrhexis invaginata (bamboo) | Loose anagen |
| Monilethrix | Pili annulati |
| Trichorrhexis nodosa | Uncombable hair (spun-glass) |
| Trichothiodystrophy | Woolly hair |
| Pili torti | Pili bifurcati |
| | Pili multigemini |
| | Acquired progressive kinking |

Adapted from Hordinsky MK. Alopecias. In: Bolognia JL, Jorizzo JL, Rapini RP. *Dermatology* Vol. 1, Mosby; London. 2003, p. 1042.

## Pull test and hair mount

1. **Pull test** – reveals telogen hairs in telogen effluvium, and anagen hairs in loose anagen syndrome. Helpful to identify active areas in cicatricial alopecia or alopecia areata.
2. **Hair mount**

| Disorder | Hair mount findings |
| --- | --- |
| Monilethrix | Beaded, pearl necklace, knots |
| Trichorrhexis nodosa | Fractures, paint brushes |
| Trichorrhexis invaginata | Bamboo/golf tee hair |
| Trichothiodystrophy | Trichoschisis, tiger-tail on polarization |
| Loose anagen | Anagen hairs with ruffled cuticles and curled ends and lacking root sheaths |
| Pili torti | Flattened, 180° irregularly spaced twists |

*continued p. 8*

| | |
|---|---|
| Uncombable hair | Pili canaliculi et trianguli, triangular in cross section |
| Pili annulati | Abnormal dark bands on polarization, air bubbles in cortex |
| Elejalde | Pigment inclusions |
| Griscelli | Pigment clumping |
| Menkes | Multiple – pili torti, trichorrhexis nodosa, trichoptilosis |

**Hair count** – helpful in quantifying hair loss

**1.** Daily hair count: collect all hairs before shampooing (Normal is <100)
**2.** 60 second hair count: comb for 60 seconds (Normally yields 10–15 hairs).

**Biopsy** – helpful in persistent alopecia, may help determine if an alopecia is cicatricial

**1.** 4 mm punch biopsy for horizontal sectioning
   **a.** Hair count: Caucasians should have ~40 total hairs (20–35 terminal, 5–10 vellus) while African Americans should have fewer (18 terminal, 3 vellus) – assess catagen vs. telogen at isthmus level and terminal vs. vellus at infundibular level.
   **b.** Look at terminal to vellus* hair ratio:

   | | |
   |---|---|
   | Normal | >4 (~7–10T: 1V) |
   | Androgenic | <2–4T: 1V |

   **c.** Look for characteristic findings:
   Alopecia areata: lymphocytes around anagen bulbs
   Trichotillomania: pigment casts, trichomalacia, catagen hairs, dermal hemorrhage
   Androgenetic alopecia: miniaturized follicles.

**Labs** – TSH, CBC, iron, TIBC, ferritin; consider RPR, ANA;
check hormones (testosterone, DHEAS, prolactin) if irregular menses, infertility, hirsutism, severe acne, galactorrhea, or virilization.

| | Hair shaft structure | Hair shaft cross section | Others |
|---|---|---|---|
| African American | Coiled, curved | Elliptical, flattened | Lowest water content, slower growth, fewer cuticular layers at minor axes (only 1–2 not 6–8), longer major axis, less dense, large follicles |
| Asian | Straight | Circular | Largest follicular diameter, fewer eyelashes with lower lift-up/curl-up angles and greater diameter |
| Caucasian | In between | In between, oval | More dermal elastic fibers anchoring hair |

* Vellus hairs – true vellus hairs (small and lack melanin) and miniaturized terminal hairs are histologically identical.

# Management of Acne

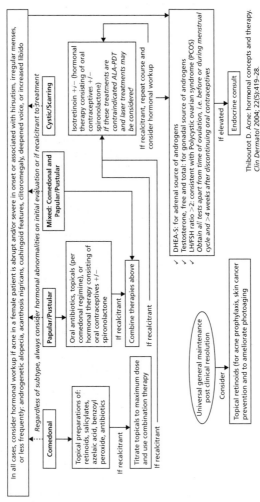

In all cases, consider hormonal workup if acne in a female patient is abrupt and/or severe in onset or associated with hirsutism, irregular menses, or less frequently: androgenetic alopecia, acanthosis nigricans, cushingoid features, clitoromegaly, deepened voice, or increased libido

*Regardless of subtype, always consider hormonal abnormalities on initial evaluation or if recalcitrant to treatment*

**Comedonal**

Topical preparations of: retinoids, salicylates, azelaic acid, benzoyl peroxide, antibiotics

If recalcitrant

Titrate topicals to maximum dose and use combination therapy

If recalcitrant

**Papular/Pustular**

Oral antibiotics, topicals (per comedonal regimen), or hormonal therapy consisting of oral contraceptives +/− spironolactone

If recalcitrant

Combine therapies above

If recalcitrant

**Mixed: Comedonal and Papular/Pustular**

**Cystic/Scarring**

Isotretinoin +/− (hormonal therapy consisting of oral contraceptives +/− spironolactone)
*If these treatments are contraindicated ALA-PDT and laser treatments may be considered*

If recalcitrant, repeat course and consider hormonal workup

➤ DHEA-S: for adrenal source of androgens
➤ Testosterone, free and total: for gonadal source of androgens
➤ LH/FSH ratio >2: consistent with Polycystic ovarian syndrome (PCOS)
➤ *Obtain all tests apart from time of ovulation, i.e. before or during menstrual cycle and >4 weeks after discontinuing oral contraceptives*

If elevated

Endocrine consult

Universal general maintenance post clinical resolution

Consider

Topical retinoids (for acne prophylaxis, skin cancer prevention and to ameliorate photoaging)

Thiboutot D. Acne: hormonal concepts and therapy.
*Clin Dermatol* 2004; 22(5):419–28.

# Aphthosis Classification and Workup

## Morphologic classification
- **Minor aphthae**: single to few, shallow ulcers (<1 cm) which spontaneously heal in 1–2 weeks
- **Major aphthae** (Sutton's, periadenitis mucosa necrotica recurrens): single to few, deep ulcers (>1 cm) which heal over weeks–months and scar
- **Herpetiform aphthae**: 10–100, clustered, small ulcers (3 mm) which heal in days–weeks, may scar (not associated with HSV)

## Classification by cause
- **Simple aphthae**: recurrent minor, major, or herpetiform aphthae, often in healthy, young patients
- **Complex aphthae**: >3, nearly constant, oral aphthae *or* recurrent genital and oral aphthae, *and* exclusion of Behçet and MAGIC syndromes
  - Primary: idiopathic
  - Secondary: IBD, HIV, cyclic neutropenia, FAPA (fever, aphthous stomatitis, pharyngitis, adenitis), gluten sensitivity, ulcus vulvae acutum, vitamin deficiencies (B1, B2, B6, B12, folate), iron, and zinc deficiencies, drugs (NSAIDS, alendronate, beta-blockers, nicorandil).

## Work-up for complex aphthae
- HSV PCR/Cx
- CBC
- Iron, folate, vitamin B12, zinc
- Consider UA
- Consider HIV, HLA-B27, antigliadin/antiendomysial Ab
- Consider biopsy
- Consider GI, rheum, ophtho, neuro consults
- If considering dapsone, check G6PD

**Local factors promoting aphthae:** chemical/mechanical injury, sodium lauryl sulfate-containing dental products, inadequate saliva, cessation of tobacco.

## Treatment
- Topical: anesthetics, corticosteroids (or IL), tacrolimus, retinoids, rinses (chlorhexidine, betadine, salt water, hydrogen peroxide, tetracyclines)
- Systemic: colchicine, dapsone, thalidomide (HIV)

Adapted from Letsinger JA *et al.* Complex aphthosis: a large case series with evaluation algorithm and therapeutic ladder from topicals to thalidomide. *J Am Acad Dermatol* 2005; 52(3 Pt 1):500–508.

# Amyloidoses

**Stains**: PAS+/diastase resistant. Fluoresces with thioflavin T. Purple with crystal violet. Birefringence with Congo red (absent after treating with potassium permanganate in AA subtype).

| Classification | Type | Symptoms/subtypes |
|---|---|---|
| Primary systemic | AL >>AH | 40% have skin involvement: waxy skin colored papules (nose, eyes, mouth), alopecia, carpal tunnel, pinch purpura, shoulder pad sign. Also may deposit in heart, GI tract, tongue. |
| Secondary/ reactive systemic | AA | Skin NOT INVOLVED. Deposits in liver, spleen, adrenals, and kidney. Associated with chronic disease (especially TB, leprosy, Hodgkin, RA, renal cell cancer). |
| Primary cutaneous | AL | Nodular amyloid: nodule(s) on extremities, trunk. |
| | Keratin | Macular amyloid: pruritic macules interscapular region, associated with nostalgia paresthetica. |
| | Keratin | Lichen amyloid: discrete papules on shins. |
| Secondary cutaneous/ tumor associated | Keratin | Following PUVA and in neoplasms. |
| Familial syndromes | AA | Hereditary periodic fever syndromes: Familial Mediterranean Fever and TNF receptor-associated periodic syndromes (but not Hyper-IgD) |
| | AA | Cryopyrin-associated periodic syndromes: Familial cold autoinflammatory, Muckle–Wells, CINCA/NOMID |

| Amyloid subtype | Precursor protein | Association |
|---|---|---|
| AL | Ig light chain | Primary systemic, myeloma, plasmacytoma, nodular |
| AH | Ig heavy chain | Primary systemic, myeloma |
| AA | (apo) serum AA (SAA) | Reactive systemic, TRAPS, FMF, Muckle–Wells, familial cold autoinflammatory |
| ATTR | Transthyretin (prealbumin) | Familial amyloid polyneuropathy 1 and 2, familial amyloid cardiomyopathy, senile systemic |
| A $\beta_2$M | $\beta_2$-microglobulin | Hemodialysis |
| A $\beta$ | A b Precursor protein (AbPP) | Alzheimer, Down, hereditary cerebral hemorrhage with amyloidosis (Dutch) |
| Keratinocyte tonofilaments | | Macular and lichen, MEN IIa, secondary cutaneous (PUVA, neoplasms) |

| | |
|---|---|
| Apolipoprotein I | Familial amyloid polyneuropathy 3 |
| Atrial natriuretic factor | Isolated atrial |
| Calcitonin | Medullary thyroid cancer associated |
| Cystatin | Hereditary cerebral hemorrhage (Icelandic) |
| Fibrinogen α chain | Familial fibrinogen associated |
| Gelsolin | Familial amyloid polyneuropathy 4 (Finnish) |
| Islet amyloid polypeptide | Diabetes mellitus II/insulinoma associated |
| Lactoferrin | Corneal lactoferrin associated |
| Lysozyme | Familial lysozyme associated |
| Medin/lactadherin | Aortic medial |
| Prion protein/scrapie | Creutzfeld-Jacob |

## Xanthomas

| Type | Distribution /appearance | Associations |
|---|---|---|
| Xanthelasma palpebrarum | Polygonal papules esp. near medial canthus | May be associated with hyperlipidemia (50%) including any primary hyperlipoproteinemia or secondary hyperlipidemias such as cholestasis |
| Tuberous xanthomas | Multilobulated tumors, pressure areas, extensors | Hypercholesterolemia (esp. LDL), familial dysbetalipoproteinemia (type 3/broad beta disease), familial hypercholesterolemia (type 2), secondary hyperlipidemias (nephrotic syndrome, hypothyroidism) |
| Tendinous xanthomas | Subcutaneous nodules esp. extensor tendons of hands, feet, Achilles, defects, trauma | Severe hypercholesterolemia (esp. LDL), particularly type 2a, apolipoprotein B-100 secondary hyperlipidemias (esp. cholestasis, cerebrotendinous xanthomatosis, beta-sitosterolemia |
| Eruptive xanthomas | Crops of small papules on buttocks, shoulders, extensors, oral | Hypertriglyceridemia (esp. types 1, 4, and 5 hyperlipidemias), secondary hyperlipidemias (esp. DM2) |
| Plane xanthomas | Palmar creases | Familial dysbetalipoproteinemia (type 3), secondary hyperlipidemia (esp. cholestasis) |
| Generalized plane xanthomas | Generalized, esp. head and neck, chest, flexures | Monoclonal gammopathy, hyperlipidemia (esp. hypertriglyceridemia) |
| Xanthoma disseminatum | Papules, nodules, mucosa of upper aerodigestive tract | Normolipemic |
| Verucciform xanthomas | Solitary, oral or genital, adults | Normolipemic |

# Hyperlipoproteinemias: Fredrickson Classification

| Type | Name | Defect, AR/AD | Lipid profile | Xanthomas | Other clinical |
|------|------|---------------|---------------|-----------|----------------|
| I | Hyperlipoproteinemia | Lipoprotein lipase, AR | ↑ chylomicrons, chol, TG ↓ LDL, HDL | Eruptive xanthomas (2/3), lipemia retinalis | ↑ CAD, HSM, pancreatitis |
| IB | Apolipoprotein C-II deficiency | APOC2 AR | Similar to Lipoprotein lipase deficiency | | |
| IIA* | Familial hypercholesterolemia, LDL receptor disorder | LDL receptor, AD | ↑ LDL, chol, TG | Tuberous, intertriginous, tendinous, planar xanthomas, xanthelasma, corneal arcus | ↑ CAD |
| | Familial hypercholesterolemia, type B | APOB, AD | Same as IIA | | |
| IIB | Combined hyperlipoproteinemia | Heterogeneous | ↑ LDL, VLDL, chol, TG | Xanthomas rare | ↑ CAD |
| III | Familial dysbetalipoproteinemia, broad beta-lipoproteinemia | APOE, AR | ↑ chylomicron remnants/VLDL, chol, TG | Planar palmar crease, tuberous xanthomas, xanthelasma | ↑ CAD, DM2 |
| IV | Carbohydrate-inducible lipemia | AD | ↑ VLDL, TG ↓ HDL | Tuberoeruptive xanthomas | ↑ CAD, DM2, obesity, etoh, hypothyroidism, pancreatitis, uremia, myeloma, nephrotic, hypopituitarism, glycogen storage type I |
| V | Mixed hyperprebeta-lipoproteinemia and chylomicronemia | APOA5, AR/AD | ↑ chylomicrons, VLDL, TG, chol ↓ LDL, HDL | Eruptive xanthomas, lipemia retinalis | Abd pain, pancreatitis, DM2, HTN, hyperuricemia, OCPs, etoh, glycogen storage type I |

*Other familial hypercholesterolemia syndromes – AR Hypercholesterolemia (ARH/LDLR Adaptor Protein mutations), AD Hypercholesterolemia type 3 (PCSK9/PROPROTEIN CONVERTASE, SUBTILISIN/KEXIN-TYPE, 9 mutations)

Mallory SB. *An Illustrated Dictionary of Dermatologic Syndromes*, 2nd edition, Taylor & Francis; New York, London: 2006.

# Histiocytosis

| Histiocytosis | Onset | Clinical features | Associations | Pathology |
|---|---|---|---|---|
| *Langerhans cell histiocytosis* 2/3 children age 1–3 years old; 1/3 adults – usually pulmonary, often smokers. New classification by organ of involvement: | | | | |
| 1. Restricted LCH: a. Skin only | | | | • CD1a+, S100+, Placental Alk Phos+ |
| b. Monostotic lesions ± diabetes insipidus (DI), LN, rash | | | | • Reniform, 'coffee-bean' nuclei |
| c. Polyostotic lesions ± DI, LN, rash | | | | • Birbeck granules |
| 2. Extensive LCH: a. Visceral organ involvement w/o dysfunction ± DI, LN, rash | | | | |
| b. Visceral organ involvement with dysfunction ± DI, LN, rash | | | | |
| Letterer–Siwe | 0–2 years old | • Acute, disseminated, multisystem form | ALL, solid tumors | |
| | | • Resembles seb derm | | |
| | | • Fever, anemia, LAN, osteolytic lesions, HSM | | |
| Hand-Schüller-Christian | 2–6 years old | • Chronic, multisystem (skin lesions in 1/3) | | |
| | | • Classic triad: bone lesions (80%, esp. cranium), DI. exophthalmos | | |
| Eosinophilic granuloma | Older children/adults | • Localized, benign | | |
| | | • May present with spontaneous fracture or otitis | | |
| Hashimoto-Pritzker | Congenital | • a.k.a Congenital self-healing reticulocytosis | | |
| | | • W despread, red-brown papules or crusts | | |

continued p. 14

**Non-Langerhans cell histiocytosis** without malignant features

| Histiocytosis | Onset | Clinical features | Associations | Pathology |
|---|---|---|---|---|
| Juvenile xanthogranuloma | Early childhood | • Most common histiocytosis, self-limiting<br>• Solitary lesion in 25–60% of cases<br>• Head/neck > trunk > extremities<br>• May be systemic (CNS, liver/spleen, lung, eye, oropharynx)<br>• Eye = most common extracutaneous site, unilateral | • NF1<br>• leukemia<br>• NF and juvenile CML | • Small histiocytes, Touton and foreign body giant cells, foam cells<br>• CD68+, factor XIIIa+, vimentin+ |
| Benign cephalic histiocytosis | 0–3 years old | • 2–5 mm, yellow-red papules on face/neck of infant<br>• Self-limiting<br>• Spares mucous membranes and viscera | Probably same as JXG | a.k.a. Histiocytosis w/ Intracytoplasmic worm-like bodies (on EM) |
| Generalized eruptive histiocytoma | Adults>children | • Crops of small, red-brown papules. Widespread axial distribution<br>• Spontaneous resolutions | | |
| Indeterminate cell histiocytosis | Adults>children | • Clinically identical to generalized eruptive histiocytoma | | Antigenic markers of both LCH and non-LCH |
| Multicentric reticulohistiocytosis | Adults (F>M) 30–50 years old | • Joints, skin, mucous membranes (50%)<br>• Papules/nodules – head, hand, elbow, periungual 'coral beads'<br>• Often misdiagnosed as RA<br>• Waxes/wanes, spontaneously remits in 5–10 years | • 25% internal malignancies (gastric, breast, GU)<br>• 6–17% autoimmune conditions<br>• 30–60% hyperlipidemia | • Histiocytes w/ 'ground glass' appearance, oncocytic histiocytes<br>• Multinucleate giant cells<br>• CD45+, CD68+, CD11b+, HAM56+, vimentin+<br>• Usu S100−, Factor XIIIa−, CD34− |

| | | Giant cell reticulohistiocytoma, a.k.a. solitary reticulohistiocytoma = isolated, cutaneous tumor version of MRH | |
|---|---|---|---|
| Necrobiotic xanthogranuloma | 6th decade | • Usu head/neck or trunk: esp. periorbital<br>• Scleritis, episcleritis → possible blindness<br>• Mcy have anemia, leukopenia, elevated ESR, 20% HSM<br>• Often chronic, progressive | • 90% IgG paraproteinemia<br>• 40% cryoglobulinemia<br>• Hyaline necrobiosis, palisaded granuloma (cholesterol cleft)<br>• Touton and foreign body giant cells<br>• 'Touton cell panniculitis'<br>• CD15+, CD4+<br>• CD1a−, S100− |
| Xanthoma disseminatum | Any | • Proliferation of foamy histiocytes despite normal serum lipids<br>• Flexors, skin folds, mucous membranes (eyes, URT, meninges → leads to DI)<br>• Usu benign, self-limiting | • Unique scalloped histiocytes in early lesions<br>• Histiocytes, foam cells, chronic inflammatory cells, Touton and foreign body giant cells<br>• CD68+, Factor XIIIa+<br>• CD1a−, S100− |
| Rosai–Dorfman Dorfman a.k.a. sinus histiocytosis with massive lymphadenopathy | 10–30 years old, M>F | • Generally benign, self-limiting<br>• Painless, cervical LAN<br>• 40% have extranodal involvement (poor prognosis)<br>• Skin is most common extranodal site | • Expansion of LN sinuses by large foamy histiocytes, plasma cells, multinucleate giant cells<br>• Emperipolesis<br>• S100+, Factor XIIIa+,<br>• CD1a − |
| Erdheim-Chester | Middle age | • Similar to XD, but 50% mortality<br>• Symmetric sclerosis of metaphyses/diaphyses of long bones (virtually pathognomonic) → chronic bone pain | • Histiocytes, foam cells<br>• CD68+, Factor XIIIa +<br>• CD1a−<br>• Usu S100− |

continued p. 16

15

| Histiocytosis | Onset | Clinical features | Associations | Pathology |
|---|---|---|---|---|
| | | • DI, renal and retroperitoneal infiltrates, xanthoma-like skin lesions (esp. eyelids), pulmonary fibrosis, CNS | | |
| Hemophagocytic lymphohistiocytosis | Children | • Rare, life-threatening, rapidly progressive<br>• Dx Criteria: F, splenomegaly, cytopenia, hyperTG, hyper-fibrinogenemia, hemophagocytosis on tissue bx<br>• Nonspecific rashes in ~60%<br>• Median survival: 2–3 months (BM failure, sepsis)<br>• Two Types – Primary and Familial HLH (in both cases) triggered by infection, esp. EBV | • CTD, malignancies, HIV<br>*Familial HLH:*<br>• FHL1 – HPLH1<br>• FHL2 – PRF1 (cytolytic granule content)<br>• FHL3 – UNC13D (cytolytic granule secretion)<br>• FHL4 – syntaxin-11 (membr-associated, SNARE family, docking/fusion) | |
| Sea-blue histiocytosis | Inherited | • Rare<br>• BM, HSM – also lungs, CNS, eyes, skin<br>• Nodular lesions; eyelid infiltration | • APOE mutations<br>• One of the manifestations of Niemann-Pick type B<br>• Common (<1/3) in BM bx's of MDS | Large, azure blue, cytoplasmic granules with May-Gruenwald stain (yellow-brown on H&E, dark blue with toluidine or Giemsa) |

### Non-Langerhans cell histiocytosis with malignant features

| Histiocytosis | Onset | Clinical features | Associations | Pathology |
|---|---|---|---|---|
| Malignant histiocytosis | M>F 2:1 | • Very rare, life-threatening<br>• Liver, spleen, LN, BM<br>• p/w painful LAN, HSM, fever, night sweats<br>• Pancytopenia, DIC, extranodal extension<br>• 10–15% skin involvement (esp. lower legs, buttocks). | | Variable |

# Lupus Erythematosus

## Systemic lupus erythematosus criteria (4 of 11)
Adapted from the American College of Rheumatology 1982 revised criteria

**Mucocutaneous**
1. Malar rash (tends to spare nasolabial folds)
2. Discoid lesions
3. Photosensitivity
4. Oral ulcers (must be observed by physician)

**Systemic**
5. Arthritis – nonerosive arthritis of 2+ joints
6. Serositis – pleuritis, pericarditis
7. Renal disorder – proteinuria > 0.5 g/day or 3+ on dipstick
8. Neurologic – seizures or psychosis
9. Hematologic:
    a. hemolytic anemia with reticulocytosis
    b. leukopenia (<4 K) on 2 occasions
    c. lymphopenia (<1.5 K) on 2 occasions
    d. thrombocytopenia (<100 K)
10. Immunologic – anti-dsDNA, anti-Sm, false positive RPR
11. ANA+

## Acute cutaneous lupus erythematosus
Clinical findings: transient butterfly malar rash, generalized photosensitive eruption, and/or bullous lesions on the face, neck, and upper trunk.
Associated with HLA-DR2, HLA-DR3
DIF: granular IgG/IgM (rare IgA) + complement at DEJ.

## Subacute cutaneous lupus erythematosus
Clinical findings: psoriasiform or annular non-scarring plaques in a photodistribution.
Associated with:
• HLA-B8, HLA-DR3, HLA-DRw52, HLA-DQ1
• SLE, Sjögren, RA, C2 deficiency
• Medications: HCTZ, Ca+ channel blocker, ACE inhibitors, griseofulvin, terbinafine, anti-TNF, penicillamine, glyburide, spironolactone, piroxicam
DIF: granular pattern of IgG/IgM in the epidermis only (variable).

## Chronic cutaneous lupus erythematosus
### Discoid lupus
Clinical findings: erythematous plaques which progress to atrophic patches with follicular plugging, scarring, and alopecia on sun-exposed skin.

Progression to SLE: 5% if above the neck; 20% if above and below the neck
DIF:  granular IgG/IgM (rare IgA) + complement at DEJ, more likely
    positive in actively inflamed lesion present × 6–8 weeks.

### Lupus panniculitis
Clinical findings: deep painful erythematous plaques, nodules and ulcers
    involving proximal extremities and trunk.  Overlying skin may have DLE
    changes.
Progression to SLE: 50%
DIF:  rare granular deposits at the DEJ.  May have deposits around dermal
    vessels.

### Tumid lupus
Clinical findings: erythematous indurations of fat with no scale or follicular
    plugs.
DIF: nonspecific

*Lupus band: strong continuous antibody deposits at the DEJ on nonlesional
skin; found in >75% of SLE patients on sun-exposed skin and 50% SLE
patients on non-sun-exposed skin*

## Autoantibody sensitivities and specificities

| Condition | Autoantibody or target | Sensitivity (%) | Specificity (%) |
| --- | --- | --- | --- |
| SLE | ANA | 93–99 | 57 |
| | Histone | 60–80 | 50 |
| | dsDNA* | 50–70 | 97 |
| | U1-RNP | 30–50 | 99 |
| | Ribosomal-P | 15–35 | 99 |
| | Sm | 10–40 | >95 |
| | SS-A | 10–50 | >85 |
| | SS-B | 10–15 | |
| SCLE | ANA | 67 | |
| | SS-A | 60–80 | |
| | SS-B | 25–50 | |
| DLE | ANA | 5–25 | |
| | SS-A | <<10 | |
| Drug-Induced LE | ANA | >95 | |
| | Histone | >95 | |
| | dsDNA | | 1–5 |
| | Sm | 1 | |

| Condition | Antibody | | |
|---|---|---|---|
| Neonatal Lupus | SS-A** | 95 | |
| | SS-B | 60–80 | |
| MCTD | ANA | 100 | |
| | U1-RNP | >95 | |
| Localized scleroderma | Nucleosome | 80 | |
| (Morphea) | Topoisomerase II | 75 | |
| | Histone | 50 | |
| | ssDNA | 50 | |
| | ANA | 45–80 | |
| Limited SSc | ANA | 90 | |
| | Centromere | 50–90 | |
| | Scl-70 | 10–15 | |
| | RNA pol III | 2 | |
| Diffuse SSc | ANA | 90 | |
| | Scl-70 | 20–40 | |
| | RNA pol III | 25 | |
| | Centromere | ≤5 | |
| Sjögren | ANA | 50–75 | 50 |
| | SS-A | 50–90 | >85 |
| | SS-B | 40 | >90 |
| | RF | 50 | |
| Polymyositis (PM) | ANA | 85 | 60 (DM/PM) |
| | Jo-1 | 25–37 | |
| Dermatomyositis (DM) | ANA | 40–80 | 60 (DM/PM) |
| Rheumatoid arthritis | CCP | 65–70 | 90–98 |
| | RF | 50–90 | >80 |
| | ANA | 20–50 | 55 |
| | Histone | 15–20 | |
| Secondary Raynaud | ANA | 65 | 40 |

*Sensitivity and specificity for different antibiodies varies depending on the assay used. The percentage reported here are estimated averages from the referenced text below.*
\* Correlates with SLE activity and renal disease
\*\* Risk of neonatal lupus among babies of SS-A+ mothers: 2–6%
ANA titers of 1:80, 1:160, and 1:320 are found in 13, 5, and 3%, respectively of healthy individuals. Among healthy elderly patients, ANA titers of 1:160 may be seen in 15%.

Sheldon J. Laboratory testing in autoimmune rheumatic disease. *Best Pract Res Clin Rheumatol.* 2004 Jun; 18(3):249–69.
Lyons *et al.* Effective use of autoantibody tests in the diagnosis of systemic autoimmune disease. *Ann N Y Acad Sci.* 2005 Jun; 1050:217–28.
Kurien BT, Scofield RH. Autoantibody determination in the diagnosis of systemic lupus erythematosus. *Scand J Immunol.* 2006 Sep; 64(3):227–35.
Habash-Bseiso *et al.* Serologic testing in connective tissue diseases. *Clin Med Res.* 2005 Aug; 3(3):190–193.

# Antinuclear Antibodies
## (S: sensitive SP: specific)

| Pattern | Antibody target | Disease | Notes |
|---|---|---|---|
| Homogenous | Histone dsDNA | **Drug-induced LE*** (>90% S), SLE (>60% S), Chronic Disease **SLE** (60% SP), **Lupus nephritis** | IC in glomeruli = nephritis, follows disease activity, test performed on *Crithidia luciliae* |
| Peripheral nuclear (Rim) | Nuclear Lamins Nuclear Pore | **SLE**, Linear Morphea PM | |
| Centromere/ true speckled | Centromere | **CREST** (50–90% S), SSc, Primary Biliary Cirrhosis (50% S), Idiopathic Raynaud, PSS | |
| Speckled/ particulate nuclear (ENA) | U1-RNP | **Mixed connective tissue disease** (near 100% S) **SLE** (30% S), DM/PM, SSc, Sjögren, RA | Titer > 1:1600 in 95–100% MCTD |
| | Smith (snRNP) | **SLE** (99% SP but only 20% S) | |
| | Ro/SS-A (E3 ubiquitin ligase, TROVE2) | **SCLE** (75–90% S), **Sjögren**, Neonatal LE, Congenital Heart Block, C2/C4 deficient LE | Photosensitivity work-up |
| | La/SS-B (binds RNA newly transcribed by RNA Pol III) | **Sjögren, SCLE** | |
| Nucleolar | Scl-70 (Topoisomerase I) | **SSc** (diffuse > limited) | Poor prognosis |
| | Fibrillarin (U3-RNP) | SSc (diffuse > limited) | |
| | PM-Scl | PM/SSc Overlap syndromes | Machinists hands, arthritis, Raynaud, calcinosis cutis |
| | RNA Pol I | SSc | Poor prognosis, renal crisis |

**\*Drug-induced ("Dusting Pattern"):** Allopurinol, aldomet, ACE-I, chloropmazine, clonidine, danazol, dilantin, ethosuximide, griseofulvin, hydralazine, isoniazid, lithium, lovastatin, mephenytoin, mesalazine, methyldopa, MCN, OCP, *para*-amino salicylic acid, penicillamine, PCN, phenothiazine, pheylbutazone, piroxicam, practolol, procainamide, propylthiouracil, quinidine, streptomycin, sulfasalazine, sulfonamides, tegretol, TCN.

# Autoantibodies in Connective Tissue Diseases

| Autoantibody or target | Activity | Clinical association |
|---|---|---|
| LAC, β2-glycoprotein I, Prothrombin, Cardiolipin, Protein S, Annexin AV | Phospholipids | Antiphospholipid antibody syndrome* |
| Rheumatoid factor | Fc portion of IgG | Low level – nonspecific (SLE, SSc, MCTD, neoplasm, chronic disease) High level – associated with erosive RA |
| KII | DNA end-binding repair protein complex | Overlap DM/PM, SSc, LE |
| U2-RNP | | Overlap DM/PM, SSc |
| Alpha-fodrin | Actin binding protein | Specific for Sjögren |
| Jo-1/PL-1 | Histidyl-tRNA synthetase | DM/PM** (20–40% sensitive) – increased risk of interstitial lung disease, but no increased rate of malignancy |
| Mi-2 | Nuclear helicase | DM with malignancy, better prognosis than anti-synthetase |
| PDGF | | SSc, cGVHD |
| SRP | Signal recognition protein | Anti-SRP syndrome (rapidly progressive necrotizing myopathy); association with cardiac disease not confirmed |
| 155 K-EB antigen | Transcriptional intermediary factor-1 | DM (20% sensitive in adult-onset classical form), may be associated with internal malignancy |

*Antiphospholipid antibody (APA) syndrome – Primary (50%), SLE (35%); Skin: livedo reticularis, ulcers, gangrene, splinter hemorrhages.
Diagnosis requires at least one clinical criterion:
- Clinical episode of vascular thrombosis
- Pregnancy complication: unexplained abortion after week 10, premature birth at or before week 34, or ≥3 unexplained, consecutive SAB before week 10.

And at least one lab criterion: anticardiolipin, lupus anticoagulant, or anti-β2-glycoprotein I Abs on 2 occasions 6 weeks apart.

Adapted from Jacobe H et al. Autoantibodies encountered in patients with autoimmune connective diseases. In: Bolognia J, Jorizzo JL, Rapini RP. Dermatology, Vol. 1. London: Mosby, 2003. pp. 589–99.

**Polymyositis/dermatomyositis – ≥40% ANA+, 90% auto-Ab. Anti-synthetase syndrome (tRNA): interstitial lung disease, fever, arthritis, Raynaud disease, machinist hands.

# Vasculitis

**Initial work-up:** Detailed history, physical exam, ROS, skin biopsy ±
CBC, ESR, BMP, UA, consider drug-induced vasculitis.
**Further testing guided by ROS and type of vasculitis suspected:**
CRP, SPEP, UPEP, cryo, LFT, HBV, HCV, RF, C3, C4, CH50, ANA, ANCA, ASO,
CXR, guaiac, cancer screening, HIV, ENA, echo, electromyogram, nerve
conduction, biopsy (nerve, respiratory tract, kidney)

## Treatment of ANCA-associated vasculitis

- Induction: Cyclophosphamide 2 mg/kg/day, Prednisolone 1 mg/kg/day
  tapered to 0.25 mg/kg/day by 12 weeks.
- Maintenance: Azathioprine 2 mg/kg/day, Prednisolone 7.5–10 mg/day
  Frequent life severe adverse events with cyclophosphamide (Cytoxan),
  nitrogen mustard, alkylating agent:
  1. Hemorrhagic cystitis (10%) and risk of bladder cancer (5% at 10
     years, 16% at 15 years): minimize by using copious fluids, mesna,
     acetylcysteine and not using h.s. dosing.
  2. Bone marrow suppression: Onset 7 days, nadir 14 days, recovery 21
     days.
  3. Infection
  4. Infertility

# Anti-neutrophil cytoplasmic antibody

|  | Wegener syndrome | Microscopic polyangiitis | Churg–Strauss syndrome |
|---|---|---|---|
| ANCA (% sensitivity) | C-ANCA (85%) > P-ANCA (10%) | P-ANCA (45–70%) > C-ANCA (45%) | P-ANCA (60%) > C-ANCA (10%) |
| Classic features | Upper respiratory (sinusitis, oral ulcers, rhinorrhea), glomerulonephritis (GN), saddle-nose, strawberry gingiva, ocular | Necrotizing GN (segmental and crescentic), pulmonary hemorrhage (esp. lower), neuropathy | Asthma, allergies, nasal polyps, eosinophilia, PNA, gastroenteritis, CHF, mononeuritis multiplex |
| Skin | Palpable purpura, SQ nodules, pyoderma gangrenosum-like lesions | Palpable purpura | Palpable purpura, SQ nodules |
| Pathology | Perivascular necrotizing granulomas, LCV | No granulomas, LCV with few/no immune deposits | Eosinophils, extravascular granulomas, LCV |
| Respiratory | Upper and lower respiratory, fixed nodular densities | Lower respiratory, alveolar hemorrhage | Patchy, transient interstitial infiltrates |
| Treatment | High-dose corticosteroids; Cytotoxic agents if severe (no controlled trial demonstrating benefits) | High-dose corticosteroids; Cytotoxic agents if severe (no controlled trial demonstrating benefits) | High-dose corticosteroids combined with cytotoxic agent (cyclopohsphamide) with proven benefit in survival |

C-ANCA = cytoplasmic (IIF) = proteinase 3.
P-ANCA = perinuclear (IIF) = myeloperoxidase.
Other conditions which may be ANCA positive: SLE, RA, chronic infection (TB, HIV), digestive disorders (inflammatory bowel disease, sclerosing cholangitis, primary biliary cirrhosis, autoimmune hepatitis), drugs (propylthiouracil, hydralazine, methimazole, minocycline, carbimazole, penicillamine), silica/occupational solvents
Titers might indicate disease activity, relapse.

## Small vessel vasculitis

| Disease | Symptoms | Etiology/Associations | Treatment |
|---|---|---|---|
| Cutaneous small vessel vasculitis | Palpable purpura, lower legs/ankles/dependent areas, ± livedo reticularis, urticaria, edema, ulcers, ± pruritic, painful/burning, fever, arthralgias | Drugs, infections, CTD, neoplasms | Usually self-limited, rest, elevation, compression, NSAIDs, anti-histamines, corticosteroids, colchicine, dapsone, immunosuppressants |
| Henoch-Schönlein purpura | Palpable purpura on extensors and buttocks, pts 4–7 years old, polyarthralgia (75%), GI bleeding, fever, hematuria, edema, renal dysfunction, pulmonary hemorrhage, headache | 1–2 weeks after respiratory infection, allergens/food, drugs; usually unknown | Primarily supportive: corticosteroids, other immunosuppressants, dapsone, factor XII |
| Acute hemorrhagic edema of infancy | Large, annular, purpuric plaques and edema on face, ears, extremities, usually in p<2 years old | Infections (especially respiratory), drugs, vaccines; usually unknown | Self-resolving |
| Urticarial vasculitis | Painful (>pruritic), lasts >24h, post-inflammatory hyperpigmentation, ± bullae, systemic dz in hypocomplementemic version (anti-C1q precipitin, F>M, ocular, angioedema, COPD), F>M | Autoimmune/CTD (30% of Sjogren, 20% of SLE pts), drugs (serum sickness), infections (HBV, HCV, EBV), neoplasms, Schnitzler syndrome | Oral corticosteroids, anti-malarials, dapsone, colchicine, anti-histamines, NSAIDs |

| | | | |
|---|---|---|---|
| Hyperimmuno-globulinemia D syndrome | Periodic fever, arthralgia, GI sxs, LAN, erythematous macules papules/nodules/urticaria on extremities, onset <10 years old, ↑ IgD and IgA levels | AR; Mevalonate kinase deficiency | NSAIDs, anti-IL-1 Ab, corticosteroids |
| Familial mediterranean fever | Periodic fever, arthritis, serositis, erysipelas-like rash on legs, myalgias, AA amyloidosis, renal failure, PID sxs; unlike Hyper-IgD, no LAN and nl IgD level | AR; Pyrin deficiency | Colchicine, anti-IL-1 |
| Erythema elevatum diutinum | Yellow/brown/red papules, plaques, and nodules over joints | Hematologic diseases, HIV, IBD, CTD, streptococcal infections | Dapsone, niacinamide, topical/intralesional corticosteroids |
| Granuloma faciale | Brown/red plaques on face, middle-aged, M>F, Caucasian | Unknown | Treatment-resistant, intralesional steroids, dapsone, surgery |
| Serum sickness | Fever, LAN, arthralgias, urt caria, maculopapular, scarlatiniform, purpura, myalgias | Type III hypersensitivity, commonly following streptokinase, IVIG, Abx (cefaclor, PCN, MCN, rifampin, cefprozil) | Avoidance, anti-histamines, anti-pyretics, corticosteroids |

## Medium (± small) vessel vasculitis

| | | |
|---|---|---|
| Polyarteritis nodosa (systemic) | SQ nodules on legs, livedo reticularis, "punched-out" ulcers, digital gangrene, p-ANCA positive, universal multisystemic involvement: myocardial/GI/renal infarction, polyneuritis, CNS, arthralgias, weight loss, HTN, (renal) microaneurysms, orchitis (esp. with HBV) | Various infections/inflammatory conditions: streptococcus, HBV, HCV, CMV, HIV, SLE, IBD, hairy cell leukemia | Corticosteroids, cyclophosphamide |
| Polyarteritis nodosa (cutaneous) | SQ nodules, starburst pattern of livedo reticularis, mild fever, nerve and muscle involvement | As above (cPAN represents 10% but is most common form in children, more often strep) | Topical/intralesional steroids, PCN |
| Microscopic polyangitis | Palpable purpura, ulcers, splinter hemorrhages, crescentic necrotizing segmental glomerulonephritis, fever, weight loss, myalgias, neuropathy, HTN, p-ANCA (60%); c-ANCA (40%) | | Corticosteroids, cyclophosphamide |
| Wegener granulomatosis | Respiratory, renal, sinus, ocular, otologic, CNS, cardiac, joints, nasal nodules/ulcers/saddle nose, pulmonary infiltrates/ nodules, SQ nodules, c-ANCA (85%) | Unknown – distinguish from lymphomatoid granulomatosis (severe EBV+ angioinvasive B-cell lymphoma of skin and lungs) | Corticosteroids, cyclophosphamide (treat staph infection and nasal carriage to minimize relapse) |
| Churg–Strauss syndrome (allergic granulomatosis) | Asthma, sinusitis, allergic rhinitis, eosinophilia, arthritis, myositis, CHF, renal/HTN, mononeuritis multiplex, palpable purpura, infiltrated nodules, p-ANCA (60%) | Vaccination, leukotriene inhibitors, desensitization therapy, rapid steroid taper | Corticosteroids, cyclophosphamide |

## Large vessel vasculitis

| | | | |
|---|---|---|---|
| Giant cell arteritis (temporal) | Tender, temporal artery, polymyalgia rheumatica, unilateral HA, jaw claudication, blindness, F>M, Northern European | Unknown | Corticosteroids |
| Takayasu arteritis | Constitutional sxs, pulselessness, signs/sxs of ischemia, EN-like nodules, pyoderma gangrenosum-like lesions | Associations: RA, other CTD | Corticosteroids, cyclophosphamide, surgical revascularization |

**Other causes of vasculitis:** Infections (bacterial – meningococcemia, gonnococcemia, strep, mycobacterial; viral – HSV; fungal), Rheumatoid vasculitis, Drug-induced, Lupus, Paraneoplastic, Buerger, Mondor

**Lymphocytic vasculitis:** Pityriasis lichenoides, Pigmented purpuras, Gyrate erythemas, Collagen vascular disease, Degos, Perniosis, Rickettsial, TRAPS

**Neutrophilic dermatoses:** Sweet, Marshall (+ acquired cutis laxa), Behcet, Rheumatoid, Bowel-associated dermatosis–arthritis syndrome

**Vasculo-occlusive/microangiopathies:** Cryos Anti-phospholip syndrome, Atrophic blanche/Livedoid, DIC, Purpura fulminans, Coumadin necrosis, TTP, Sneddon (livedo reticularis + cerebrovascular ischemia), Cholesterol emboli, CADASIL, Calciphylaxis, Amyloid

# Cryoglobulinemia

| Cryoglobulinemia type* | Monoclonal or polyclonal | Immunoglobulins | Diseases |
|---|---|---|---|
| 1 ('Simple/Single') | Single monoclonal | IgM > IgG > IgA or light chain | **Associations:** Lymphoproliferative disorders: lymphoma, CLL, myeloma, Waldenstrom macroglobulinemia <br> **Manifestations:** Retiform necrotic lesions, acrocyanosis, Raynaud phenomenon, cold urticaria, livedo reticularis, retinal hemorrhage, arterial thrombosis |
| 2 ('Mixed') | Monoclonal and polyclonal | Monoclonal IgM (RF) complexed to polyclonal IgG | **Associations:** HCV > other autoimmune (Sjögren, SLE, RA), infections (CMV, EBV, HIV, HBV, HAV), lymphoproliferative disorders <br> **Manifestations:** LCV with palpable purpura, arthralgias/arthritis involving PIPs, MCPs, knees and ankles, diffuse glomerulonephritis |
| 3 ('Mixed') | Polyclonal | IgG and/or IgM | **Associations:** HCV, other autoimmune (Sjögren, SLE, RA), infections (CMV, EBV, HIV, HBV, HAV), lymphoproliferative disorders <br> **Manifestations:** LCV with palpable purpura, arthralgias/arthritis involving PIP, MCP, knees and ankles, diffuse glomerulonephritis |

Rheumatoid Factor = Antibody against Fc portion of IgG = Cryoglobulinemia Types 2 (monoclonal RF) and 3 (polyclonal RF).

Meltzer Triad = Purpura, arthralgia, weakness.

Work-up: Serum specimen must be obtained in WARM tubes. Immunoglobulins precipitate at cold temperature. Type 1 precipitates in 24 h, Type 3 may require 7 days.

**Cryoglobulinemia:** Immunoglobulins which reversibly precipitate on cold exposure.

**Cryofibrinogen:** Fibrinogen, fibrin, fibronectin which precipitate in the cold.

**Cold Agglutinins:** IgM antibodies which promote agglutination of RBCs on exposure to cold, triggering complement activation and lysis of RBCs.

*All 3 groups cause occlusive syndromes in the skin triggered by cold exposure.

# CTCL Classification

| | Relative frequency (%) | 5-Year survival (%) |
|---|---|---|
| Indolent cutaneous T-cell and NK-cell lymphoma | | |
| Mycosis fungoides | 44 | 88 |
| Follicular MF | 4 | 80 |
| Pagetoid reticulosis | <1 | 100 |
| Granulomatous slack skin | <1 | 100 |
| Cutaneous anaplastic CD30+ large cell lymphoma | 8 | 95 |
| Lymphomatoid papulosis | 12 | 100 |
| Subcutaneous panniculitis-like T-cell lymphoma | 1 | 82 |
| CD4+ small/medium pleomorphic T-cell lymphoma | 2 | 75 |
| Aggressive cutaneous T-cell and NK-cell lymphoma | | |
| Sézary syndrome | 3 | 24 |
| Cutaneous aggressive CD8+ T-cell lymphoma | <1 | 18 |
| Cutaneous γ/δ T-cell lymphoma | <1 | – |
| Cutaneous peripheral T-cell lymphoma unspecified | 2 | 16 |
| Cutaneous NK/T-cell lymphoma, nasal-type | <1 | – |

Modified from: Willemze R *et al.* WHO-EORTC classification for cutaneous lymphoma. *Blood* 2005;105,3798. Based on 1905 patients with primary cutaneous lymphoma registered at the Dutch and Austrian Cutaneous Lymphoma Group 1986–2002.

## Mycosis fungoides variants

**Alibert-Bazin** – classic type of MF

**Follicular MF** – 10% of MF, folliculotropic infiltrates, follicular mucinosis, favors head and neck (esp. eyebrow), alopecia, mucinorrhea, pruritic, stage as if classical tumor stage. Less responsive to skin directed therapies due to the deep follicular localization of MF infiltrate. *Follicular Mucinosis (Alopecia Mucinosa) Classification:

- Primary localized – pediatric, H/N, upper trunk, usu resolve within several months-years
- Primary chronic, generalized – adults, concerning for malignant progression
- Secondary – benign (lupus, LSC, ALHE, drug – adalimumab, imatinib), malignant (MF, KS, Hodgkin)

**Woringer-Kolopp/Pagetoid Reticulosis** – <1% of CTCL, localized, solitary hyperkeratotic patch/plaque, slowly progressive. Good prognosis – No reports of extracutaneous dissemination or disease-related deaths.

**Ketron-Goodmann** – disseminated pagetoid reticulosis, aggressive

**Granulomatous Slack Skin** – pendulous atrophic lax skin, esp. axillae and groin. Associated with MF or Hodgkin lymphoma in 1/3 of cases. Usually indolent, very rare.

**Sezary** – 5% of MF cases, triad of exfoliative erythoderma, lymphadenopathy, and atypical circulating ("Sezary," "Lutzner," or "mycosis") cells. MF-like immunophenotype but characteristically CD26- and CD3+ but diminished. Change from Th1 to Th2 profile may drive progression to Sezary.

## Clonality studies

- Suspected B-cell lymphomas: Flow cytometry (provides $\kappa{:}\lambda$ ratio, requires fresh tissue in cell culture), immunoglobulin heavy chain gene rearrangement studies (can use paraffin-embedded tissue), immunohistochemistry for kappa or lambda restriction has low sensitivity (normally $\kappa{:}\lambda$ ratio $\sim 3$)
- Suspected T-cell lymphomas: $\alpha\,\beta$ TCR gene rearrangement studies (more sensitive than $\gamma\,\delta$ TCR gene rearrangement studies, can use paraffin-embedded tissue), flow cytometry (less useful for suspected T-cell lymphomas)
- For detecting CTCL, specificity can be increased by performing TCR rearrangement studies on biopsy specimens from $\geqslant 2$ anatomic locations looking for a shared clone

## MF (TNMB) staging

| T (Skin) | N (Nodes) | M (Viscera) | B (Blood) |
|----------|-----------|-------------|-----------|
| T1= Patch/plaque <10% | N0= None | M0= None | B0= <5% Sezary cells |
| T2= Patch/plaque >10% | N1= Palpable nodes, path (−) | M1= Visceral involvement | B1= >5% Sezary cells |
| T3= Tumor(s) | N2= No palpable nodes, path (+) | | |
| T4= Erythroderma | N3= Palpable nodes, path (+) | | |

| Stage | Clinical involvement | Clinically enlarged nodes | Histologically + nodes | TNMB | 5-Year survival (%)* |
|-------|----------------------|---------------------------|------------------------|------|----------------------|
| IA | Patch/plaque < 10% | | | T1 N0 M0 | 96 |
| IB | Patch/plaque > 10% | | | T2 N0 M0 | 73 |
| IIA | Patch/plaque | + Nodes | − Path | T1-2 N1 M0 | 73 |
| IIB | Tumor(s) | ± Nodes | − Path | T3 N0-1 M0 | 44 |
| IIIA | Erythroderma | ± Nodes | − Path | T4 N0 M0 | 44 |
| IIIB | Erythroderma | + Nodes | − Path | T4 N1 M0 | |
| IVA | | + Nodes | + Path | T1-4 N2-3 M0 | 27 |
| IVB | Visceral involvement | | | T1-4 N0-3 M1 | |

Kim YH. Mycosis fungoides and the Sezary syndrome. *Semin Oncol.* 1999; 26: 276–89.
*Adapted from Kim YH *et al.* Long-term outcome of 525 patients with mycosis fungoides and Sezary syndrome. *Arch Dermatol.* 2003; 139: 857–66.

## MF treatment algorithm

| Stage | First line | Second line | Experimental |
|---|---|---|---|
| IA | SDT or no therapy | | |
| IB, IIA | SDT<br>PUVA, NB/BB-UVB | TSEB<br>Radiotherapy<br>IFN-α<br>PUVA + IFN-α,<br>Retinoids, or<br>Bexarotene<br>Low-dose MTX | Cytokines (i.e. Il-2, IL-12,<br>IFN-γ)<br>Pegylated Liposomal<br>Doxorubicin<br>Chlorodeoxyadenosine |
| IIB | TSEB + Superficial<br>radiotherapy<br>combination<br>(2 of 3) tx w/<br>IFN-α, PUVA, or<br>Retinoids | Denileukin diftitox<br>Bexarotene<br>IFN-α<br>Chemotherapy<br>Vorinostat | Autologous PBSCT,<br>mini-allograft<br>Zanolimumab |
| III | PUVA ± IFN-α or<br>Retinoids<br>ECP ± IFN-α<br>MTX<br>IFN-α | TSEB<br>Denileukin diftitox<br>Bexarotene<br>Chemotherapy<br>Alemtuzumab<br>Vorinostat | Autologous PBSCT,<br>mini-allograft<br>Zanolimumab |
| IVA, IVB | TSEB or<br>Radiotherapy,<br>Chemotherapy | IFN-α<br>Bexarotene<br>Denileukin Diftitox<br>Low-dose MTX<br>Alemtuzumab<br>Vorinostat<br>Palliative | Autologous PBSCT,<br>mini-allograft<br>Zanolimumab |

**SDT:** Skin-Directed Therapy: Emollients, Topical Steroids, Nitrogen Mustard
(Mechlorethamine/HN$_2$, Carmustine/BCNU), Bexarotene Gel, Imiquimod, Topical-MTX
**ECP:** Extracorporeal Photopheresis
**TSEB:** Total Skin Electron Beam
**PBSCT:** Peripheral Blood Stem Cell Transplant
Denileukin Diftitox = IL-2/Diptheria Toxin Fusion
Bexarotene = Retinoid X Receptor Specific
Vorinostat = Suberoylanilide Hydroxamic Acid, SAHA (Histone Deacetylase Inhibitor)
Alemtuzumab = anti-CD52
Zanolimumab = HuMax-CD4

Modified from: Whittaker SJ *et al.* Joint British Association of Dermatologists and UK
Cutaneous Lymphoma Group guidelines for the management of primary cutaneous
T-cell lymphomas. *Br J Dermatol.* 2003 Dec; 149(6):1095–107 and Trautinger F *et al.*
EORTC consensus recommendations for the treatment of mycosis Fungoides/Sézary
syndrome. *Eur J Cancer.* 2006; 42:1014–30.

# Cutaneous B-cell Lymphoma

| Type | Clinical | Immunophenotype | 5-Year survival (%) |
|---|---|---|---|
| Marginal zone | Often solitary lesions on trunk or extremities, possible Borrelia association, tattoo association | BCL2+ BCL6− CD10− IRTA1+ | >95 |
| Primary follicle center | Often solitary/ grouped plaques on scalp/forehead or trunk | BCL2− BCL6+ CD10± * | >95 |
| Diffuse large B-cell | 80% on leg of elderly patients, F>M | BCL2+ BCL6+ CD10− MUM1/ IRF4+ | 50 |

Other B-cell lymphomas – Intravascular large B-cell lymphoma, Lymphomatoid granulomatosis, CLL (ZAP-70+), Mantle cell lymphoma, Burkitt lymphoma, B-lymphoblastic lymphoma
*Secondary cutaneous follicle center lymphoma – BCL2+ BCL6+ CD10+ with t(14;18).
PREVALENCE: 20–25% of primary cutaneous lymphomas are B-cell lymphomas, each of the 3 major types representing ≤10% of cutaneous lymphomas.


## Leukemia cutis
- Affects children > adults
- Skin involvement rarely precedes systemic disease.
- Except for congenital leukemia, leukemia cutis is a poor prognostic sign, esp. with myeloid leukemia
- Frequently associated with extramedullary involvement
- Usually p/w asx papules and nodules
- Other presentations – CLL and HTLV-1-associated leukemia may be pruritic; greenish tumors = chloromas, aka granulocytic sarcomas (due to myeloperoxidase); gingival hypertrophy in AML-M4 and AML-M5; rarely leonine facies
- Histologically, often grenz zone (grenz zone DDx = granuloma faciale, lepromatous leprosy, lymphoma/leukemia/pseudolymphoma, acrodermatitis chronica atrophicans, AFX)
- Common Types:
  - AML – 10% of affected patients develop leukemia cutis (esp. AML-M4 and -M5)

- CLL and Hairy Cell Leukemia – 5–10% of affected patients develop leukemia cutis
- HTLV-1-associated leukemia – very rare type of leukemia (except in Caribbean, Japan) but 50% of patients may develop leukemia cutis (also get "infective dematitis")

## Monoclonal Gammopathies

- Types of monoclonal gammopathies by frequency: monoclonal gammopathy of undetermined significance (MGUS) (65%), multiple myeloma (15%), AL amyloidosis (10%), others (10%): plasmacytoma, Waldenstrom, lymphoma
- Ig produced by monoclonal gammopathies: IgG (60%), IgM (20%), IgA (15%), extremely rarely IgD or IgE

| Disease | Ig type |
| --- | --- |
| Direct cutaneous infiltration of cells causing monoclonal gammopathy or deposition of cell products | |
|   Waldenstrom | IgM |
|   AL amyloidosis | IgG |
|   Multiple myeloma | IgG |
|   Plasmacytoma | IgA |
|   Cryoglobulinemia | IgM |
| Disorders associated with monoclonal gammopathies | |
|   Scleromyxedema | IgG $\lambda$ |
|   Schnitzler | IgM $\kappa$ |
|   POEMS | IgA > IgG |
|   Scleredema | IgG $\kappa$ |
|   Plane xanthoma | IgG |
|   EED | IgA |
|   NXG | IgG $\kappa$ |
|   Pyoderma gangrenosum | IgA |
|   Sneddon-Wilkinson | IgA |
|   IgA pemphigus | IgA |
|   Sweet | IgG |

Source: Daoud MS *et al.* Monoclonal gammopathies and associated skin disorders. *J Am Acad Dermatol.* 1999; 40(4):507–35.

# Melanoma – Classification

## T classification

| Tx | 1° tumor cannot be assessed | |
|---|---|---|
| T0 | No evidence of 1° tumor | |
| Tis | Melanoma *in situ* | |
| T1 | ≤1.0 mm | a: no ulceration and Clarks level II/III |
| | | b: + ulceration or Clarks level IV/V |
| T2 | 1.01–2.0 mm | a: no ulceration |
| | | b: + ulceration |
| T3 | 2.01–4.0 mm | a: no ulceration |
| | | b: + ulceration |
| T4 | >4.0 mm | a: no ulceration |
| | | b: + ulceration |

## N classification

| Nx | Nodes cannot be assessed | |
|---|---|---|
| N0 | No regional lymphadenopathy | |
| N1 | 1 node | a: micrometastasis |
| | | b: macrometastasis |
| N2 | 2–3 nodes | a: micrometastasis |
| | | b: macrometastasis |
| | | c: satellite or in transit metastasis *without* metastatic nodes |
| N3 | ≥4 nodes or matted nodes, or in transit mets/satellites *and* metastatic nodes | |

**Micrometastases**: patients without clinical or radiologic evidence of LN mets (clinically occult) but with pathologically + nodal mets after sentinel or elective lymphadenectomy

**Macrometastases**: patients with clinically detectable of nodal metastases confirmed by therapeutic lymphadenectomy or when nodal mets exhibit gross extracapsular extension

Adapted from Balch CM *et al*. Final version of the AJCC staging system for cutaneous melanoma. *J Clin Oncol*. 2001; 19:3635–48.

## M classification

| Mx | Distant mets cannot be assessed |
|---|---|
| M0 | No distant metastases |
| M1a | Distant skin, subcutaneous, nodal metastases |
| M1b | Lung metastases |
| M1c | Other visceral metastases or distant metastasis at any site with elevated LDH |

| Clark level | |
|---|---|
| Level I | Confined to the epidermis (MIS) |
| Level II | Invasion past basement membrane into the papillary dermis |
| Level III | Tumor filling papillary dermis to the junction of the superficial reticular dermis |
| Level IV | Invasion into the reticular dermis |
| Level V | Invasion into the subcutaneous tissue |

## Breslow depth

Breslow tumor thickness is measured in mm from the top of the granular layer of the epidermis (or the base of an ulcer) to the deepest point of tumor invasion using an ocular micrometer.

## Melanoma – staging and survival

| | Clinical staging | | | Pathologic staging | | | Survival (%) | |
|---|---|---|---|---|---|---|---|---|
| | T | N | M | T | N | M | 5-Year | 10-Year |
| IA | T1a | 0 | 0 | T1a | 0 | 0 | 95 | 88 |
| IB | T1b | 0 | 0 | T1b | 0 | 0 | 91 | 83 |
| | T2a | | | T2a | | | 89 | 79 |
| IIA | T2b | 0 | 0 | T2b | 0 | 0 | 77 | 64 |
| | T3a | | | T3a | | | 79 | 64 |
| IIB | T3b | 0 | 0 | T3b | 0 | 0 | 63 | 51 |
| | T4a | | | T4a | | | 67 | 54 |
| IIC | T4b | 0 | 0 | T4b | 0 | 0 | 45 | 32 |
| IIIA | Any T* | N1–3 | 0 | T1-4a | N1a | 0 | 70 | 63 |
| | | | | T1-4a | N2a | | 63 | 57 |
| IIIB | | | | T1-4b | N1a | 0 | 53 | 38 |
| | | | | T1-4b | N2a | | 50 | 36 |
| | | | | T1-4a | N1b | | 59 | 48 |
| | | | | T1-4a | N2b | | 46 | 39 |
| | | | | T1-4a/b | N2c | | | |
| IIIC | | | | T1-4b | N1b | 0 | 29 | 24 |
| | | | | T1-4b | N2b | | 24 | 15 |
| | | | | Any T | N3 | | 27 | 18 |
| IV | Any T | Any N | Any M | Any T | Any N | M1a | 19 | 16 |
| | | | | | | M1b | 7 | 3 |
| | | | | | | M1c | 10 | 6 |

*There are no Stage III subgroups in clinical staging.

Adapted from Balch CM *et al*. Final version of the AJCC staging system for cutaneous melanoma. *J Clin Oncol* 2001; 19:3635–648.

# Melanoma – treatment guidelines

| Breslow depth (mm) | Margin (cm) | SLN* | Physical exam** | Work-up*** | Adjuvant Treatment |
|---|---|---|---|---|---|
| *In situ* | 0.5 | No | q6months × 1 year then yearly | • Symptom specific (CT, PET, MRI) | – |
| <1 | 1 | No* | q3–12 months | • Symptom specific (CT, PET, MRI) | – |
| 1.01–2.00 | 1–2 | Yes | q3–6 months × 3 years, q4–12 months × 2 years, then yearly | • CXR, LDH, CBC, LFT q3–12 months (optional) | – |
| 2.01–4.00 | 2 | Yes | | • Symptom specific (CT, PET, MRI) | • Clinical Trial<br>• Observe |
| >4 | 2 | Yes | | | • Clinical Trial<br>• Observe<br>• IFN α |
| Stage III SLN +, micromet | WLE (as above) | LNC or clinical trial | q3–6 months × 3 years, q4–12 months × 2 years, then yearly | • CXR, LDH, CBC, LFT q3–12 months (optional)<br>• Symptom specific (CT, PET, MRI) | • Clinical Trial<br>• Observe<br>• IFN α |

continued p. 38

GENERAL DERMATOLOGY

| Breslow depth (mm) | Margin (cm) | SLN* | Physical exam** | Work-up*** | Adjuvant treatment |
|---|---|---|---|---|---|
| Stage III Clinical + nodes, macromet | WLE | FNA or bx of +LN, then LND | | | • Clinical Trial<br>• Observe<br>• IFN α<br>• ±RT to nodal basin if Stage IIIC |
| Stage III in-transit | WLE + FNA or Bx of in-transit lesions | Yes | q3–6 months × 3 years, q4–12 months × 2 years, then yearly | • CXR, LDH, CBC, LFT q3–12 months (optional)<br>• Symptom specific (CT, PET, MRI) | • Intralesional BCG, IL-2<br>• CO$_2$ ablation<br>• Limb perfusion with melphalan<br>• Clinical Trial<br>• Radiation tx<br>• Systemic tx |
| Stage IV | FNA or bx | Yes | q3–6 months × 3 years, q4–12 months × 2 years, then yearly | • Baseline CXR, Chest CT, LDH<br>• Abd/pelvic CT, MRI brain, PET as indicated | • See NCCN Guidelines<br>• Clinical trial<br>• Dacarbazine<br>• Temozolomide<br>• High Dose IL2 |

*Sentinel Lymph node should be performed at time of Wide Local Excision. Consider in tumor <1mm if initial bx with Clark IV/V, ulceration, positive deep margin, or extensive regression. The yield and clinical significance of SLNBx in Stage IA is unknown.

**Follow-up: At least annual skin exam for life, educate patient in monthly self skin and lymph noce exam. No evidence to support specific follow-up interval. AAD Task force recommends q3–12 months × 2 years, then q6–12 months. (Sober et al. AAD Guidelines: Care for primary cutaneous melanoma. J AM Acad Dermatol 2001; 579–86.)

***Evaluation: Strong evidence that routine CXR and blood work have limited value in patients with Stage 0/IA disease (Sober et al. AAD Guidelines: Care for primary cutaneous melanoma. J Am Acad Dermatol 2001; 579–86.) CT, PET, MRI may be performed to evaluate specific sxs.

Adapted from NCCN Practice Guideline in Oncology- v.2.2007 Melanoma.

# Infectious Disease

## Viruses and diseases

| | Family | Examples | Replication site | Genome (+ sense; − antisense) |
|---|---|---|---|---|
| DNA | Poxviridae | Molluscipox: Molluscum<br>Orthopox: Vaccinia, smallpox, cowpox<br>Parapox: Orf, milker's nodule ("pseudo-cowpox") | Cytoplasm | dsDNA |
| | Papillomaviridae | Human papilloma virus | Nucleus | dsDNA |
| | Herpesviridae | HHV1: HSV1<br>HHV2: HSV2<br>HHV3: VZV<br>HHV4: EBV<br>HHV5: CMV<br>HHV6: Roseola infantum, reactivation increases<br>   drug-induced hypersensitivity syndrome severity<br>HHV7: ? Pityriasis rosea<br>HHV8: Kaposi sarcoma | Nucleus | dsDNA for all |
| | Hepadnaviridae | HBV | Nucleus w/ RNA intermediate* | Gapped dsDNA |

continued p. 40

|  | Family | Examples | Replication site | Genome (+ sense; − antisense) |
|---|---|---|---|---|
|  | Adenoviridae | Human adenovirus | Nucleus | dsDNA |
|  | Parvoviridae | Erythema infectiosum | Nucleus | ssDNA |
| RNA | Paramyxoviridae | Measles, Mumps | Nucleus | −ssRNA |
|  | Togaviridae | Rubella, Chikungunya | Cytoplasm | +ssRNA |
|  | Rhabdoviridae | Rabies | Nucleus | −ssRNA |
|  | Retroviridae | HIV, HTLV | Nucleus | +ssRNA (dsDNA intermediate) |
|  | Picornaviridae | Enterovirus (coxsackie; HAV) | Nucleus | +ssRNA |
|  | Flaviviridae | HCV, West Nile, Yellow Fever, Dengue | Cytoplasm | +ssRNA |
|  | Filoviridae | Ebola, Marburg | Cytoplasm | −ssRNA |
|  | Bunyaviridae | Hantavirus, Rift valley, Congo-Crimean | Cytoplasm | −ssRNA |
|  | Arenaviridae | Lassa | Cytoplasm | −ssRNA |

*Therefore, HBV is susceptible to anti-HIV medications.

# Human papillomavirus

| Disease | Description | Associated HPV type |
|---|---|---|
| Verruca vulgaris | Common warts | 1, 2, 4 |
| Myrmecia | Large cup-shaped palmoplantar warts | 1 |
| Verruca plantaris/palmaris | Plantar warts | 1, 2, 27, 57 |
| Butcher's wart | Warty lesions from handling raw meat | 2, 7 |
| Verrucous carcinoma, foot | Epithelioma cuniculatum | 2, 11, 16 |
| Verruca planae | Flat warts | 3, 10 |
| Epidermodysplasia verruciformis | Inherited disorder of HPV infection and SCCs | 3, 5, 8, 12, many others |
| Buschke and Löwenstein | Giant condyloma | 6, 11 |
| Condyloma acuminata | Genital warts | LOW RISK: 6, 11 HIGH RISK: 16, 18, 31 Flat condyloma: 42 Oral condyloma: 6, 11 |
| Oral florid papillomatosis (Ackermann) | Oral/nasal, multiple lesions, smoking/irradiation/chronic inflammation | 6, 11 |
| Recurrent respiratory papillomatosis | Laryngeal papillomas | 6, 11 |
| Heck disease (Focal epithelial hyperplasia) | Small white and pink papules in mouth | 13, 32 |
| Bowen disease | SCCIS | 16, 18 |
| Bowenoid papulosis | Genital papules and plaques resembling Bowen disease | 16, 18 |
| Cervical cancer | | 16, 18, 31, 33, 35, 39 Guardasil: 6, 11, 16, 18 |
| Stucco keratoses | White hyperkeratotic plaques on legs | 23b, 9, 16 |
| Ridged wart | Wart with preserved dermatoglyphics | 60 |

## Other viral diseases

| Viral disease | Description | Cause |
|---|---|---|
| Boston exanthem | Roseola-like morbilliform eruption on face and trunk, small oral ulcerations | Echovirus 16 |
| Castleman disease (associated w/ POEMS and paraneoplastic pemphigus) | (Angio)lymphoid hamartoma: hyaline-vascular type, plasma cell, and multicentric/ generalized types | HHV-8 |
| Dengue fever (virus may cause Dengue fever, Dengue hemorrhagic fever, or Dengue shock syndrome) | Rash in 50% of patients, flushing erythema within 1–2 days of symptom onset, then 3–5 days later a generalized often asx maculopapular eruption with distinct white "islands of sparing," 1/3 mucosal lesions, may be ecchymotic or petechial, incubation 3–14 days | Dengue flavivirus |
| Eruptive pseudoangiomatosis | Fever, transient hemangioma-like lesions, usually children, often with halo | Echovirus 25 & 32 |
| Erythema infectiosum (Fifth disease) | Children aged 4–10 years, "slapped cheeks," reticular exanthem, usually extremities, arthropathy in adults, anemia/ hydrops in fetus, persistent in Sickle Cell | Parvovirus B19 |
| Gianotti-Crosti syndrome (Papular acrodermatitis of childhood) | Children (often ≤4 years old) with acute onset of often asymptomatic, lichenoid papules on face and extremities, less on trunk | Various: HBV most common worldwide, EBV most common in U.S. |
| Hand-foot-and-mouth | Brief mild prodrome, fever, erosive stomatitis, acral and buttock vesicles, highly contagious, mouth hurts, skin asymptomatic | Various Coxsackie viruses, Coxsackie Virus A16, Enterovirus 71 |
| Herpangina | Fever, painful oral vesicles/ erosions, no exanthem | Coxsackie Groups A and B, various echoviruses |

| Viral disease | Description | Cause |
|---|---|---|
| Hydroa vacciniforme | Vesiculopapules, photosensitivity, pediatric with resolution by early adulthood | EBV (when severe, EBV-associated NK/T-cell lymphoproliferative disorders) |
| Infectious mononucleosis (Glandular fever) | 2 peaks: 1–6 years old and 14–20 years old; fever, pharyngitis, (cervical) lymphadenopathy, HSM, eyelid edema, 5% rash, leukocytosis, elevated LFTs; 90% get maculopapular exanthema with ampicillin/amoxicillin | EBV (also causes nasopharyngeal carcinoma, post-transplant lymphoproliferative disorder, African Burkitt lymphoma) |
| Kaposi sarcoma | Vascular tumors | HHV-8 |
| Kaposi varicelliform eruption (Eczema herpeticum) | Often generalized, crusted, vesiculopustular dermatitis; may be umbilicated*; fever, malaise, lymphadenopathy | HSV, may also occur with coxsackie, vaccinia, and other dermatitidis |
| Lichen planus | Purple, polygonal, planar, pruritic, papules | HCV |
| Measles (Rubeola) | Prodrome – cough, coryza, conjunctivitis, Koplik spots. Then maculopapular rash spreads craniocaudally. Incubation 10–14 days | Paramyxovirus |
| Milker's nodules | Similar to Orf From infected cows | Paravaccinia/ Parapoxvirus |
| Molluscum contagiosum | Umbilicated papules in children and HIV, or as STD | Poxvirus; 4 MCV subtypes: MCV 1 is most common overall, MCV 2 in immunocompromised |
| Monkeypox | Smallpox-like but milder and lesions may appear in crops, with prominent lymphadenopathy, and without centrifugal spread | Monkeypox /Orthopoxvirus (smallpox vaccination is protective) |
| Oral hairy leukoplakia | Non-painful, corrugated white plaque on lateral tongue in HIV or other immunosuppressed patients, + smoking correlation | EBV |

continued p. 44

| Viral disease | Description | Cause |
|---|---|---|
| Orf (Ecthyma contagiosum) | Umbilicated nodule after animal contact, 6 stages; sheep, goats, reindeer; self-limiting in ~5 weeks | Orf/Parapoxvirus |
| Papular/Purpuric stocking-glove syndrome | Young adults, mild prodrome, enanthem, edema, erythema, petechiae, purpura, burning, pruritus on wrists/ankles | Various: Parvovirus B19, Coxsackie B6, HHV-6 |
| Pityriasis rosea | Usually asymptomatic papulosquamous exanthem | Possibly HHV-7 |
| Ramsey Hunt | Vesicular lesions following geniculate ganglion on external ear, tympanic membrane, with ipsilateral facial paralysis and deafness, tinnitus, vertigo, oral lesions | VZV |
| Roseola infantum (Exanthum subitum, sixth disease) | Infants with high fever (x3 days) followed by morbilliform rash, 15% have seizure | HHV-6B, rarely HHV-6A or HHV-7 |
| Rubella (German measles) | Mild prodrome, tender LAN, pain with superolateral eye movements, morbilliform rash, spreads craniocaudally, petechial enanthem (Forschiemer spots), incubation 16–18 days | Togavirus |
| Smallpox | 7–17 days incubation, 2–4 days prodrome (fever, HA, malaise), then centrifugal vesiculopustular rash, lesions are all the same stage, respiratory spread | Variola/Orthopoxvirus |
| STAR complex | Sore throat, elevated Temperature, Arthritis, Rash | Various: HBV, Parvovirus B19, Rubella |
| Unilateral laterothoracic exanthem | Age <4 years, morbilliform or eczematous, often starts in axilla, unilateral then spreads | Various: EBV, HBV, Echovirus 6 |

*Umblicated lesions DDx: molluscum, pox viruses, HSV, histoplasmosis, cryptococcosis, penicilliosis, perforating disorders, leprosy, GA.

Adapted from Benjamin A. Solky, MD and Jennifer L. Jones, MD. Boards' Fodder – Viruses

## Mycoses
## Laboratory tests
*Direct Microscopy*
KOH: softens keratin, clearing effect can be accelerated by
gentle heating
DMSO: softens keratin more quickly than KOH alone in the absence
of heat
Chlorazole Black E: chitin specific, stains hyphae green
Parker Black Ink: stains hyphae, not chitin specific
Calcofluor White: stains fungal cell wall (chitin) and fluoresces blue/white
or apple/green using fluorescent microscopy
India Ink: capsule excludes ink (halo effect) – best for Cryptococcus
neoformans
Gram Stain: stains blue
PAS: stains red
GMS: stains black
Mucicarmine: pink = capsule; red = yeast
AFB: + if nocardia
Lactophenol Cotton Blue: use for mounting and staining fungal colonies

*Cultures*
Sabouraud's Dextrose Agar: standard medium for fungal growth
> + chloramphenicol: inhibits bacteria
> + cycloheximide: use to recover dimorphic fungi and dermatophytes.
> Inhibits crypto, candida (*not albicans*), Prototheca, Scopulariopsis,
> Aspergillus

Dermatophyte Test Medium (DTM): use to recover dermatophytes
> Turns medium from yellow to red (pH indicator)

## Superficial mycoses
**White piedra:** Trichosporon. Soft mobile nodules, face, axilla,
pubic, tropical.
> Tx: Shave hair. Systemic antifungal if relapse.

**Black piedra:** Piedraia hortae. Hard non-mobile nodules, face, scalp,
pubic, temperate.
> Tx: Shave hair. Systemic antifungal if relapse.

**Tinea nigra:** Phaeoannellomyces (Hortaea) werneckii. Brown macules
on the palms.
> Tx: Topical iodine, azole antifungal, terbinafine for 2–4 weeks
> beyond resolution to prevent relapse. Resistant to griseofulvin.

**Tinea versicolor:** Malassezia furfur/Pityrosporum ovale. Hypo/
hyperpigmented macules on trunk and extremities.

> KOH: 'spaghetti and meatballs' – hyphae and spores
>
> Tx: Topical ketoconazole cream, selenium sulfide shampoo, oral
> ketoconazole.

## DDx superficial bacterial infection

> Erythrasma: Corynebacterium minutissima (coproporphyrin III)
>
> Trichomycosis axillaris: Corynebacterium tenuis
>
> Pitted keratolysis: Micrococcus sedentarius

## Cutaneous mycoses
## Dermatophytes by sporulation characteristics

|  | **Trichophyton** | **Microsporum** | **Epidermophyton** |
|---|---|---|---|
| Macroconidia | Rare | Many | Many, grouped |
| Shape | Cigar/pencil | Spindled/tapered | Club/blunt |
| Wall | Thin/smooth | Thick/echinulate | Thin/smooth |
| Microconidia | Many | Few | None |

## Dermatophytes by mode of transmission
*Zoophilic and geographic dermatophytes elicit significant inflammation*

| Anthrophilic | Humans | T. rubrum, T. tonsurans, E. floccosum, T. concentricum, T. mentagrophytes var. interdigitale |
|---|---|---|
| Zoophilic | Animals | T. mentagrophytes var. mentagrophytes, M. canis, T. Verrucosum |
| Geographic | Soil | M. gypseum |

## Most common dermatophytes

| Tinea corporis, tinea cruris, tinea mannum, tinea pedis | T. rubrum, T. mentagrophytes, E. floccosum |
|---|---|
| Tinea pedis | **Moccasin:** T. rubrum, E. floccosum |
|  | **Vesicular:** T. mentagrophytes var. mentagrophytes |
| Onychomycosis | **Distal subungual:** T. rubrum |
|  | **Proximal white subungual (HIV):** T. rubrum |
|  | **White superficial:** T. mentagrophytes (adults); T. rubrum (children). Also molds: Aspergillus, Cephalosporium, Fusarium, Scopulariopsis |

| Tinea barbae | Usually zoophilic dermatophytes (esp. T. mentagrophytes var. mentagrophytes and T. verrucosum) or T. rubrum |
|---|---|
| Tinea capitis | **US:** T. tonsurans > M. audouinii, M. canis |
| | **Europe:** M. canis, M. audouinii |
| | **Favus:** T. schoenleinii > T. violaceum, M. gypseum |
| Tinea imbricata/ Tokelau | T. concentricum |
| Majocchi granuloma | Often T. rubrum > T. violaceum, T. tonsurans |

## Dermatophytes invading hair

| Ectothrix | Fluorescent (pteridine) | M. canis, M. audouinii, M. distortum, M. ferrugineum, M gypseum |
|---|---|---|
| | Non-fluorescent | T. mentagrophytes, T. rubrum, T. verrucosum, T. megninii, M. gypseum, M. nanum |
| Endothrix (black dot) | | T. rubrum, T. tonsurans, T. violaceum, T. gourvilli, T. yaoundie, T. soudanense, T. schoenleinii (fluoresces) |

M. gypseum may or may not be fluorescent; T. rubrum may be ecto- or endothrix
E. floccosum and T. concentricum do not invade scalp hair.

## Subcutaneous mycoses

| Disease | Etiology | In vivo/KOH (Tissue phase) | Culture (Mold phase) | Clinical | Tx |
|---|---|---|---|---|---|
| Sporotrichosis | Sporothrix schenckii | Cigar-shaped budding yeast, Splendore–Hoeppli phenomenon | Hyphae with daisy sporulation | Florist, gardener, farmer: (rose thorn, splinter), Zoonotic (cats) Sporotrichoid spread (fixed if prior exposure) Sporotrichoid DDx: leish, atypical mycobacteria, tularemia, nocardia, furunculosis | Itraconazole, SSKI |
| Chromoblastomycosis | Fonsecaea (most common), Cladosporium, Phialophora, Rhinocladiella | Copper pennies/Medlar bodies/sclerotic bodies | | Small pink warty papule expands slowly to indurated verrucous plaques with surface black dots | Itraconazole, surgical excision |
| Phaeohyphomycosis | Exophiala jeanselmei, Wangiella dermatitidis, Alternaria, Bipolaris, Curvularia, Phialophora | Like chromo but with hyphae | | Solitary subcutaneous draining abscess | Surgical excision, itraconazole |
| Lobomycosis (Keloidal blastomycosis) | Loboa loboi (Lacazia loboi) | Lemon-shaped cell chains with narrow intracellular bridges Maltese crosses-polarized light | Not cultured | Bottle nose dolphins and rural men in Brazil Confluent papules/verrucous nodules that ulcerate/crusts Fibrosis may resemble keloids | Surgical excision |

| Disease | Organism | Diagnostic feature | | Clinical features | Treatment |
|---|---|---|---|---|---|
| Zygomycosis | Conidiobolus coronatus | | | Rhinofacial subcutaneous mass | Surgical excision |
| Rhinosporidiosis (protozoan) | Rhinosporidium seeberi | Giant sporangia (raspberries) Stains with mucicarmine | Not cultured | Stagnant water, endemic in India and Sri Lanka Nasopharyngeal polyps may obstruct breathing | |
| Protothecosis (algae) | Prototheca wickerhamii | Morula (soccer ball) | | Olecranon bursitis | |
| Actinomycotic mycetoma (bacterial) | Actinomadura pelletieri (red) Actinomadura madurae (white) Streptomyces (yellow) Actinomyces israeli Botryomycosis Nocardia (white-orange) | | | Volcano-like ulcer and sinus tracts Sulfur grains – yellow, white, red, or brown Tissue swelling Early bone and muscle invasion | Antimicrobial |
| Eumycotic mycetoma (fungal) | Pseudallescheria boydii (most common, white-yellow) Madurella grisea Madurella mycetomi (brown-black) Exophiala jeanselmei Acremonium spp. (white-yellow) | | | Small ulcer with sinus tracts Sulfur grains (white or black) Tissue swelling Lytic bone changes occur late; rare muscle invasion | Antifungal rarely effective, surgical excision |

## Systemic mycoses

| Disease | Etiology | *In vivo*/KOH (Tissue phase) | Culture (Mold phase) | Clinical | Tx |
|---|---|---|---|---|---|
| Coccidiomycosis (San Joaquin Valley fever) | *Coccidioides immitis/C. posadasii* | Large spherules, Splendore-Hoeppli phenomenon | Boxcars: barrel-shaped arthroconidia alternating with empty cells | Southwestern US, Mexico, Central America Primary pulmonary infection (60% asx) Dissemination to CNS, bone Skin lesions more verrucous. May develop EN or EM lesions | Itraconazole, fluconazole, amphoB |
| Paracoccidiomycosis (South American blastomycosis) | *Paracoccidioides brasiliensis* | Mariner's wheel (thin-walled yeast with multiple buds) | Oval microconidia indistinguishable from Blastomyces | South America, Central America Chronic granulomatous pulmonary disease Disseminates to liver, spleen, adrenals, GI, nodes Skin: granulomatous oral/ perioral lesions * Men >> women: estrogen may inhibit growth | Ketoconazole |
| Blastomycosis (Gilchrist disease, North American blastomycosis) | *Blastomyces dermatitidis* | Broad-based budding yeast with thick walls | Lollipop spores | Southeast US and Great Lakes Primary pulmonary infection Disseminates to CNS, liver, spleen, GU, long bones Skin: verrucous lesion with "stadium edge" borders | Itraconazole, amphoB |
| Histoplasmosis (Darling disease) | *Histoplasmosis capsulatum/H. duboisii* | Intracellular yeasts in macrophages (parasitized histiocytes, may see halo unlike Leish) | Tuberculate macroconidia | Mississippi/ Ohio river valley basin- bird/bat droppings Most common: pulmonary infection (80–95%) Dissemination to liver, BM, spleen, CNS Skin: molluscum-like lesions in AIDS | Itrazconazole, amphoB |

## Opportunistic mycoses

| Disease | Etiology | *In vivo*/KOH (Tissue phase) | Culture (Mold phase) | Clinical |
|---------|----------|------------------------------|----------------------|----------|
| Candidiasis | *Candida albicans* | Pseudohyphae or true septate hyphae | Part of normal enteric flora<br>Infection is due to predisposing factors: impaired epithelial barrier: burns, maceration, wounds, occlusion, foreign bodies (dentures, catheters), antibiotics<br>Constitutional disorders: DM2, polyendocrinopathy, malnutrition<br>Immunodeficiency: cytotoxic agents, neutropenia, agranulocytosis, HIV, chronic granulomatous disease | Topicals: nystatin, miconazole, clotrimazole<br>Systemic: SAF |
| Cryptococcosis | *Cryptococcus neoformans* | Encapsulated yeasts with surrounding clear halo, "tear drop budding"<br>Stain with mucicarmine, PAS, GMS, or India ink | Bird droppings — usually via pulmonary infection then hematogenous spread to lungs, bones, and viscera. Predilection for CNS.<br>Skin: nasopharygeal papules/pustules, SQ ulcerated abscess | AmphoB<br>fluconazole |
| Aspergillosis | *Aspergillus flavus*<br>*A. fumigatus*<br>*A. niger* | Phialides with chains of conidia (broom brush)<br>Septate hyphae 45° branching | Infection from inhalation of conidia → pulmonary aspergillosis<br>Allergic bronchopulmonary aspergillosis: hypersensitivity, no tissue invasion<br>Invasive/ Disseminated aspergillosis: angioinvasive | Allergic: steroid<br>Invasive: SAF |
| Zygomycosis/<br>Mucormycosis | *Rhizopus*<br>*Mucor*<br>*Absidia* | Hyphae broad ribbon-like with 90° branching<br>Rhizoid opposite sporangia<br>No rhizoids<br>Rhizoids between sporangia | Most commonly respiratory portal of entry → rhinocerebral infection<br>Associated with diabetic ketoacidosis | AmphoB, surgical excision |
| Penicilliosis | *Penicillium marneffei* | Histo-like intracellular yeasts | Southeast Asia<br>Umbilicated lesions, 85% of affected patients have skin lesions | AmphoB, fluconazole |

SAF: Systemic Antifungal: amphoB, liposomal amphoB, flucorazole, itraconazole, voriconazole, caspofungin.

## Vector-borne diseases

| Disease | Cause | Vector/Transmission | Treatment |
|---|---|---|---|
| Acrodermatitis chronica atrophicans (Pick-Herxheimer disease) | *Borrelia afzelii*, *Borrelia garinii* | *Ixodes ricinus, Ixodes hexagonus, Ixodes persulcatus* | Amoxicillin, doxycycline, cefotaxime, penicillin G |
| African Tick-Bite fever | *Rickettsia africae* | *Amblyomma hebraeum*, *Amblyomma variegatum* | Doxycycline |
| African Trypanosomiasis (sleeping sickness) | *Trypanosoma brucei gambiense* (West Africa) | Tsetse fly (*Glossina morsitans*) | Pentamidine isethionate (hemolytic stage) |
| – Winterbottom's sign (posterior cervical LAN) | | | Melarsoprol or eflornithine (CNS involvement) |
| – Kerandel's sign (hyperesthesia) | *Trypanosoma brucei rhodesiense* (East Africa) | Tsetse fly (*Glossina morsitans*) | Suramin (hemolytic stage)<br>Melarsoprol (CNS involvement) |
| Bacillary angiomatosis | *Bartonella henselae, Bartonella quintana* | Cat flea (*Pediculus humanus*) | Erythromycin, doxycycline |
| Brazilian spotted fever | *Rickettsia rickettsii* | *Amblyomma cajennense*<br>RESERVOIR: Capybara | Doxycycline |

| Disease | Organism | Vector/Source | Treatment |
|---|---|---|---|
| Carrion disease (Bartonellosis, Oroya fever, Verruga peruana) | *Bartonella bacilliformis* | Sandfly (*Lutzomyia verrucarum*) | Chloramphenicol (due to frequent superinfxn with salmonella) |
| Cercarial Dermatitis (Swimmer's itch) | Cercariae of animal schistosomes | Snail | Topical corticosteroids |
| Chagas Disease (American trypanosomiasis) | *Trypanosoma cruzi* | Reduviid bug (assassin bug, kissing bug) | Benznidazole, nifurtimox |
| Cutaneous Larva Migrans (Creeping eruption) | *Ancylostoma brasiliense, Ancylostoma caninum* | Animal feces | Albendazole, ivermectin, thiabendazole topically |
| Cysticercosis | *Taenia solium* | Contaminated pork | Albendazole, praziquantel |
| Dengue fever | Flavivirus | *Aedes aegypti* or *albopticus* | Supportive Tx |
| Dracunculiasis | *Dracunculus medinensis* (Guinea fire worm) | Cyclops water flea ingestion | Slow extraction of worm + wound care Oral metronidazole facilitates removal |
| Ehrlichiosis, human monocytic (HME) | *Ehrlichia chaffeensis* | *Amblyomma americanum* | Doxycycline, rifampin (pregnancy) |
| Ehrlichiosis, human granulocytic (HGE) and human granulocytic anaplasmosis (HGA) | *Ehrlichia ewingii* (HGE), *Anaplasma phagocytophilum* (HGA) | *Ixodes persulcatus* and *Dermacentor variabilis* | Doxycycline, rifampin (pregnancy) |

*continued p. 54*

53

| Disease | Cause | Vector/Transmission | Treatment |
|---------|-------|---------------------|-----------|
| Elephantiasis tropica (lymphatic filariasis) | *Wuchereria bancrofti, Brugia malayi, Brugia timori* | *Culex, Aedes,* and *Anopheles* mosquitos | Diethylcarbamazine |
| Erysipeloid (of Rosenbach) | *Erysipelothrix rhusiopathiae* | Fish, shellfish, poultry, meat | Penicillin G, cipro, erythromycin/rifampin |
| Glanders (Farcy) | *Burkholderia (Pseudomonas) mallei* | Horses, mules, donkeys | Augmentin, doxycycline, TMP-SMX |
| Kala-azar (visceral leishmaniasis) | *L. donovani; L. infantum* (Old World) *L. chagas* (New World) | *Phlebotomus* sand fly *Lutzomyia* sand fly | Pentavalent antimony (sodium stibogluconate) or amphotericin |
| Leishmaniasis, New World (muco)cutaneous (Chiclero ulcer, Uta, Espundia, Bay sore) | *L. mexicana, L. brasiliensis* | *Lutzomyia* sand fly | Pentavalent antimony (sodium stibogluconate) or amphotericin |
| Leishmaniasis, Old World cutaneous (Oriental/Baghdad/Dehli sore) | *L. tropica; L. major, L. aethiopia, L. infantum* | *Phlebotomus* sand fly RESERVOIR: Rodents | Pentavalent antimony (sodium stibogluconate) |
| Loiasis (Calabar, Fugitive swelling) | *Loa loa* | *Tabanid* (horse/mango) fly, *Chrysops* (red, deer) fly | Diethylcarbamazine |
| Lyme disease | US: *Borrelia burgdorferi* EUROPE: *B. garinii & B. afzelli* | NE/GREAT LAKES: *Ixodes scapularis/dammini* WEST US: *I. pacificus* EUROPE: *I. ricinus* | Doxycycline Amoxicillin if pregnancy or <9 years old |
| Mediterranean spotted fever (Boutonneuse fever) | *Rickettsia conorii* | *Rhipicephalus sanguineous* (dog tick) | Doxycycline, chloramphenicol, floroquinolone |

| | | |
|---|---|---|
| Melioidosis (Whitmore disease) | *Burkholderia (Pseudomonas) pseudomallei* | IV ceftazidime (high intensity phase) then TMZ-SMX and Doxycycline |
| Myiasis | *Dermatobia hominis* (botfly), *Cordylobia anthropophaga* (tumbu fly), *Phaenicia sericata* (green blowfly) | Mosquito (for *Dermatobia hominis*) | Removal of larvae and treatment with abx for superinfection |
| Onchocerciasis (River blindness) | *Onchocerca volvulus* | *Simulium* species (black fly) | Ivermectin |
| Plague (Bubonic) | *Yersinia pestis* | *Xenopsylla cheopis* (rat flea) | Streptomycin, gentamicin |
| Q Fever | *Coxiella burnetii* | Dried tick feces inhalation | Doxycycline |
| Rat-Bite Fever (Haverhill, Sodoku) | *Spirillum minus* (Asia/Africa), *Streptobacillus moniliformis* (US) | Rat bite, scratch, excrement, contaminated food | Penicillin |
| Relapsing Fever – Louse-borne | *Borrelia recurrentis* (Africa, South America) | *Pediculosis humanus,* | Doxycycline |
| Relapsing Fever – Tick-borne | *Borrelia duttonii, Borrelia hermsii* (Western US) | *Ornithodorus* genus (soft-bodied ticks) | Doxycycline |
| Rickettsialpox | *Rickettsia akari* | *Allodermanyssus (Liponyssoides) sanguineus* (house mouse mite) RESERVOIR: *Mus musculus*- domestic mouse | Doxycycline |
| Rift valley fever | Phlebovirus, bunyavirus | *Aedes* | Supportive Tx, ribavirin (investigational) |

*continued p. 56*

| Disease | Cause | Vector/Transmission | Treatment |
|---|---|---|---|
| Rocky Mountain spotted fever | *Rickettsia rickettsii* | *Dermacentor andersoni, Dermacentor variabilis* | Doxycycline |
| Schistosomiasis/bilharziasis (Cercarial dermatitis, Katayama fever, late allergic dermatitis, perigenital granulomata, extragenital infiltrative) | *Schistosoma mansoni* (GI), *S. japonicum* (GI), *S. haematobium* (urinary system) | Snail | Praziquantel |
| Scrub typhus (Tsutsugamushi fever) | *Rickettsia/Orientia tsutsugamushi* | Larval stage of trombiculid mite (chigger, *Trombicula/Leptotrombidium akamushi*) | Doxycycline |
| South African tick-bite fever | *Rickettsia conorii* | *Rhipicephalus simus, Haemaphysalis leachii, Rhipicephalus mushamae* | Doxycycline |
| Sparganosis | *Spirometra* (dog and cat tapeworm larvae) | Application/ingestion of infected frog, snake, or fish | Surgical removal |
| Toxoplasmosis | *Toxoplasma gondii* | Cat feces, undercooked meat, milk | Pyrimethamine and sulfadiazine 1st trimester: spiramycin |
| Trench (Quintana) fever | *Bartonella quintana* | *Pediculus humanus corporis* | Doxycycline, erythromycin |
| Trichinosis | *Trichinella spiralis* | Undercooked pig, wild game | Steroids for severe symptoms and mebendazole or albenazole |

| | | |
|---|---|---|
| Tularemia (deer fly fever, Ohara disease) | *Francisella tularensis* | Rabbit, *Dermacentor andersonii*, *Amblyomma americanum*, *Chrysops discalis* (deer fly), domestic cats | Streptomycin |
| Typhus, endemic; murine/flea-borne typhus | *Rickettsia typhi* | *Xenopsylla cheopis* (rat flea) | Doxycycline |
| Typhus, epidemic; Brill-Zinsser disease/ relapsing louse-borne typhus) | *Rickettsia prowazekii* | *Pediculus humanus*, squirrel fleas RESERVOIR: *Glaucomys volans*-flying squirrel | Doxycycline |
| Weil Disease (leptospirosis) | *Leptospira interrogans icterohaemorriagiae* | Rat urine | Doxycycline, penicillin, ampicillin, amoxicillin |
| West Nile fever | Arbovirus | *Aedes, culex, anopheles* | Supportive Tx |
| Yellow fever | Arbovirus | *Aedes aegypti* | Supportive Tx |

Adapted from Solky BA, Jones JL, Boards' Fodder – Bugs and their Vectors. Treatment adapted from *The Medical Letter*. 2004; 46:1189.

## Creatures in dermatology

| Creature | Scientific name | Special features |
|---|---|---|
| **SPIDERS** | | |
| Brown Recluse spider | *Loxosceles reclusa* | • VENOM: Sphingomyelinase-D, hyaluronidase<br>• Violin-shaped marking on back<br>• Painless bite but with extensive necrosis<br>• Red, white, and blue sign<br>• Viscerocutaneous loxoscelism: fever, chills, vomit, joint pain, hemolytic anemia, shock, death<br>• Tx: steroid, ASA, antivenom. Avoid debridement |
| Black Widow spider | *Latrodectus mactans* | • VENOM: A-lactotoxin<br>• Hourglass-shaped red marking on abdomen<br>• Painful bites but no necrosis<br>• Neurotoxin causes chills, GI sxs, paralysis, spasm, diaphoresis, HTN, shock<br>• Tx: IV Ca gluconate, muscle relaxant, antivenom |
| Jumping spider | *Phidippus formosus* | • VENOM: Hyaluronidase<br>• Dark body hairs and various white patterns<br>• Very aggressive spider<br>• Painful with toxin venom but no systemic sxs |
| Wolf spider | *Lycosidae* | • VENOM: Histamine<br>• Lymphangitis, eschar |
| Sac spider | *Chiracanthium* | • VENOM: Lipase<br>• Yellow colored |
| Hobo spider | *Tegenaria agrestis* | • Herringbone-striped pattern on abdomen<br>• Painless bite with fast onset induration then eschar<br>• Aggressive spider<br>• Funnel-shaped web |
| Green Lynx spider | *Peucetia viridans* | • Green with red spots<br>• Painful bite with tenderness and pruritus |
| Tarantula | *Theraphosidae* | • Hairs cause urticaria<br>• Ophthalmia nodosa – if hair gets into eyes → chronic granuloma formation |

| Creature | Scientific name | Special features |
|---|---|---|
| **CATERPILLARS *Lepidoptera*** (urticaria after contact with hairs) | | |
| Puss/Asp | *Megalopyge opercularis* | • Brown woolly flat<br>• Checkerboard eruption |
| Iomoth | *Automeris io* | • Green with lateral white strip from head to toe |
| Gypsy/Tent moth | *Lymantria dispar* | • Histamine in lance-like hair<br>• Windborne can cause air-borne dermatitis |
| Saddleback | *Sibine stimulea* | • Bright green saddle on the back |
| Hylesia moth | *Hylesia metabus* | • Caparito/ Venezuela itch |
| Lonomia caterpillar | *Lonomia achelous/ obliqua* | • Latin America moth, fatal bleeding diathesis |
| **FLIES** | | |
| Black fly | *Simulium* | • VECTOR: Onchocerciasis |
| Sand fly | *Phlebotomus*<br>*Lutzomyia* | • VECTOR: *L. donovani, L. tropica, L. infantum, L. major, L. aethiopia*<br>• VECTOR: *L. mexicana, L. braziliensis*, Bartonellosis |
| Tsetse fly | *Glossina* | • VECTOR: African trypanosomiasis |
| Deer fly | *Chrysops* | • VECTOR: Loiasis, tularemia |
| Botfly larvae | *Dermatobia hominis,<br>Callitroga americana* (US) | • Myiasis when larvae (maggot) infest skin<br>• Other flies whose larvae cause myiasis: *Cordylobia anthropophaga* (tumbu fly, moist clothing) and *Phaenicia sericata* (green blowfly, US) |
| **MOSQUITOES *Culicidae*** | | |
| | *Anopheles* | • VECTOR: Malaria, filariasis |
| | *Aedes* | • VECTOR: Yellow fever, dengue, filariasis, chikungunya |
| | *Culex* | • VECTOR: Filariasis, West Nile |
| **FLEAS *Siphonaptera*** | | |
| Human flea | *Pulex irritans* | • May play role in plague, affects other mammals |
| Cat flea | *Ctenocephalides felis* | • VECTOR: Bartonella henselae → cat scratch disease and bacillary angiomatosis<br>• PARINAUD: oculoglandular syndrome—granulomatous conjunctivitis and preauricular LAN |
| Rat flea | *Xenopsylla cheopis* | • VECTOR: R. typhi → endemic typhus<br>*Yersinia pestis* → bubonic plaque |

*continued p. 60*

| Creature | Scientific name | Special features |
|----------|----------------|------------------|
| Sand /Chigoe Flea | *Tunga penetrans* | • Tungiasis<br>• Give tetanus px when tx (surgery or ivermectin) |

**BEETLES**

| | | |
|----------|----------------|------------------|
| Rove beetle | *Paederus eximius* | • Nairobi eye<br>• TOXIN: Pederin |
| Blister beetle | *Lytta vesicatoria*/Spanish fly | • Source of cantharadin<br>• Blister if squished on skin |
| Carpet beetle | *Attagenus megatoma* and *A. scrophulariae* | • ACD with larvae |

**LICE**

| | | |
|----------|----------------|------------------|
| Pubic (crab) | *Pthirus pubis* | • Shortest and broadest body with stout claws<br>• Maculae ceruleae (blue macules) on surrounding skin from louse saliva on blood products |
| Head lice | *Pediculus capitis* | • Six legs, long narrow body |
| Body lice | *Pediculus humanus corporis* | • Narrow, longest body<br>• Lives in folds of clothing not directly on host<br>• VECTORS: Bartonella quintana → trench fever Borellia recurrentis → relapsing fever Rickettsia prowazekii → epidemic typhus |

**MITES**

| | | |
|----------|----------------|------------------|
| Scabies | *Sarcoptes scabiei hominis* | • Classic burrows along webspaces, folds<br>• Skin scraping for eggs, feces, mites<br>• Tx: Permethrin, lindane, ivermectin |
| Straw itch mite | *Pyemotes tritici* | • Found on grain, dried beans, hay, dried grasses<br>• Salivary enzymes are sensitizing<br>• May cause systemic sx: fever, diarrhea, anorexia |
| Demodex | *Demodicidae* | • Associated with acne rosacea, demodex folliculitis<br>• Lives in human hair follicles |
| Grain mite | *Acarus siro* | • Causes baker's itch |
| Cheese mite | *Glyciphagus* | • Causes grocer's itch<br>• Papular urticaria or vesicopapular eruption |

| Creature | Scientific name | Special features |
|---|---|---|
| Grocery mite | *Tyrophagus* | • Papular urticaria or vesicopapular eruption |
| Harvest mite (Chigger) | *Trombicula alfreddugesi* | • Intense pruritus on ankles, legs, belt line<br>• VECTOR: *R. tsutsugamushi* → scrub typhus |
| Dust mite | *Dermatophagoides Euroglyphus* | • Atopy |
| House mouse mite | *Allodermanyssus sanguineus* | • VECTOR: *R. akari* → rickettsialpox |
| Walking dander | *Cheyletiella* | • Walking dandruff on dogs/cats<br>• Pet is asx; human gets pruritic dermatitis |
| Fowl mite | *Ornithonyssus,* | • Bird handlers most commonly bitten |
| | *Dermanyssus* | • VECTOR: Western equine encephalitis |
| Copra itch | *Tyrophagus putrescentiae* | • Causes itching to dried coconut handlers<br>• Resembles scabies on hand but no burrows |

**OTHERS**

| | | |
|---|---|---|
| Scorpions | *Centruroides sculturatus* and *C. gertschi* | • Neurotoxin causes numbness distally<br>• Systemic: convulsion, coma, hemiplegia, hyper/hypothermia, tremor, restlessness<br>• Arrhythmia, pulmonary edema, hypertension<br>• Local wound care, ice packs, antihistamine |
| Bedbugs | *Cimex Lectularius* | • Flat with broad bodies, 4–5 mm in length |
| Bees, wasps, hornets, ants | *Hymenoptera* | • May cause angioedema<br>• VENOM of honeybee: Phospholipase A |
| Fire ant | *Solenopsis* | • VENOM: Solenopsin D (piperidine derivative) |
| Reduviid bug | *Hemiptera* | • Kissing/ Assassin bugs<br>• VECTOR: *Trypanosoma cruzi* → Chagas disease<br>• Primary lesion: chagoma<br>• Romana's sign: unilateral eyelid swelling<br>• Acute: 1–2 weeks, fever, LAN, arthralgia, myalgia |

*continued p. 62*

| Creature | Scientific name | Special features |
|----------|----------------|------------------|
| Centipedes | *Chilopoda* | • Chronic: progressive heart, megacolon<br>• Carnivores: venomous claws cause painful bites with two black puncture wounds 1 cm apart |
| Millipedes | *Deplopoda* | • Vegetarians, emit toxin which burns, blister |

**WATER CREATURES**

| | |
|--|--|
| Leeches | • Medicinal use associated with Aeromonas hydrophila wound infection |
| Sea urchin | • Foreign body reaction to spines, use hot water and vinegar for pain relief and inactivating toxins<br>• Black sea urchin = *Diadema setosa* |
| Sea cucumber | • Toxin holothurin causes conjunctivitis |
| Dolphins | • Lobomycosis – keloidal blastomycosis, *Loboa loboi* |
| *Schistosomes* (flukes) –nonhuman host | • **Swimmer's itch/clam digger's itch (uncovered** skin)<br>• Cercarial forms of flatworm penetrates skin in fresh or salt water (Northern US/Canada), causes allergic reaction<br>• Schistosomes of ducks and fowls (nonhuman) |
| *Schistosomes* (flukes) –human host | • *S. mansonii, S. japonicum, S. hematobium →* Schistosomiasis<br>• Cercarial forms penetrates skin and enters the portal venous system to the lungs, heart, and mesenteric vessels |
| *Stronglyoides stercoralis* (threadworm) | • **Cutaneous Larva Currens**<br>• Serpiginous **urticarial** burrow on buttocks, groin, truck<br>• May penetrate basement membrane to affect lungs and GI tract (chronic strongyloidiasis, Loefler's syndrome)<br>• FAST migration (5–10 cm/h)<br>• Tx: Ivermectin |
| *Ancylostoma caninum, A. braziliense* (hookworm) | • **Cutaneous Larva Migrans**<br>• Hookworm penetrates skin on foot on sandy beaches<br>• Cannot penetrate basement membrane (dead-end host)<br>• Larvae deposited by dogs and cat feces<br>• Serpiginous **vesicular** burrow<br>• SLOW migration (2–10 mm/h)<br>• Tx: Thiabendazole or ivermectin |

- **Cnidarian** – Jellyfish, Portuguese man of war, sea anemone, coral, and hydroids. Stingers (nematocytes) break through skin causing pain and potential systemic symptoms. For jellyfish other than Portuguese man of war, use 3–10% acetic acid or vinegar to fix nematocytes to prevent firing and toxin release.

| | |
|---|---|
| Box jellyfish | • Toxic stings may lead to shock |
| Portuguese man of war | • Painful stings may cause hemorrhagic lesions with vesicles |
| Sea anemone (*Edwardsiella lineate*) | • **Seabather's eruption** (pruritic papules in areas **covered** by swimwear) |
| Thimble jellyfish (*Linuche unguiculata*) | • Contact with **cnidarian larvae** in salt water (Southern US/Caribbean), larvae trapped beneath swimsuit |

**EXOTIC PETS, OTHERS**

| | |
|---|---|
| Iguana | • Salmonella, *Serratia marcescens*, Herpes-like virus |
| Hedgehog | • *Trichophyton mentagrophytes*, *Salmonella*, atypical mycobacteria |
| Cockatoo, pigeon | • Cryptococcus neoformans, avian mites |
| Chinchilla | • *Trichophyton mentagrophytes*, *Microsporum gypseum*, *Klebsiella*, *Pseudomonas* |
| Fish/fish tank/swimming pool | • *Mycobacterium marinum*<br>• Treat with TMP-SMX, clarithromycin, doxycycline |
| Flying squirrel | • *Rickettsia prowazekii*, *Toxoplasma gondii*, Staphylococcus |
| Lambs (lambing) | • Lambing ears: farmers develop blistering, itching, painful rash at pinnae (resembles juvenile spring eruption/PMLE) |

# Immunology

## Complement

| Complement type | Action |
|---|---|
| C1q | Binds antibody, activates C1r |
| C1r | Activates C1s |
| C1s | Cleaves C2 and C4 |
| C2 | Cleaves C5 and C3 |
| C3a | Basophil and mast cell activation |
| C3b | Opsonin, component at which classical and alternative pathways converge |
| C4a | Basophil and mast cell activation |
| C4b | Opsonin |
| C5a | Basophil and mast cell activation |
| C5b, 6, 7, 8, 9 | Membrane attack complex |
| C5, 6, 7 | PMN chemotaxis |
| C5b | Basophil chemotaxis |

**Classical pathway:** C1qrs, C1 INH, C4, C2, C3
> Activated by: antibody–antigen complex
> IgM > IgG (except IgG4 does not bind C1q)

**Alternative pathway:** C3, Properdin, factor B, D
> Activated by: pathogen surfaces

**Lectin pathway:** Mannan-binding lectin and ficolins serve as opsonins, analogous to C1qrs. Leads to activation of the classical pathway without antibody.
> Activated by: pathogen surfaces

**Membrane attack complex:** C5-9

**C3NeF:** Autoantibody that stabilizes bound C3 convertase (C3Bb). IgG isotype against Factor H inhibits its activity to also drive complement activation. Associated with mesangiocapillary glomerulonephritis and/or partial lipodystrophy.

## Complement deficiencies

Most are AR, except hereditary angioneurotic edema (HAE) which is AD

| Complement deficiency | Disease |
|---|---|
| Early classical pathway (C1, C4, C2) | SLE without ANA, increased infections (encapsulated organisms) |
| C1 esterase | HAE |
| Decreased C1q | SCID |
| C2 | Most common complement deficiency, SLE (sometimes HSP, JRA) |
| C3 | Infections, SLE, partial lipodystrophy, Leiner disease |
| C4 | SLE with PPK |
| C3, C4, or C5 | Leiner disease (diarrhea, wasting, seborrheic dermatitis) |
| C5-9 | Recurrent neisseria infections |

## Angioedema and complement levels

|  | C1 | C1 INH | C2 | C3 | C4 |
|---|---|---|---|---|---|
| HAE – 1 | Nl | ↓ | ↓ | Nl | ↓ |
| HAE – 2 | Nl | Nl/↑ (but non-functional) | ↓ | Nl | ↓ |
| HAE – 3* | Nl | Nl | Nl | Nl | Nl |
| AAE – 1** | ↓ | ↓ | ↓ | Nl/↓ | ↓ |
| AAE – 2*** | ↓ | ↓ | ↓ | Nl/↓ | ↓ |
| ACEI-induced | Nl | Nl | Nl | Nl | Nl |

Tx: C1-INH concentrate/FFP, epi, steroids, antihistamines, androgens, antifibrinolytics (epsilon-aminocaproic acid or tranexamic acid).

*HAE-3 = estrogen-dependent form.

**AAE-1 = associated w/ B-cell lymphoproliferation.

***AAE-2 = autoimmune form, Ab against C1-INH.

## Th profiles

| Th Profile | Cytokines | Associated diseases |
|---|---|---|
| Th1 | IL-2, IFN-γ, IL-12 | Tuberculoid leprosy, Cutaneous leishmaniasis, Erythema nodosum, Sarcoidosis, Behcet, MF, Delayed type (IV) hypersensitivity reaction |
| Th2 | IL-4, IL-5, IL-6, IL-10, IL-9, IL-13 | Atopic dermatitis, Lepromatous leprosy, Disseminated leishmaniasis, Sezary, Pregnancy (flares Th2 diseases, helps Th1 diseases), Tissue fibrosis (i.e. SSc), Papular urticaria to fleabite |
| Th17* | IL-6, IL-15, IL-17, IL-21, IL-22, IL-23, TGF-β | Psoriasis, ACD, Hyper-IgE |
| T regulatory | IL-10 or TGF-β (also CD25+ and FOXP3+) | IPEX |

*Th17 and Treg differentiation are both TGFβ dependent, but retinoic acid inhibits Th17 and promotes Treg differentiation.

## Bullous Disorders

### Intracorneal/subcorneal

- Impetigo – PMNs + bacteria
- SSSS – Epidermolytic/exfoliative toxins cleave Dsg 1 (160 kd) (ETA – chromosomal, ETB – plasmid-derived), strain type 71 of phage group II, organisms not usu present on bx, kids <6 years or immunosuppressed/ renally insufficient adults
- Staphylococcal toxic shock – superantigens activate T-cell receptor through Vβ
- Streptococcal toxic shock   group A including (strep pyogenes), 60% have + blood cx (unlike Staphylococcal toxic shock)
- P. foliaceous – Dsg 1 (160 kd) (upper epidermis), may have dyskeratotic cells (resemble 'grains') in granular layer of older lesions
  - Endemic – fogo selvagem
  - DIF – intercellular IgG/C3
- P. erythematosus (Senear–Usher) – features of lupus + PF
  DIF – intercellular IgG/C3 + lupus band
- Subconeal pustular dermatosis (SPD) (Sneddon–Wilkinson) – rule-out IgA pemphigus – IgA Pemphigus has 2 variants: SPD variant (Ab's to desmocollin 1) and intraepidermal neutrophilic (IEN) variant (AB's to Dsg 1 or 3), 20% IgA monoclonal gammopathy, intercellular IgA (upper epidermis in SPD type but less restricted in IEN type)

- Infantile acropustulosis
- Erythema toxicum neonatorum – eosinophils, may be intraepidermal
- Eosinophilic pustular folliculitis
- Transient neonatal pustular melanosis – neutrophils
- AGEP – β-lactams, cephalosporins, macrolides, mercury
- Miliaria crystallina.

## Intraepidermal blisters

- Palmoplantar pustulosis
- Viral blistering diseases
- Friction blister – acral, Just beneath SG
- EBS – may be suprabasilar
- Amicrobial pustulosis associated with autoimmune disease (APAD)
- Coma blisters – may be subepidermal, sweat gland necrosis (EM-like)

## Suprabasilar blisters

Acantholysis – P. vulgaris, P. vegetans, Hailey-Hailey, acantholytic AK

Acantholysis + dyskeratosis – Darier, Grover, paraneoplastic pemphigus, warty dyskeratoma

Other blistering diseases with acantholysis – SSSS, P. foliaceous

- P. vulgaris – Dsg 3 (130 kd), ~50% also have Ab to Dsg 1 (160 kd), "tombstoning" with adnexal involvement unlike Hailey–Hailey, DIF: intercellular IgG/C3, IIF: 80–90% positivity, fishnet on monkey esophagus (more sensitive than guinea pig)
- P. vegetans – Dsg 3 (130 kd), Dsg 1 (160 kd), Histo: eos > pms (esp. in early pustular lesions), DIF = P. vulgaris, Two types of P. vegetans:
  - Neumann type – more common, starts erosive and vesicular, then becomes vegetating
  - Hallopeau type – starts pustular, more benign course

  Should distinguish P. vegetans from pyodermatitis–pyostomatitis vegetans – associated with IBD, DIF-
- Hailey–Hailey (Benign familial pemphigus) – dilapidated brick wall, DIF negative
- Darier – acantholytic (more than PV) dyskeratosis (less than H–H)
- Grover – 4 histo patterns: Darier-like, H–H-like, PV-like, spongiotic
- EBS
- Pemphigus-like blisters + PPK – case report with Ab to Desmocollin 3, BPAg1, LAD

## Subepidermal with little inflammation

- EB
  - EBS – fragmented basal layer at base of blister, floor: BP Ag, Col IV, laminin, PAS+ BM
  - JEB – subepidermal, cell-poor, roof: BP Ag; floor: Col IV, laminin, PAS+ BM

- DEB – subepidermal, cell-poor, roof: BP Ag, Col IV, laminin, PAS+ BM
- EB types may also demonstrate supepidermal blisters with eos
- EBA – Ab to Col VII (290 kd), DIF: linear IgG/C3 at BMZ, EBA variant may also demonstrate subepidermal blisters with PMNs
- PCT/pseudo-PCT
- Burns and cryotherapy
- PUVA-induced
- TEN
- Suction blisters
- Bullous amyloidosis
- Kindler (now classified as major EB type with "Mixed"/Variable level of cleavage)
- Vesiculobullae over scars
- Bullous drug

## Subepidermal with lymphocytes

- EM
- Paraneoplastic pemphigus – can demonstrate suprabasaliar acantholysis or subepidermal clefting, dyskeratosis, basal vacuolar change, band-like dermal infiltrate, DIF: intercellular IgG/C3 + IgG/C3 at BMZ (~P. erythematosus), IIF: intercellular staining on rat bladder
- LS&A
- LP pemphigoides
- Fixed drug
- PMLE
- Bullous tinea

## Subepidermal with eosinophils

- BP – DIF: linear BMZ IgG/C3, Abs to BPAg1 (230 kd, 80% of patients) and/or BPAg2 (180 kd, contains Col 17 and NC16A domain, 30% of patients)
- Pemphigoid gestationis (herpes gestationis) – DIF similar to BP, BPAg2 – placental matrix antigen
- Arthropod bite – esp. with chronic lymphocytic leukemia

## Subepidermal with neutrophils

- DH – IgA endomysial ab, DIF: IgA at the dermal papillae (perilesional and uninvolved skin)
- Linear IgA –Various antigens including 97 kd (ladinin) or 120 kd (LAD-1) = BPAg2 degradation products (in lamina lucida form), DIF: linear IgA at BMZ (non-lesional skin)
- CP (benign mucosal pemphigoid)
  Brunsting-Perry = localized form, head/neck, w/o mucosa
- Deep lamina lucida (anti-P105) pemphigoid
- Anti-P200 pemphigoid

## 'Laminated' model of the epidermal basement membrane

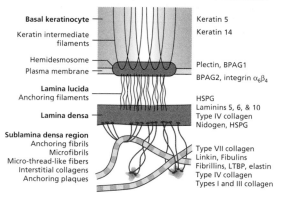

| | |
|---|---|
| **Basal keratinocyte** | Keratin 5 |
| Keratin intermediate filaments | Keratin 14 |
| Hemidesmosome | Plectin, BPAG1 |
| Plasma membrane | BPAG2, integrin $\alpha_6\beta_4$ |
| **Lamina lucida** Anchoring filaments | HSPG Laminins 5, 6, & 10 |
| **Lamina densa** | Type IV collagen Nidogen, HSPG |
| **Sublamina densa region** Anchoring fibrils Microfibrils Micro-thread-like fibers Interstitial collagens Anchoring plaques | Type VII collagen Linkin, Fibulins Fibrillins, LTBP, elastin Type IV collagen Types I and III collagen |

From Yancey KB, Allen DM. The biology of the basement membrane zone, In: Bolognia JL, Jorizzo JL, Rapini RP (eds). *Dermatology*, Vol. 1. London: Mosby, 2003. p. 436, with permission from Elsevier.

- Bullous LE – Clinically, may be similar to DH or have large hemorrhagic bullae, Ab to Col VII (like EBA), Histo: like DH and often lacks vacuolar change of other forms of LE
- Sweet
- Orf – May have eos, DIF: C3/IgG at DEJ, IIF: anti-BMZ IgG (binding dermal side of SSS)

## Subepidermal with mast cells
- Bullous mastocytosis

## Epidermolysis bullosa
**Simplex** ("epidermolytic EB") – split basal layer (tonofilament clumping in basal layer on EM, 40% of EB patients, sxs worse in summer/heat, typically no scarring and not severe (except Dowling–Meara and AR forms)
>    **Mutations:** KRT5 or 14, plectin, mainly AD (99%)
>    **IF:** Col IV, laminin, BPAg on floor of blister

### Localized forms:
1. Weber–Cockayne (AD) – most common, hyperhidrosis, palms/soles, usually due to KRT5 or 14 mutations, rarely may be due to ITGB4 (integrin β4) mutations
2. Kallin (AR) – anodontia/hypodontia, hair/nail anomalies
3. Autosomal Recessive EBS (AR) – KRT14

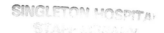

**Generalized forms:**

1. Koebner (AD) – mild, (−) Nikolsky, mucous membrane and nails are nl
2. Dowling-Meara (AD) – herpetiform pattern, hemorrhagic bullae, milia, oral involvement, dystrophic/absent nails, alopetic areas, confluent PPK, improves at ~10-years old and in adulthood (becomes more restricted to acral/pressure sites)
3. Ogna (AD) – hemorrhagic blister & bruising, *plectin* defect but no MD, closely linked to glutamic pyruvic transaminase
4. Mottled pigmentation (AD) – reticulated hyperpigmentation
5. Muscular dystrophy (AR) – *plectin* defect, blisters at birth with scarring, neuromuscular disease
6. Pyloric atresia (AD, AR) – *plectin* defect, may be lethal, single family reported (Pfendner E and Uitto J. Plectin gene mutations can cause epidermolysis bullosa with pyloric atresia *J Invest Dermatol.* 2005 January 124(1):111–15).

**Junctional** – split lamina lucida, defect in hemidesmosome, <10% of EB patients, oral lesions, absent/dystrophic nails, dysplastic teeth, usually no scarring/milia

    **Mutations:** Laminin 5 (=Laminin 332), $\alpha 6\beta 4$ (ITGA6, ITGB4), BPAg2, CD151/MER2, all AR except Traupe-Belter-Kolde-Voss

    **IF**: Col IV, laminin on floor; BPAg on roof.

1. Herlitz (EB letalis or gravis) – defect: laminin 5, very severe generalized desies – may be fatal (often during infancy or childhood), manifest at birth, stereotypical stridor/cry, non-healing erosions (often large and zygomatic), GI, gallbladder, corneal, vaginal, laryngeal (>esophageal), and bronchial lesions, dystrophic/absent nails, exuberant granulation tissue and bleeding
2. Non-herlitz (non-lethal) – defect: laminin 5, moderately severe generalized disease worse pretibially, bullae smaller and healing, dystrophic nails, risk of SCC, large acquired melanocytic nevi (seen in JEB > DEB or EBS; asymmetric, irregular)
3. JEB with Pyloric Atresia – defect: $\alpha 6\beta 4$, severe mucocutaneous fragility & gastric outlet obstruction, manifest at birth, polyhydramnios during pregnancy
4. Generalized Atrophic Benign EB – defect: COL XVIIA1 (BPAg2), moderately severe generalized disease + enamel defects/oral lesions and atrophic alopecia (~ male-pattern), survive to adulthood, dystrophic nails, 'Localized Atrophic' variant also due to COL XVII mutations
5. JEB Letalis with Congenital Muscular Dystrophy – Doriguzzi C *et al.* Congenital muscular dystrophy associated with familial junctional epidermolysis bullosa letalis. *Eur Neurol.* 1993; 33(6):454–60.
6. Laryngo-Onycho-Cutaneous/laryngeal and ocular granulation tissue in children from the Indian subcontinent (LOGIC)/Shabbir – hoarse cry as newborn, erosions, and bleeding at traumatic sites, onychodystrophy,

conjunctival and laryngeal chronic granulation tissue, symblepharon, blindness, dental enamel hypoplasia, anemia

7. Pretibial EB with nephropathy and deafness – defect: CD151/MER2
8. Others: Acral, inversa, cicatricial, late-onset/progressiva

**Dystrophic** ("dermolytic EB") – split sublamina densa (papillary dermis), >50% of EB patients, defective anchoring fibers, scars, and milia
   **Mutation:** Col VII*
   **IF:** Col IV, laminin, BPAg on roof

**Dominant Dystrophic EB:** manifest at birth, bullae on extensor surfaces, (+) Nikolsky, (onion) scars and atrophy, milia on ears, hands, arms, and legs, mucous membrane/esophagus involved, nail dystrophy, scarring tip of tongue, improve w/time

1. Albopapuloid (Pasini, Pretibial with Lichenoid Features) – white papules on trunk not preceded by bullae, more severe, present in adolescence
2. Cockayne–Touraine – hypertrophic scars, more limited
3. Bart – aplasia cutis (legs), blisters, and nail deformities, rarely with JEB
4. Dominant transient bullous dermolysis of the newborn – vesiculobullae at birth, recover by 4 months, no scars
5. Pruriginosa – pruritis, prurigo-like lesions, nail dystrophy, and may have albopapuloid lesions, may be AR
6. EBD with subcorneal cleavage = EBS-superficialis

**Recessive Dystrophic EB**

1. Generalized – mitis (non-Hallopeau-Siemens) – severe blisters, generalized, esophageal strictures, ± digital cicatricial pseudosyndactyly
2. Generalized – gravis (Hallopeau-Siemens) – very severe, generalized, skin and mucous membrane bullae as newborn, high risk of SCC (primary cause of death), mitten deformity, esophageal stricture, anemia, cardiomyopathy, fatal amyloidosis (AA type)
3. Others – Inversa (axilla, groin), Centripetal, Recessive Transient Bullous Dermolysis of the Newborn

* Tumorigenesis in RDEB is increased with production/retention of Col VII containing the NC1 domain (in laminin 5-dependent process).
Non-EB genodermatoses with infantile bullae: Ichthyosis Bullosa of Siemens, BCIE, Gunther

## Major bullous diseases – clinicopathologic findings

| Disease | Manifestation | Antigen(s) | Size (kD) | Path | DIF | Rx |
|---|---|---|---|---|---|---|
| **Pemphigus foliaceus** | Crusted, scaly erosions, seborrheic distribution, positive Nikolsky, non-mucosal | Dsg 1 Plakoglobin | 160 85 | Acantholysis in upper epidermis, split in SG or right below SC | Intercellular IgG/C3, often superficial, may be throughout epidermis | Topical steroids if mild, systemics similar to PV if generalized |
| **Pemphigus vegetans** | Flaccid bullae, erosions, fungoid vegetations, intertriginous, head, mucous membrane, 2 subtypes: Neumann – severe Hallopeau – mild | Dsg 3 Dsg 1 Plakoglobin | 130 160 85 | Like PF | Like PF | Like PF |
| **Pemphigus vulgaris** Drug-induced (usually PF-like): penicillamine, IL-2, PCN, thiopurine, rifampin, ACE-I | Flaccid bullae, mucous membrane, + Nikolsky, + Asboe-Hansen | Dsg 3–100% Dsg 1–50% Plakoglobin | 130 160 85 | Suprabasilar acantholysis can follow hair, + tombstones | Intercellular IgG (also C3, IgM, IgA) throughout epidermis. Follow progression with IIF (Dsg 3) (monkey esophagus) | Prednisone, azathioprine, cyclophosphamide, mycophenolate mofetil, CSA |

continued p. 72

| Disease | Manifestation | Antigen(s) | Size (kD) | Path | DIF | Rx |
|---|---|---|---|---|---|---|
| IgA pemphigus | Flaccid vesicles, superficial pustules in annular/serpentine patterns, trunk (axilla, groin), proximal extremities | SPD variant – Desmocollin 1; IEN variant – Dsg 1/3 | 105, 115 | Pustules: subcorneal or suprabasilar, no acantholysis, PMNs | IgA in upper epidermis (intercellular), no IgG | Dapsone, sulfapyridine, etretinate, UV, steroids |
| Pemphigus erythematosus (Senear–Usher) | Erythematous, crusted, erosions, often malar, originally PE = PV + LE | Dsg 1<br>Plakoglobin | 160<br>85 | Like PF | Intercellular and DEJ<br>IgG/C3 + lupus band sometimes | Prednisone |
| Paraneoplastic pemphigus<br>Associations: NHL, CLL, Castleman, sarcoma, thymoma | Bullae, erosions, EM-like, lichenoid, SJ-like in mucous membranes | Plectin<br>Desmoplakin 1<br>BPAg1<br>Envoplakin<br>Desmoplakin 2<br>Periplakin<br>?<br>Dsg 1,3 | 500<br>250<br>230<br>210<br>210<br>190<br>170<br>160, 130 | Suprabasilar acantholysis, dyskeratotic keratinocytes, sometimes basal layer degeneration/band-like infiltrate | Intercellular IgG/C3 in epidermis and at BMZ<br>IIF: IgG rat bladder | Treat associated neoplasm<br>May die from bronchiolitis obliterans |
| Epidermolysis bullosa acquista<br>Associations: myeloma, colitis, DM2, leukemia, lymphoma, amyloid, cancer | Fragile skin, blisters with trauma, atrophic scars, milia, nail dystrophy | Col VII (also an antigen in bullous LE) | 290/145 | Non-inflammatory subepidermal bullae, PMN>Eos | IgG/C3 linear BMZ<br>IIF anti-BMZ<br>Salt split skin: immunoreactants on dermal side, type IV collagen on roof | Immunosuppression, wound care |

| | | | | | |
|---|---|---|---|---|---|
| **Bullous pemphigoid**<br>Drug-induced: lasix, PCN, ACE-I, sulfasalzine, nalidixic acid | Large, tense bullae on trunk and extremities | BPAg1<br>BPAg2 | 230<br>180 | Subepidermal bullae, eosinophils in superficial dermis (more likely acral in infants) | Linear IgG/C3 at BMZ<br>Salt split skin: immunoreactants on epidermal side, type IV collagen on base | Topical steroids, prednisone, MTX, mycophenolate mofetil, azathioprine, nicotinamide, TCN, sulfapyridine, dapsone |
| **Herpes gestationis/ gestational pemphigoid**<br>Associations: HLA-DR 3,4, B8 | Pruritic, urticarial plaques on trunk, starts near umbilicus, flares with delivery/OCP, increased risk of prematurity/SGA, 10% of newborns with skin lesions | BPAg1<br>BPAg2<br>*BPAg2 worse prognosis | 230<br>180 | Subepidermal bullae, eosinophils, perivascular infiltrate | Linear C3 ± IgG at BMZ IIF: anti-BMZ IgG by complement-added IIF. | Topical/oral steroids |
| **Dermatitis herpetiformis** | Grouped, pruritic papules and vesicles on extensors, HLA-B8, DR3, DQ2 | Endomysial Ag (tissue transglutaminase)<br>Anti-gliadin | | Subepidermal bullae, PMNs in dermal papillae | Granular IgA ± C3 (tips of papillae) | Gluten-free diet, dapsone, sulfapyridine, TCN, nicotinamide, colchicine |

continued p. 74

| Disease | Manifestation | Antigen(s) | Size (kD) | Path | DIF | Rx |
|---|---|---|---|---|---|---|
| **Linear IgA**<br>Drug-induced: vancomycin, lithium, amiodarone, ACE-I, PCN, PUVA, lasix, IL-2, oxaprozin, IFN-γ, dilantin, diclofenac, glibenclamide | DH-like vesicles (crown of jewels), BP-like bullae, 50% mucous membrane involvement, children: self-limited | Ladinin<br>LAD-1<br>BPAg1<br>BPAg2<br>Col VII | 97<br>120<br>230<br>180<br>290/145 | Subepidermal bullae, PMNs in dermal papillae ± Eos | Linear IgA at BMZ, maybe IgG, no C3 | Dapsone, steroids, TCN, nicotinamide, IVIg, colchicine |
| **Cicatricial pemphigoid (benign mucosal pemphigoid)**<br>Drug-induced: penicillamine, clonidine | Primarily mucous membrane, vesicles, erosions, ulcers, scars, erosive gingivitis, chronic | BPAg1<br>BPAg2<br>Laminin-6<br>Epiligrin (Lam-5)<br>Integrin β4 | 230<br>180<br>165, 220, 200<br>165, 140, 105<br>200 | Like BP plus scarring in upper dermis | C3/IgG at BMZ n 80%; IIF+ in 20%, usually IgG | Topical steroids, dapsone, cyclophosphamide, oral steroids, surgery. |

# Glands

| Glands | Apocrine | Eccrine | Sebaceous |
|---|---|---|---|
| Derivation | Ectodermal (~week 16–24) | Ectodermal (~week 14) | Ectodermal (~week 14) |
| Secretion | Decapitation | Merocrine | Holocrine |
| Innervation | Sympathetic adrenergic | Sympathetic cholinergic and cholinergic | Androgenic hormones (not innervated) |
| Purpose | Pheromones | Temperature regulation | Lubricate, waterproof |
| Locations | Axillary, breast (mammary), external ear (ceruminous), anogenital, eyelid (Moll) nevus sebaceous | Widespread (esp. soles) excluding vermilion border, labia minora, glans, nail beds, inner prepuce | Everywhere except palms and soles<br>Associated with hair follicles except on mucosa<br>Montgomery tubercles – nipples, areola<br>Meibomian – deep eyelid; granuloma<br>Glands of Zeis – superficial eyelid<br>Tyson – foreskin, labia minora<br>Fordyce spots – vermilion, buccal |
| Secretion contents | Fatty acids, cholesterol, triglycerides, squalene, androgens, ammonia, iron, carbohydrates, antimicrobial peptides | NaCl, potassium, bicarbonate, calcium, glucose, lactate, urea, pyruvate, glucose, ammonia, enzymes, cytokins, Igs | Ceramides, triglycerides, free fatty acids, squalene, sterol and wax esters, free sterols |

continued p. 76

| Glands | Apocrine | Eccrine | Sebaceous |
|---|---|---|---|
| Stains* | GCDFP, EMA, CEA, keratins | CEA, S100, EMA, keratins (CAM 5.2, AE1) | EMA, CK15, lipid stains |
| Non-neoplastic conditions | • Fox Fordyce (apocrine miliaria)<br>• Apocrine chromhidrosis – ochronosis, stained undershirts<br>• Axillary bromhidrosis – (E)-3-methyl-2-hexanoic acid, Micrococcus or Corynebacterium, M>F, post-puberty, more common than eccrine bromhidrosis except during childhood | • Neutrophilic eccrine hidradenitis: chemo, palmoplantar (pediatric), pseudomonas<br>• Syringolymphoid hyperplasia with alopecia<br>• Miliaria<br>• Lafora – PAS+ granules<br>• Bromhidrosis – drugs (bromides, PCN), food, metabolic, or bacterial degradation of softened keratin<br>• Uremia – small eccrine glands<br>• PAS+ granules in hypothyroidism<br>• Degeneration in lymphoma, heat stroke, coma blister<br>• Ebola particles | • Acne<br>• Vernix caseosa<br>• Juxtaclavicular beaded lines<br>• Chalazion – granuloma involving Meibomian glands<br>• Internal hordeolum (stye) – infection/inflammation of Meibomian glands<br>• External hordeolum (stye) – infection/inflammation of Zeiss or Moll (apocrine) |

*Specificity of apocrine vs. eccrine stains is controversial.

# Disorders or drugs associated with skeletal, ocular, and/or nail findings

| | Ocular | Skeletal/oral | Nail |
|---|---|---|---|
| 5-FU, AZT, phenophthalein, anti-malarials, hydroxyurea, MCN | | | Blue lunulae (also argyria, Wilson, Hgb M disease) |
| Acitretin | | | Koilonychia, onychocryptosis (ingrown/unguis incarnatus, granuloma) |
| Acne fulminans | | Osteolytic lesions (clavicle, sternum, long bones, ilium) | |
| Albright hereditary osteodystrophy | | Short stature, brachydactyly, subcutaneous ossifications | |
| Alkaptonuria | | Arthritis, blue/gray ear cartilage, calcified cartilage | |
| Alezzandrini | Unilateral retinitis pigmentosa, retinal detachment | | |
| Alopecia areata | Ask punctate lens opacities | | Pitting, trachyonychia, red spotted lunulae |
| Antimalarials | Retinopathy | | Blue lunulae |

continued p. 78

| | Ocular | Skeletal/oral | Nail |
|---|---|---|---|
| Apert | Hypertelorism, exophthalmos | Craniosynostosis | Brittle nails, fusion of nails |
| Argyria | Blue/gray sclera | Blue/gray gums | Azure lunulae |
| Arsenic | | Garlic breath, intra-abdominal radio-opacities (acute) | Mees lines |
| Ataxia-telangiectasia (Louis-Bar) | Bulbar telangiectasia, strabismus, nystagmus | | |
| Behçet | Retinal vasculitis, uveitis, hypopyon, optic disk hyperemia, macular edema | Arthritis, oral ulcers | |
| Buschke-Ollendorff | | Osteopoikolosis | |
| Carbon monoxide poisoning, polycythemia, CTD, CHF, | | | Red lunulae |
| CHIME | Retinal colobomas | | |
| Cicatricial pemphigoid | Conjunctivitis, symblepharon, synechiae, ankyloblepharon | Oral ulcers, hoarseness, dysphagia | |
| Cirrhosis, CHF | | | Terry nails |
| Cholesterol emboli | Hollenhorst plaque | | |
| Cockayne | Salt and pepper retinal pigmentary degeneration, optic atrophy, cataracts, strabismus, nystagmus, sunken eyes | Dwarfism, dental caries, osteoporosis, overcrowded mouth | |

| | | | |
|---|---|---|---|
| Coffin-Siris | Bushy eyebrows | Hypoplastic/absent fifth distal phalanges, microcephaly | Hypoplastic/absent fifth nail |
| Congenital erythropoietic porphyria | Conjunctivitis, scleromalacia perforans | Erythrodontia, acro-osteolysis, osteoporosis | Nail dystrophy |
| Congenital syphilis | Keratitis | Osteochondritis, saddle nose, mulberry molars, Hutchinson teeth, saber shins | |
| Connective tissue disease, trauma | | Pterygium inversum unguis | |
| Conradi–Hünermann syndrome | Striated cataracts, microphthalmus, optic nerve atrophy | Asymmetric limb shortening, chondrodysplasia punctata – stippled epiphyses (also in CHILD) | |
| Cooks syndrome | | Absent/hypoplastic distal phalanges, brachydactyly fifth finger | Anonychia/onychodystrophy |
| Darier–White | | | Longitudinal red and white bands and ridging, V-shaped notches, subungual hyperkeratosis |
| Dermochondrocorneal dystrophy (Francois) | Corneal dystrophy, central opacities | Acral osteochondrodystrophy, contractures, subluxations, gingival hyperplasia | |
| Drug (azidothymidine, tetracycline), ethnicity, Laugier–Hunziker, Peutz–Jeghers | | | Longitudinal melanonychia |
| Dyskeratosis congenita | Blepharitis, conjunctivitis, epiphora | Dental caries, loss of teeth, premalignant leukoplakia, dysphagia | Longitudinal ridging, thinning, pterygium |

continued p. 80

| | Ocular | Skeletal/oral | Nail |
|---|---|---|---|
| Ehlers–Danlos VI | Fragile sclerae/cornea, keratoconus, hemorrhage, retinal detachment, blue sclerae, angioid streaks | Kyphoscoliosis | |
| Ehlers–Danlos VIII | | Periodontitis, loss of teeth | |
| Ehlers–Danlos IX | | Occipital horns, elbow, and wrist defects | |
| Endocarditis, trauma, trichinosis, cirrhosis, vasculitis | | | Splinter hemorrhages |
| Epidermal nevus syndrome | Lipodermoids, colobomas, choristomas | Kyphoscoliosis, abnormal skull shape, limb hypertrophy/asymmetry, rickets | |
| Fabry disease | Circular corneal opacities (cornea verticillata), tortuous vasculature, spoke-like cataracts | Oral angiokeratoma (tongue), osteoporosis | |
| Fanconi anemia | Strabismus, retinal hemorrhages | Radius and thumb defects | |
| Fever, stress, meds (chemo) | | | Beau lines |
| Gardner | Congenital hypertrophy of retinal pigmented epithelium | Osteomas, dental abnormalities | |
| Gaucher | Pingueculae | Erlenmeyer flask deformity, osteopenia, osteonecrosis | |

| Syndrome | | | |
|---|---|---|---|
| Goldenhar (Facioauriculovertebral sequence) | Epibulbar choristomas, blepharoptosis or narrow palpebral fissures, eyelid colobomas, lacrimal drainage system anomalies | Ipsilateral mandibular hypoplasia, ear anomalies, vertebral anomalies | |
| Goltz | Retinal colobomas, microphthalmia, nystagmus, strabismus | Osteopathia striata, lobster claw deformity, cleft lip/palate, hypo/oligodontia, oral papilloma, enamel hypoplasia | |
| Gorlin | Cataracts, strabismus, iris colobomas | Odontogenic cysts, fused/bifid ribs, spina bifida occulta, kyphoscoliosis, calcified falx cerebri, frontal bossing | |
| Hallerman–Streiff syndrome | Microphthalmia, congenital cataracts, strabismus | Bird-like facies, natal teeth, hypodontia | |
| Hemochromatosis | Angioid streaks | | Koilonychia |
| Homocystinuria | Ectopia lentis (downward) | Marfanoid habitus, genu valgum, osteoporosis | |
| Huriez | | Scleroatrophy of hands, sclerodactyly, lip telangiectasia | Hypoplasia, ridging, white, clubbing |
| Hyperimmunoglobulin E syndrome | | Osteopenia, fractures, scoliosis, hyperextensible joints, candidiasis | Chronic candidiasis |
| Hypoalbuminemia | | | Muehrcke lines |

continued p. 82

| | Ocular | Skeletal/oral | Nail |
|---|---|---|---|
| HSV, varicella | Dendritis, keratitis | | |
| Incontinentia Pigmenti (Bloch–Sulzberger) | Strabismus, cataracts, optic nerve atrophy, retinal vascular changes, detached retina, retinal/iris colobomas | Peg/conical teeth, partial adontia, late dentition | Nail dystrophy, grooving, painful subungual dyskeratotic tumors |
| Iron deficiency, syphilis, thyroid disease | | | Koilonychia |
| Iso-Kikuchi | | Index finger hypoplasia, brachydactyly | Hypoplastic index finger nail |
| JXG | Ocular JXG, hyphema, glaucoma | | |
| KID | Keratoconjunctivitis, blepharitis, photophobia, corneal defects | | Nail dystrophy |
| Kindler | | Cicatricial pseudosyndactyly (between MCP and PIP), leukoplakia, caries | Nail dystrophy |
| Lamellar ichthyosis | Ectropion, corneal damage | Phalangeal reabsorption | |
| LCH: Hand–Schuller–Christian | Exophthalmos | Bone lesions (esp. cranium) | |
| LEOPARD | Hypertelorism | | |
| Leprosy | Madarosis, lagophthalmos, keratitis, episcleritis, corneal anesthesia, blindness | Digital resorption, malaligned fractures, diaphyseal whitting, saddle nose | Longitudinal melanonychia, longitudinal ridging, subungual hyperkeratosis, rudimentary nail |
| Lichen planus | | | Pterygium |
| Linear morphea | | Melorheostosis (of Leri; "flowing candle wax") | |

| | |
|---|---|
| Lipoid proteinosis (Urbach–Wiethe) | Eyelid beading/moniliform blepharosis | Calcifications in hippocampus (suprasellar, "bean-shaped"), thick tongue, hoarseness |
| Mafucci | | Enchondromas, chondrosarcoma |
| Marfan | Ectopia lertis (upward) | Marfanoid habitus |
| McCune–Albright | | Polyostotic fibrous dysplasia |
| MEN IIb | Conjunctival neuroma | Plexiform neuromas (oral mucosa, tongue), nodular lips, marfanoid habitus |
| Menkes | Blue irides, strabismus, aberrant eyelashes, iris stromal hypoplasia | Wormian bones of skull, metaphyseal spurring of long bones |
| Multicentric reticulohistiocytosis | | Mutilating arthritis |
| Myxoid cyst, verruca vulgaris | | Median canaliform dystrophy |
| Naegeli–Franceschetti–Jadassohn | Periocular hyperpigmentation | Enamel defects, perioral hyperpigmentation |
| Nail-patella | Lester iris, heterochromia irides | Patella aplasia, posterior iliac horns, elbow arthrodysplasia |
| | | Malaligned great toenails |
| | | Triangular lunulae, micro/ anonychia |
| Necrobiotic xanthogranuloma | Scleritis, episcleritis | |
| NF-1 | Lisch nodules, congenital glaucoma, optic glioma | Sphenoid wing dysplasia |
| NF-2 | Cataracts, retinal hamartomas | |

continued p. 84

83

| | Ocular | Skeletal/oral | Nail |
|---|---|---|---|
| Nicotine, chemotherapy, potassium permanganate, podophyllin, hydroxyurea (streaks) | | | Brown nails |
| Niemann–Pick | Cherry red spots, macular haloes | | |
| Noonan | Hypertelorism, ptosis, epicanthic folds, downward palpebral fissures, epicanthic folds, refractive errors, strabismus, amblyopia | Pectus carinatum superiorly, pectus excavatum inferiorly, scoliosis, short stature, cubitus valgus, joint hyperextensibility | |
| Old age | | | Diminished or absent lunulae, longitudinal ridging, onychogryphosis |
| Olmsted | Corneal anomalies | Osteoporosis, joint laxity, leukoplakia, periorificial keratotic plaques | Nail dystrophy |
| Orofaciodigital 1 | Colobomas | Bifid tongue, accessory frenulae, lip nodules/ pseudoclefting, supernumerary teeth, frontal bossing, syndactyly | |
| Osteogenesis imperfecta | Blue sclera | Brittle bones | |
| Pachyonychia congenita | Corneal dystrophy | Oral leukokeratosis, natal teeth | Thickened nails, pincer nails, paronychia |

| | | |
|---|---|---|
| Papillon–Lefévre | Dural calcifications, periodontitis, gingivitis (+ acro-osteolysis and onychogryphosis in Haim–Munk) | |
| Phenylketonuria | Blue irides | |
| Porphyria cutanea tarda | Osteopenia | Photo-onycholysis |
| Progeria | Delayed/abnormal dentition, high-pitched voice, acro-osteolysis, short stature, osteoporosis, persistent open fontanelles | |
| Pseudomonas (pyocyanin) | | Green nails |
| Psoriasis | | Nail pits, oil spots |
| PXE (Gronblad–Strandberg) | Angioid streaks (also Paget's disease of bone, sickle cell, thalassemia, Pb poisoning, HFE, ED6) | |
| Refsum | Salt and pepper retinitis pigmentosa | |
| Relapsing polychondritis | Conjunctivitis, scleritis, uveitis, corneal ulceration, optic neuritis | Oral yellow papules |
| Renal disease | Epiphyseal dysplasia | |
| | Arthritis (truncal), aphthosis | |
| | | Lindsay nails |
| Retinoids, indinavir, estrogen | Isotretinoin – DISH-like hyperostotic changes (bones spurs, calcified tendons, ligaments) | Pyogenic granuloma |

continued p. 86

| | Ocular | Skeletal/oral | Nail |
|---|---|---|---|
| Richner–Hanhart | Pseudoherpetic keratitis | Tongue leukokeratosis | |
| Rothmund–Thomson | Cataracts (juvenile zonular) | Anomalies of radius and hands, hypodontia | Nail dystrophy |
| Rubinstein–Taybi | Long eyelashes, thick eyebrows, strabismus, cataracts | Broad thumb–great toe, clinodactyly of fourth toe and fourth to fifth fingers, short stature | Racquet nails |
| SAPHO | | Osteomyelitis | |
| Schnitzler | | Bone/joint pain (iliac/tibia), hyperostosis, osteosclerosis | |
| Schopf–Schulz–Passarge | Eyelid hidrocystomas | Hypodontia | Nail hypoplasia, dystrophy |
| Sjögren–Larsson | Retinitis pigmentosa, glistening dots | Short stature | |
| Sturge–Weber | Glaucoma, retinal malformations | Tram-track calcifications (skull x-ray) | |
| Sweet syndrome | Conjunctivitis, episcleritis, iridocyclitis | Arthritis, arthralgias | |
| Tricho-dento-osseus | | Caries, periodontitis, small teeth, enamel defects, tall stature, frontal bossing | Brittle nails |
| Trichorhinophalangeal | | Cone-shaped epiphyses, shortened phalanges and metacarpals, thin upper lip | Nail dystrophy |
| Trichothiodystrophy | Cataract, conjunctivitis, nystagmus | Osteosclerosis, short stature | Koiloynchia, ridging, splitting, leukonychia |
| Tuberous sclerosis | Retinal hamartomas (mulberry appearing), hypopigmented spots on iris | Dental p ts, gingival fibromas, bone cysts, osteosclerosis | Koenen tumor |

| Condition | | | |
|---|---|---|---|
| Vitamin A deficiency | Night blindness, unable to see in bright light, xerophthalmia, Bitot spots, keratomalacia | Growth retardation, excessive periosteal bone (decreased osteoclastic activity) | Brittle nails |
| Vitamin B2 (riboflavin) deficiency (Oral–ocular–genital) | Eye redness, burning, fatigue, sandiness, dryness, photosensitivity to light, cataracts | Cheilosis, red sore tongue | |
| Vitiligo | Uveitis, depigmented retina | | |
| Von Hippel Lindau | Retinal hemangioblastoma | | |
| Waardenburg | Dystopia canthorum, heterchromia irides | Caries, cleft lip/palate, scrotal tongue | |
| Werner | Cataract, glaucoma | Sclerodactyly, osteoporosis, high-pitched voice | |
| Wilson | Kayser–Fleischer ring | | Blue lunulae |
| Witkop | | Retained primary teeth | Nail dystrophy (toe>finger) |
| X-linked ichthyosis | Posterior comma-shaped corneal opacities (Descemet's membrane) | | |
| Yellow nail syndrome | | | Yellow nails, thick, slowed growth (yellow lunulae – consider insecticides/weed killers (dinitro-orthocresol, diquat, and paraquat), tetracycline, smoking |

Adapted from Solky BA, Jones JL. Boards' Fodder – Bones, Eyes, and Nails (http://www.aad.org/members/resident/fodder.html)

# Dermatoses of Pregnancy

| Condition | Frequency | Synonyms | Onset | Course | Description | Path/labs | Treatment |
|---|---|---|---|---|---|---|---|
| Polymorphic eruption of pregnancy | 1:160 | PUPPP, Toxic erythema/ rash of preg, Late-onset prurigo of pregnancy | Late third trimester or immediately post-partum | Often primiparous, no maternal/ fetal risk, rarely recurs, resolves 1–2 weeks post-partum | Urticarial papules/plaques in abdominal striae, spares umbilicus, spares face/palms/ soles; rapid weight gain may be risk factor | Non-specific | Topical steroids, antihistamines |
| Pemphigoid gestationis | 1:50,000 | Herpes gestationis | Late pregnancy or immediately post-partum | Often recurs w/ subsequent preg, menstruation, and OCP, increased prematurity and SGA, <10% of neonates have skin lesions, BP2 Ag, assoc w/ Graves, resolves weeks–months post-partum | Intensely pruritic, vesiculobullous, trunk, 75% flare w/ delivery, spares face/palms/soles/ oral, HLA-DR3/DR4 associated | Subepi vesicle, perivasc lymphs/eos, DIF: linear C3 ± IgG along BMZ of perilesional skin | Systemic steroids |

| | Incidence | Synonyms/Associations | Timing | Features/Risks | Diagnosis | Treatment |
|---|---|---|---|---|---|---|
| Atopic eruption of pregnancy | 1:300 | Prurigo of pregnancy, Prurigo gestationis, Early-onset prurigo, Papular derm of pregnancy, Pruritic folliculitis of pregnancy | Usu first or second trimester | No fetal/maternal risk, some have h/o atopic dermatitis, may recur w/ subsequent pregnancy, resolves weeks–months post-partum | 2/3 eczematous, 1/3 papular or prurigo | Diagnosis of exclusion, non-specific path | Emollients, urea, topical steroids. If severe, systemic steroids, antihistamines, UVB |
| Intrahepatic cholestasis of pregnancy | 1:100–1000, higher incidence with twins, + FH | Pruritus/prurigo gravidarum, Obstetric cholestasis, Jaundice of pregnancy | Third trimester | Increased rates of prematurity, fetal distress/death, and meconium staining, pruritus resolves within days post-partum, malabsorption → Vit K def, 2/3 recur w/ subsequent preg, often recurs w/ OCP | Intensely pruritic, ± jaundice, no primary lesions, UTI in 50%, sxs worse at night and on trunk and palms/soles | Increased serum bile salts, Liver US nl, Biopsy: centrilobular cholestasis | Urodeoxycholic acid, UVB, vit K |
| Impetigo herpetiformis | Rare | May represent acute generalized pustular psoriasis | Third trimester | Increased rates of placental insufficiency, stillbirth, fetal abnormality, hypocalcemia, vitamin D deficiency, often remits with delivery, recurs next preg | Sterile crusted pustules in flexures and inguinal, spreading centrifugally, fever, cardiac/renal failure possible | Pustular psoriasis-like path, DIF neg, hypocalcemia | Systemic steroids |

# Neonatal Vesiculopustular Eruptions

| Condition | Population | Onset | Duration | Description | Diagnosis | Treatment |
|---|---|---|---|---|---|---|
| **NON-INFECTIONS** | | | | | | |
| Erythema toxicum neonatorum | 1/3–2/3 of Fullterm | Usu 1–2 days | 1 week–1 month | Erythematous macules, papules, (subcorneal or intraepi) pustules, wheals, usu on trunk, spares palms/soles | Smear – eos | None needed |
| Transient neonatal pustular melanosis | 4% of Black, <1% in White; Fullterm | Birth | Pustules – days; PIH – months | Fragile (subcorneal) pustules at birth → resolve with collarette of scale → PIH | Smear – PMNs | None needed |
| Neonatal cephalic pustulosis/ Neonatal acne | 10% | Variable w/i first month | Within 6 months | Inflammatory papules/pustules on head/neck, no comedones, may scar, controversial pathogenesis – may be 2/2 hormones and/or malassezia | Smear – malassezia, PMNs | Self-limited, topical imidazole or BP/erythromycin |
| Miliaria crystallina | 4%; high in tropics | Birth or first few weeks | Resolves w/i days when precipitants removed | Superficial clear noninflammatory vesicles; forehead, upper trunk (sub/intra-corneal eccrine duct obstruction) | Smear – negative | Avoid overheating and swaddling |
| Miliaria rubra | 4%; high in tropics | Usu after first week | Resolves w/i days when precipitants removed | Pruritic, erythematous papules and pustules usu on forehead, upper trunk (eccrine duct obstruction at malpighian layer) | Smear – negative | Avoid overheating and swaddling |

| | | | | | |
|---|---|---|---|---|---|
| Infantile acropustulosis | <1%, increased in Black males | Up to 18 months, usu 3–6 months | Pruritic acral (subcorneal) pustules/vesicles in crops (q2–4 weeks), eosinophilia, no burrows | Smear – eos (early), PMNs (late); Scabies prep neg | Midpotency topical steroids, antihistamines |
| Eosinophilic pustular folliculitis/Ofuji's | M>F | Birth or first few weeks | Pruritic, crusted, erythematous follicular papules/pustules/vesicles in crops (q2–4 weeks), mainly on scalp, eosinophilia | Smear – eos | Topical steroids, systemic abx |
| Congenital self-healing langerhans/Hashimoto–Pritzker | Unknown, likely underreported | Weeks–months | Widespread red-brown nodules, skin-limited | Bx – CD1a +, S100 + | None needed |
| Incontinentia pigmenti/Block–Sulzberger | 1:300,000, XLD | Birth or days | Linear and whorled; Stages: Vesicular/Bullous (birth – 1 year) →; Verrucous (months – 3 years) →; Hyperpigmented (1–20 years) →; Hypopigmented/Atrophic (adulthood) | Bx: Bullous – eos spong; Verrucous – eos dysk; Hyperpig – dermal melanin; Hypopig – epi atrophy, no appendages | Referrals: ophtho, audiology, neuro, dental |

continued p. 92

| Condition | Population | Onset | Duration | Description | Diagnosis | Treatment |
|---|---|---|---|---|---|---|
| **VIRAL** | | | | | | |
| HSV – congenital/intrauterine | 5% of newborn HSV | Birth | | Generalized vesicles, pustules, scars, erosions, microcephaly, chorioretinitis, hydranencephaly, microphthalmia | Tzank – multinucleated giant cells; DFA, PCR, Cx, IgG serology | IV acyclovir |
| HSV – primary neonatal | 95% of newborn HSV (usu peri- not postnatal infxn); ~1:3200 deliveries | Birth (30%) to several weeks | 30–50% mortality if disseminated | 40% Skin–Eye–Mucosal disease, 35% CNS, 25% disseminated (sepsis, hepatitis, resp, coag); Primary maternal infxn has 10× the risk of perinatal infxn vs. recurrent maternal infxn | Tzank – multinucleated giant cells; DFA, PCR, Cx, IgG serology | IV acyclovir |
| VZV – congenital | ~10% risk with exposure (<20 weeks gestation) | Birth | | LBW, scars, limb hypoplasia, microcephaly encephalitis, cortical atrophy, optho, MSK, GI, GU | Tzank – multinucleated giant cells; DFA, Cx | VZIG/acyclovir w/i 5 days to exposed mom |

| | | | | | | |
|---|---|---|---|---|---|---|
| VZV – neonatal | 20–60% risk with materna exposure 5 days before or 2 days post-partum | Birth to 2 weeks | 30% mortality | Pustules, vesicles → may ulcerate, necrose; pneumonitis, encephalitis, hepatitis | Tzank – multinucleated giant cells; DFA, Cx | VZIG/acyclovir w/i 5 days to exposed mom and to neonate |
| VZV – infantile zoster | 2% of patients w/ intrauterine exposure by 20 weeks gestation | First year | | Dermatomal papules, vesicles | Tzank – multinucleated giant cells; DFA, Cx | Consider iv acyclovir |
| **FUNGAL** | | | | | | |
| Candidiasis – congenital/intrauterine | <1% | Birth | Several weeks | Widespread erythematous papules/pustules, thrush, rarely systemic; Risk factors – prematurity, cervical/uterine foreign bodies | KOH: budding yeast, pseudohyphae | Topical nystatin or imidazole unless severe or disseminated |
| Candidiasis – neonatal | 5% | Few days or weeks | Several weeks | Red plaques, satellite papules/pustules, more common and may disseminate in LBW babies | KOH: budding yeast, pseudohyphae | IV fluconazole if preterm/LBW |
| Aspergillosis | Premature/LBW/ immunodef | Days or weeks | | Necrotic papules, pustules, ulcers | Bx: branching hyphae at 45°; Cx | Debridement, ampho |

continued p. 94

| Condition | Population | Onset | Duration | Description | Diagnosis | Treatment |
|---|---|---|---|---|---|---|
| **Parasites** | | | | | | |
| Scabies | Rare in neonates | | | Excoriated vesicles, pustules, papules, nodules, burrows | KOH/Mineral oil – mites, feces/ scybala, eggs | Permethrin 5% 1 week apart, treat linens/family; sulfur; lindane contraindicated |
| **BACTERIAL** | | | | | | |
| Impetigo neonatorum | | Anytime | | Erythematous pustules, vesicles, tense bullae, honey-colored crust, oozing, glazed, central clearing, satellite lesions, fever, adenopathy, diarrhea | Gram stain and cx; Staph – Gram + cocci in clusters; Strep – Gram + cocci in chains | Mupirocin, oral abx, nursery isolation |
| Rare, life-threatening bacterial infxns: *Listeria monocytogenes, Chlamydia trachomatis, E. coli, H. influenzae, Pseudomonas* | | Onset: Birth, days, or weeks | | | Systemic involvement; Risk factors: prematurity, LBW, immunodef, maternal fever | Gram – rods: *Pseudomonas, H. influenzae, E. coli* Gram + rods: *Listeria monocytogenes* |

Other neonatal vesiculopustular eruptions: Pustular leukemoid rxn in Down syndrome, Hyper IgE, Neonatal Behcet, Pustular Psoriasis, Syphilis.

Adapted from Van Praag MC *et al.* Diagnosis and treatment of pustular disorders in the neonate. *Pediatr. Dermatol.* 1997 March–April; 14(2):131–43; Johr RH and Schachner LA. Neonatal dermatologic challenges. *Pediatrics in Review.* 1997; 18:86–94. Pauporte M and Frieden I. Vesiculobullous and erosive diseases in the newborn, In: Bolognia Jorizzo JL, Rapini RP. *Dermatology*, Vol. 1. London: Mosby, 2003.

# Genital Ulcers

| Infection | Organism | Incubation | Presentation | Treatment | Notes |
|-----------|----------|------------|--------------|-----------|-------|
| Chancroid | *Haemophilus ducreyi* | 3–10 days | Painful, soft, ragged edges; tender and unilateral LAN | Azithromycin, ceftriaxone, ciprofloxacin, erythromycin | "School of fish" Gram stain |
| Primary syphilis (chancre) | *Treponema pallidum* | 2–4 weeks | Painless, indurated, sharp and raised edges; bilateral and nontender LAN | Penicillin | Rubbery, "ham-colored base" |
| Genital HSV | HSV | 3–7 days | Painful, grouped | Antivirals | |
| Lymphogranuloma venereum | *Chlamydia trachomatis* serovars L1-3 | 3–12 days | Painless; soft; tender LAN | Doxycycline | "Groove sign" – tender nodes around Poupart's ligament |
| Donovanosis/granuloma inguinale | *Calymmatobacterium/ Klebsiella granulomatis* | 2–12 weeks | Non- or mildly painful, beefy red, bleeding | TMP-SMX, doxycycline, erythromycin, ciprofloxacin | "Safety pin" Donovan bodies |

Other infectious causes of genital ulcers: EBV, Amebiasis, Candida, TB, Leishmaniasis.
Non-Infectious causes of genital ulcers: Behcet/Apthous, Crohn, Lichen Planus, Tumor, Lichen Sclerosis, Contact, Trauma, Factitial, Fixed Drug (NSAIDs, metronidazole, sulfonamide, acetaminophen, TCN, phenytoin, OCPs, phenolphthalein, barbiturates), Other Meds (all-trans-retinoic acid, foscarnet), MAGIC Syndrome, Cicatricial/Bullous Pemphigoid, Hemangioma, EM/SJS/TEN.

# Common Contact Allergens

| Allergen | Uses/products/cross reactions (X-RXN) | Test |
|---|---|---|
| **METAL** | | |
| Nickel | • Jewelry, watches, coins, buckles, eyelash curlers, kitchen utensils, canned food | Dimethylglyoxime – to detect nickel; TRUE test #1 |
| Gold | • Jewelry, dentistry, electronics<br>X-RXN: nickel, cobalt | |
| Chromates/potassium dichromate | • Tanned leather, cement, mortar, matches, anti-rust products, paint, plaster, GREEN dyes/tattoos (pool/card table felt)<br>X-RXN: nickel, cobalt | TRUE test #4 |
| Cobalt | USES: mixed with metals for strength<br>• Cement, cosmetics, vitamin B12 injections, pigment in porcelain, paint, crayon, glass, pottery<br>X-RXN: nickel, chromates | TRUE test #12 |
| **RESIN** | | |
| p-tert-Butylphenol (PTBP) formaldehyde resin | USES: Resin for adhesive<br>• Glues, shoes/watchband/handbag (glued leather products), plywood, disinfectants, rubber, varnish, printer inks, fiberglass; depigmenting | TRUE test #13 |
| Epoxy resin (bisphenol A) | USES: Resin for adhesive<br>Allergens: bisphenol A, epichlorohydrin<br>• Glues, plastics, adhesives, PVC products, electrical insulation | TRUE test #14 |
| Rosin (colophony, abietic acid) | Adhesives, cosmetics, epilation wax, polish, paint, chewing gum, paper products; from conifer | TRUE test #7 |
| **RUBBER COMPOUND** | | |
| Carba mix | USES: Rubber stabilizer<br>• Elastic bands, condoms, shoes, cements<br>X-RXN: thiurams | TRUE test #15 |
| Black rubber mix | USES: Rubber stabilizer<br>Isopropyl PPD, cyclohexyl PPD, diphenyl PPD<br>• Black and gray rubber products: tires, rubber boots, eyelash curlers, scuba suits, balls | TRUE test #16 |

| Allergen | Uses/products/cross reactions (X-RXN) | Test |
|---|---|---|
| Thiuram mix | USES: Rubber additives<br>• Gloves, adhesive, latex, condoms, fungi- and pesticides, disulfiram | TRUE test #24 |
| Mercapto mix | USES: Rubber accelerator<br>MOR: morpholinyl mercapto-benzothiazole<br>CBS: N-cyclohexyl-2-benzothiazyl sulfenamide MBTS: dibenzothiazyl disulfide<br>• Rubber products: gloves, makeup sponges, undergarments, tires | TRUE test #22 |
| Mercapto-benzothiazole (MBT) | USES: Rubber accelerator<br>• Rubber shoes, tires, undergarments, shoes | TRUE test #19 |
| **MEDICAMENTS** | | |
| Lanolin/wool alcohol | USES: Emulsifier<br>From: sheep sebum (wool wax/alcohol/fat)<br>• Cosmetics, soaps, adhesives, topical agents<br>X-RXN: Aquaphor, Eucerin (cetyl or stearyl alcohols) | TRUE test #2 (wool alcohols) |
| Neomycin sulfate | Aminoglycoside group<br>• Topical creams, ear/eye drops<br>X-RXN: aminoglycosides<br>Co-sensitivity: bacitracin | TRUE test #3 |
| Benzocaine/tetracaine | PABA derivative, ester anesthetic<br>X-RXN: procaine, cocaine, PABA, sulfa meds, thiazide, PPD | TRUE test #5: Caine mix |
| Dibucaine | Amide anesthetic<br>X-RXN: lidocaine, bupivicaine | TRUE test #5: Caine mix |
| Corticosteroids | Four classes based on structure:<br>A – HC/Prednisone<br>B – TMC acetonide<br>C – Betamethasone<br>D – Hydrocortisone-17-butyrate and clobetasone-17-butyrate<br>Tixocortol pivalate – test for class A; Budesonide – test for classes B and D | |
| Ethylenediamine | Stabilizer<br>• Topical antibiotic/steroid creams (Mycolog cream); dye, rubber, resin, waxes<br>X-RXN: hydroxyzine, aminophylline, phenothiazine | TRUE test #11 |

continued p. 98

| Allergen | Uses/products/cross reactions (X-RXN) | Test |
|---|---|---|
| Propylene glycol | Dimer alcohol to increase drug solubility<br>• Vehicle base in topical meds, valium, lubricant jelly; brake fluid, antifreeze | |
| Bacitracin<br>Clioquinol | Risk groups: leg ulcers, post-op, chronic otitis externa<br>Topical antibacterials and antifungals | |
| **FRAGRANCES** | | |
| Fragrance mix (8 fragrances) | α-amyl cinnamic aldehyde, cinnamic alcohol, cinnamic aldehyde (toothpaste, gum, lipstick) hydroxycitronellal – synthetic, floral isoeugenol, eugenol – clove oak moss absolute – lichen extract, cologne geraniol – geranium<br>X-RXN: colophony, wood tars, turpentine, propolis, benzoin, storax | TRUE test #6 |
| Balsam of peru (myroxylon pereirae) | Cinnamic acid, cinnamyl cinnamate, benzyl benzoate, benzoic acid, vanillin<br>• Fragrances, spices (cloves, cinnamon, Jamaican pepper), flavoring agent (wine, tobacco, vermouth, cola), mild antimicrobial properties<br>X-RXN: Colophony, turpentine, benzoin, wood tar | TRUE test #10 |
| **PRESERVATIVES** | | |
| Formaldehyde | • Ubiquitous – fabric finishes (waterproof, anti-wrinkle), cosmetics, cleansers, paper products, paint<br>Formaldehyde-releasing preservatives: quaternium-15, imidazolidinyl urea, diazolidinyl urea, DMDM-hydantoin | TRUE test #21 |
| Quaternium-15 (Dowicil 200) | Formaldehyde-releasing preservative Sensitivity may be to formaldehyde<br>• Soaps, shampoos, moisturizers | TRUE test #18 |
| Methyl-choloro-isothiazinolone (Kathon CG) | Cosmetics, hair/skin products (Eucerin), household products (toilet paper), permanent waves, latex emulsions | TRUE test #17 |
| Paraben mix | USES: preservatives<br>• Topical pharmaceutical products, cosmetics<br>X-RXN: PABA, PPD | TRUE test #8 |
| Thimerosal (Merthiolate) | Preservative/antiseptic/vaccine/eye drops<br>Two components: thiosalicylic acid and ethyl mercuric chloride<br>X-RXN: piroxicam, mercury | TRUE test #23 |

| Allergen | Uses/products/cross reactions (X-RXN) | Test |
|---|---|---|
| Imidazolidinyl urea (Germall 115, Tristat) | Formaldehyde-releasing preservatives<br>• Cosmetics, skin/hair products, adhesive, latex emulsions | |

### OTHERS

| Allergen | Uses/products/cross reactions (X-RXN) | Test |
|---|---|---|
| Paraphenylenediamine (PPD) | Blue-black aniline dye<br>• Permanent hair dyes, tattoos, photography solutions, printer inks, oils, gasoline<br>X-RXN: pro/benzocaine, PABA, azo- and aniline dyes, sulfas, para-aminosalicylic acid | TRUE test #20 |
| Ammonium persulfate | Bleaching agent<br>• Hair bleach, flour<br>Contact urticaria, anaphylactoid rxn | |
| Disperse blue dyes | Fabrics; waistbands, thighs, axillae | |
| Glyceryl monothioglycolate | Acidic perming solutions<br>Chemical remains in hair shaft for months | |
| Latex | Sap from the rubber tree *Hevae brasiliensis*<br>• Gloves, condom, balloon<br>High risk: children with spina bifida, health care workers<br>X-RXN: avocado, banana, chestnut, kiwi, papaya | RAST test, prick test |
| Cocamidopropyl betaine | Nonionic surfactant from coconut oil<br>Antigens: amidoamine, DMAPA, CAPB<br>• Shampoo, liquid soaps<br>Usually facial pattern rash | |
| Ethyl cyanoacrylate | "Superglue"<br>• Artificial nails glue, liquid bandage | |
| Methyl methacrylate | • Artificial nails, dental work, glue for surgical prostheses | |
| Gluteraldehyde | Cold sterilizing solution<br>Health care workers, embalming fluid, electron microscopy, hand cleansers | |
| Limonene | • Citrus peels, fragrance additive, sanitizers, cleansers, degreasers | |
| Propolis | Dimethylallyl ester of caffeic acid<br>• Bee glue, lipstick, ointments, mascara | |

*continued p. 100*

| Allergen | Uses/products/cross reactions (X-RXN) | Test |
|---|---|---|
| Thioureas | Rubber antioxidant<br>• Wet suits, shoe insoles, adhesives, copy paper, photography | |
| Euxyl K-400 | Methyldibromo glutaronitrile phenoxyethanol<br>• Cosmetic/personal care products | |
| Toluene-sulfonamide (tosylamide) formaldehyde resin | Nail lacquer/ hardener: eyelid, face, neck, finger dermatitis | |
| Benzyl alcohol | Solvent, preservative, anesthetic<br>• Plants, essential oils, foods, cosmetics, medications, paints/ lacquers | |

## Features suggestive of specific irritant/toxin

| | |
|---|---|
| Acne/folliculitis | Arsenic, oils, glass fibers, asphalt, tar, chlorinated naphthalenes, polyhalogenated biphenyls |
| Miliaria | Occlusion, aluminum chloride, UV, infrared |
| Alopecia | Borax, chloroprene dimers |
| Granulomatous | Silica, beryllium, keratin, talc, cotton |

## Plants and dermatoses

### Plants causing non-immunologic contact urticaria
Urticaceae family (nettle):
• *Urtica* spp. (dioica) – stinging nettle
• *Dendrocnide* spp. – Australian stinging nettle, may be fatal
Euphorbiaceae family (spurge):
• *Acidoton* and *Cnidosculus* spp.
• Croton plant
Hydrophyllaceae family (water-leaf)

### Plants causing mechanical irritant dermatitis
*Hedera helix* – Araliaceae – common ivy
*Opuntia* spp. – Cactaceae – prickly pear
*Tulipa* spp. – Liliaceae – tulip
*Ficus* and *Morus* spp. – Moraceae – fig, mulberry
*Carduus* and *Cirsium* spp. – Asteraceae – thistle
*Bidens tripartite* – Asteraceae – bur marigold
*Other Asteraceae* – dandelion, lettuce, chicory (irritant latex)

**GENERAL DERMATOLOGY**

## Plants causing chemical irritant dermatitis

| Chemical | Plant | Scientific name |
|---|---|---|
| Calcium oxalate | Daffodil | *Narcissus* spp. (Amaryllidaceae) |
| | Century plant | *Agave americana* (Agavaceae) |
| | Dumb cane | *Dieffenbachia picta* and *Philodendron* |
| | Philodendron | spp. (Araceae) |
| | Pineapple | *Ananas cosmosus* (Bromeliaceae) |
| | Hyacinth | *Hyacinthus orientalis* (Liliaceae) |
| | Rhubarb | *Rheum rhaponticum* (Polygonaceae) |
| Thiocyanates | Garlic | *Allium sativum* (Alliaceae) |
| | Black mustard | *Brassica nigra* (Brassicaceae) |
| | Radish | *Raphanus sativus* (Brassicaceae) |
| Cashew nut shell oil | Cashew tree | *Anacardium occidentale* (Anacardiaceae) |
| Bromelin | Pineapple | *Ananas comosus* (Bromeliaceae) |
| Phorbol esters, diterpenes (latex) | Poinsettia | *Euphorbia pulcherrima* (Euphorbiaceae) |
| Protoanemonin | Buttercup | *Ranunculus* spp. (Ranunculaceae) |
| Capsaicin | Chili pepper | *Capsicum anuum* (Salanaceae) |

## Phytophotodermatoses

Apiaceae: hogweed (*Heracleum sphondylium*), celery (*Apium gaveolens*), parsley (*Petroselinum*), parsnips, fennel (*Foeniculum vulgare*)

Rutaceae: lime, orange, lemon, garden rue, Hawaiian lei, gas plant/burning bush

Moraceae: mulberry, fig tree

Fabaceae/Leguminosae: bavachee/scurf-pea (vitiligo tx)

## Plant allergic contact dermatitis

| Allergen | Family | Plant (scientific name) |
|---|---|---|
| Urushiol | Anacardiaceae | Poison ivy/oak/sumac (*Toxicodendron vernix*) Cashew nut tree (*Anacardium occidentale*) Mango (*Mangifera indica*) |
| | Cross-reactions: *Ginko biloba*, Grevillea | Brazilian pepper tree (*Schinus terebinthifolius*, Florida Holly) Indian marking tree nut (*Semecarpus anacardium*) Japanese lacquer tree (*Toxicodendron verniciflua*) |

*continued p. 102*

| Allergen | Family | Plant (scientific name) |
|---|---|---|
| | | Rengas tree (*Gluta* spp.) |
| | | Poisonwood tree (*Metopium toxiferum*) |
| Sesquiterpene lactones | Asteraceae (Compositae) | Feverfew (*Tanacetum parthenium*) |
| | | Chrysanthemum (*X Dendranthema*) |
| | | Dandelion (*Taraxacum officinale*) |
| | | Sunflower (*Helianthus annuus*) |
| | | Scourge of India (*Parthenium hysterophorus*, wild feverfew) |
| | | Daisy (*Leucanthemum* spp.) |
| | | Ragweed (*Ambrosia* spp.) |
| | | Marigold (*Tagetes* spp.) |
| | | Artichoke (*Cynara scolymus*) |
| | | Lettuce (*Lactuca sativa*) |
| | | Endive (*Cichorium endiva*) |
| | | Chicory (*Cichorium intybus*) |
| | | Chamomile, mugwort (*Artemisia* spp.) |
| | | Yarrow (*Achillea millefolium*) |
| Diallyl disulfide | Alliaceae | Onion (*A. cepa*) |
| | | Garlic (*A. sativum*) |
| | | Leek (*A. porrum*) |
| | | Chive |
| Tuliposide A | Alstromeriaceae and Lillaceae | Tulip, Peruvian lily (*A. auriantiaca* and *A. ligtu*) |
| Primin | Primulaceae | Primrose (*Primula obconica*) |
| | Lamiaceae | Peppermint (*menthol*), spearmint (*carvone*), lavender, thyme |
| d-limonene | Myrtaceae | Tea tree (*Melaleuca* spp.) |
| Colophony and turpentine/ carene | Pinaceae | Pine tree (*Pinus* spp.) |
| | | Spruce tree (*Picea* spp.) |
| Ricin | Castor bean | *Ricinus communis* |
| Abrin | Jequirity bean | *Abrus precatorius* |
| Usnic acid, evenic acid, atronorin | Lichens | |

# Vitamin Deficiencies/Hypervitaminoses

### Vitamin A
Vitamin A supplementation helpful in rubeola
Deficiency = Phrynoderma (toadskin)

- Due to fat malabsorption, diet; found in animal fat, liver, milk
- Night blindness, poor acuity in bright light, Bitot spots, keratomalacia, xerophthalmia, xerosis, follicular hyperkeratosis, fragile hair, apathy, mental and growth retardation

Hypervitaminosis A

- Similar to medical retinoid treatment: dry lips, arthralgias, cheilitis, alopecia, onychodystrophy/clubbing, hyperpigmentation, impaired bone growth, hyperostosis, pseudotumor cerebri, lethargy, anorexia

### Vitamin B1 – Thiamine
Deficiency = Beriberi

- Due to diet (polished rice), pregnancy, alcoholism, GI disease
- Glossitis, edema, glossodynia, neuropathy, Wernicke-Korsakoff, CHF

### Vitamin B2 – Riboflavin
Deficiency

- Alcoholics, malabsorption, neonatal phototherapy, chlorpromazine
- Oral-ocular-genital syndrome: cheilits, seborrheic dermatitis-like rash, tongue atrophy, belpharitis, conjunctivitis, photophobia, genital and peri-nasal dermatitis, anemia

### Vitamin B3 – Niacin/Nicotinic Acid
Deficiency = Pellagra

- May be due to precursor (tryptophan, Hartnup) deficiency, alcoholism, carcinoid tumor, INH, 5-FU, azathioprine, GI disorders, anorexia
- Casal necklace eruption, photosensitivity, shellac-like appearance, acral fissures, perineal rash, cheilitis, diarrhea, dementia
- Below granular layer (stratum malpighii): vacuolar changes

### Vitamin B6 – Pyridoxine
Deficiency

- Due to cirrhosis, uremia, isoniazid, hydralazine, OCP, phenelzine, penicillamine
- Rash resembling seborrheic dermatitis, intertrigo, cheilitis, glossitis, conjunctivitis, fatigue, neuropathy, disorientation, N/V

### Vitamin B12– Cyanocobalamin
Deficiency

- Due to diet (found in animal products), pernicious anemia, malabsorption
- Glossitis, hyperpigmentation, canities, neurologic symptoms

### Vitamin C
Deficiency = Scurvy

- Alcoholics, diet
- Water-soluble, fruits/vegetables
- Perifollicular hyperkeratosis and petechiae, corkscrew hairs, hemorrhagic gingivitis, epistaxis, hypochondriasis, subperiosteal hemorrhage (pseudoparalysis), soft teeth, gingivitis, hematologic changes, weakness

### Vitamin D
Physiology

- Vit $D_2$ and $D_3$ in the diet are transported to the liver in chylomicrons and Vit $D_3$ from the skin and Vit $D_2$ and $D_3$ from fat cell stores are bound to Vit D-binding protein for transport to the liver
- In the liver, Vit D-25-hydroxylase turns Vit D into 25-hydroxyvitamin D, or 25(OH)D, the main circulating form of Vit D
- 25(OH)D is biologically inactive until it is converted to 1,25-dihydroxyvitamin D, or $1,25(OH)_2D$, by 25-hydroxyvitamin D-1$\alpha$-hydroxylase in the kidneys
- $1,25(OH)_2D$ is inactivated by 25-hydroxyvitamin D-24-hydroxylase and turned into calcitroic acid, which is excreted in the bile
- In osteoblasts, $1,25(OH)_2D$ increases RANKL which bind RANK on preosteoclasts, leading to activation
  In intestinal cells, $1,25(OH)_2D$ binds VDR-RXR, leading to increased calcium channel TRPV6 and calcium binding protein calbindin 9K
- Calcium-phosphate product: saturation product = $60 \, mg^2/dl^2$; between 42 and $52 \, mg^2/dl^2$ is desirable in the ESRD population $60 \, mg^2/dl^2$; between 42 and $52 \, mg^2/dl^2$ is desirable in the ESRD population.

Deficiency

- Poor diet (Vit D is fat soluble – found in oily fish, eggs, butter, liver, cod-liver oil), insufficient sun (need UVB to convert 7-dehydrocholesterol to previtamin $D_3$, which is quickly turned into vitamin $D_3$), anticonvulsants, fat malabsorption, old age, chronic kidney disease, breastfeeding (human milk has low Vit D)
- Requirements: controversial, ~800 IU/day of vitamin D3
- Alopecia, rickets/osteomalacia, osteoporosis, cancer (colon, breast, prostate, hematologic), autoimmune disease, muscle weakness

Hypervitaminosis D

- Hypercalcemia, calcinosis, anorexia, headache, N/V

**Vitamin K**
Deficiency

- Due to diet (fat-soluble, meat, green leafy vegetables; GI flora produces 50% of requirements), anorexia, CF, liver disease, malabsorption, coumadin, cephalosporins, salicylates, cholestyramine
- Hemorrhage

**Zinc deficiency**

- Due to AR genetic defect, diet (low zinc, excess fiber), malabsorption, CRF, alcoholism, TPN, cancer
- Typically when wean breastfeeding but zinc in human breastmilk does have lower bioavailability than cowmilk and may sometimes be low; premature infants have reduced zinc stores, poor GI absorbance, and higher zinc needs
- Acrodermatitis enteropathica (acral, periorificial, periungual, cheilitis), diarrhea, alopecia, candida/staph superinfection, paronychia, irritable, photophobia, blepharitis, failure to thrive
- Resembles biotin deficiency, essential fatty acid deficiency, CF, Crohn, necrolytic migratory erythema
- Low alkaline phosphatase
- Histo: epidermal pallor ± psoriasiform hyperplasia, necrosis, subcorneal/intraepidermal vesicle (similar to necrolytic migratory erythema, necrolytic acral erythema, genetic deficiency of M subunit of LDH)
- Zinc-responsive diseases: necrolytic acral erythema, amicrobial pustulosis of the flexures and scalp

**Biotin deficiency**

- Due to short gut (gut bacteria make biotin), malabsorption, avidin (raw egg white) consumption, biotinidase deficiency (infantile), multiple carboxylase synthetase or holocarboxylase synthetase defects (neonatal)
- Rash like zinc deficiency, alopecia, conjunctivitis, fatigue, paresthesias

**Essential fatty acid deficiency**

- Due to GI abnormalities/surgery, diet, chronic TPN
- Rash resembling biotin and zinc deficiencies, alopecia, leathery skin, intertrigo
- Eicosatrienoic acid: Arachidonic acid ratio > 4

### Copper

- Deficiency in Menkes, Wilson
- Local, exogenous excess – green hair (copper in water)

### Selenium deficiency

- Component of glutathione peroxidase
- Due to TPN, low soil content
- Weakness, cardiomyopathy, elevated transaminases and CK, hypopigmentation (skin/hair), leukonychia

### Lycopenemia

- Excess consumption of red fruits/vegetables (tomatoes, papaya) → reddish skin

### Carotenemia

- Carotene-containing foods: carrots, squash, oranges, spinach, corn, beans, eggs, butter, pumpkins, papaya, baby foods
- Yellow soles/palms, central face (sebaceous area)

### Kwashiorkor

- Protein deficiency
- Due to diet, GI surgery, HIV
- Dyschromia, pallor, flaky paint desquamation, sparse, hypopigmented hair, flag sign, potbelly, edema, moon facies, cheilitis, soft nails, irritable, infections

### Marasmus

- Protein and caloric deficiency
- Due to diet neglect, anorexia, malabsorption, HIV, liver/kidney failure
- Xerotic, lax, thin skin, follicular hyperkeratosis, broken lanugo-like hair, monkey/aged facies, no edema/hypoproteinemia

# Genodermatoses

## Gene list

| Disease | Gene | Protein | Comment |
|---|---|---|---|
| Acral peeling skin syndrome | TGM5 | Transglutaminase-5 | AR |
| Acrodermatitis enteropathica | SLC39A4 | Intestinal zinc-specific transporter | AR Defective zinc absorption from the gut |
| Acrokeratosis verruciformis of hopf | ATP2A2 | ATPase, Ca$^{2+}$ transporting | AD Allelic to darier |
| AEC | P63 | P63 | AD Tumor suppressor; Allelic to EEC, Rapp–Hodgkin, limb-mammary syndrome, split-hand and split-foot malformation type 4, and acro-dermatoungual-lacrimal-tooth (ADULT) |
| Albright hereditary osteodystrophy | GNAS1 | G protein, alpha stimulating | AD G protein subunit of adenylate cyclase; Allelic to McCune–Albright and progressive osseus heteroplasia |
| Alagille | JAG1 | Jagged-1 | AD Jagged-1 is a ligand for NOTCH |
|  | | NOTCH2 | |
| Alkaptonuria | HGO | Homogentisate 1,2-dioxygenase | AR Deficient homogentisic acid oxidase causes homogentisic acid to accumulate in tissues |
| Alport | COL4A3 | Collagen 4 | AR XL form may be associated with leiomyomatosis |
|  | COL4A4 | | AR (esophageal, tracheo-bronchial, female genital) |
|  | COL4A5 | | XL |

continued p. 108

| Disease | Gene | Protein | | Comment |
|---|---|---|---|---|
| Anhidrotic ectodermal dysplasia (Christ–Siemens–Touraine; hypohidrotic) | EDA | Ectodysplasin-A | XLR | Similar to AD form due to ectodysplasin anhidrotic receptor (EDAR) mutation; Similar to AR form due to either EDAR or EDAR-associated death domain (EDARADD) mutations |
| Anhidrotic ectodermal dysplasia with immune deficiency ± osteoporosis and lymphedema | NEMO | NF–κB essential modulator/IKK-gamma | XLR | Allelic to IP |
| Anonychia congenita | RSPO4 | R-spondin 4 | AR | Wnt/β-catenin signaling pathway (no bone hypoplasia unlike Cooks) |
| Apert | FGFR2 | Fibroblast growth factor receptor 2 | AD | Allelic to Beare–Stevenson and Crouzon |
| Argininosuccinic aciduria | ASL | Argininosuccinate lyase | AR | Urea cycle defect |
| Arrhythmogenic right ventricular dysplasia/cardiomyopathy | DSP PLK2 DSG2 DSC2 | Desmoplakin Plakophilin-2 Desmoglein-2 Desmocollin-2 | AR | |
| Atrichia with papular lesions | HR | Hairless | AR | Zinc finger protein |
| Ataxia–telangiectasia | ATM | Ataxia telangiectasia mutated | AR | Phosphatidyl inositol 3 kinase-like domain |
| Autoimmune polyendocrinopathy | AIRE | Autoimmune regulator | AD AR | Candidiasis, ectodermal dysplasia |
| Bannayan–Riley–Ruvalcaba | PTEN | Phosphatase and tensin homolog | AD | Tumor suppressor; Allelic to Cowden and Lhermitte–Duclos |

| | | | |
|---|---|---|---|
| Bart–Pumphrey | GJB2 | Connexin 26 | AD | Knuckle pads, leukonychia, and sensorineural deafness; Allelic to KID and classic Vohwinkel |
| Basal cell nevus syndrome (Gorlin) | PTCH | Patched | AD | Tumor suppressor, SHH transmembrane receptor, inhibits SMOH |
| Beare–Stevenson Cutis Gyrata | FGFR2 | Fibroblast growth factor receptor 2 | AD | Allelic to Apert and Crouzon |
| Beckwith–Wiedemann | CDKN1C/ KIP2 P57; NSD1; 11p15 imprinting | Cyclin-dependent kinase inhibitor 1C | Sp > AD | Deregulation of imprinted growth regulatory genes; 11p15 imprinting region also involved in Russell–Silver |
| Birt–Hogg–Dube | FLCN | Folliculin | AD | Interacts with AMPK and FNIP1 in mTOR signaling |
| Bloom | RECQL3 | RecQ protein-like 3 | AR | DNA helicase |
| Brooke–Spiegler | CYLD | Cylindromatosis | AD | Tumor suppressor |
| Bruton agammaglobulinemia | BTK | Bruton agammaglobulinemia tyrosine kinase | XLR | Tyrosine kinase |
| Bullous congenital ichthyosiform Erythroderma (epidermolytic hyperkeratosis) | KRT 1, 10 | Keratin 1, 10 | AD | Intermediate filaments |
| Buschke–Ollendorff | LEMD3/MAN1 | LEM domain-containing protein 3 | AD | Inner nuclear membrane protein; Allelic to familial cutaneous collagenoma syndrome |
| Capillary malformation-arteriovenous malformation | RASA1 | RAS family, GTPase activating protein | AD | |

continued p. 110

109

| Disease | Gene | Protein | | Comment |
|---------|------|---------|---|---------|
| Caridiofaciocutaneous | KRAS<br>BRAF<br>MEK1<br>MEK2 | Kirsten rat sarcoma virus oncogene homolog | Sp | All proteins in RAS-ERK pathway |
| Carney complex (NAME, LAMB) | PRKAR1A | Protein kinase A regulatory subunit 1α | AD | |
| Carney complex with distal arthrogryposis | MYH8 | Myosin heavy chain 8 | AD | Variant associated with trismus and pseudocamptodactyly |
| Cartilage hair hypoplasia | RMRP | Mitochondrial RNA-processing endoribonuclease | AR | |
| Carvajal | DSP | Desmoplakin | AR | Dilated cardiomyopathy with woolly hair and keratoderma; Allelic to keratosis palmaris striata II, lethal acantholytic EB, skin fragility-wooly hair syndrome |
| CEDNIK (cerebral dysgenesis, neuropathy, ichthyosis, PPK) | SNAP29 | Synaptosomal-associated protein 29 | AR | |
| Cerebral capillary malformations, familial | CCM1/KRIT1 | Krev-interaction trapped 1 | AD | Hyperkeratotic AVMs |
| Cerebrotendinous xanthomatosis | CYP27 | Cytochrome p450, subfamily 27A, polypeptide 1 (sterol-27-hydroxylase) | AR | |
| Chédiak-Higashi | LYST | Lysosomal trafficking regulator | AR | Lysosomal transport – transfer of melanosomes |

| | | | | |
|---|---|---|---|---|
| CHILD | NSDHL | NADP steroid dehydrogenase-like | XLD | Cholesterol biosynthesis (aka 3β-hydroxysteroid dehydrogenase) |
| Chondrodysplasia punctata 1 | ARSE | Arylsulfatase E | XLR | |
| Chondrodysplasia punctata 2 (Conradi–Hünermann) | EBP | Emopamil-binding protein | XLD | Sterol isomerase – cholesterol biosynthesis |
| Chondrodysplasia punctata, rhizomelic, type 1 | PEX7 | Peroxisomal type 2 targeting signal receptor (PTS2) | AR | Allelic to refsum |
| Chondrodysplasia punctata, rhizomelic, type 2 | DHAPAT | Acyl-CoA:dihydroxyacetone phosphate acyltransferase | AR | |
| Chronic granulomatous disease Cytochrome, X-linked | CYBB | p91-Phagocyte oxidase (cytochrome b-245 beta subunit) | XLR | Cytochrome b is part of NADPH oxidase – need oxidative burst to kill catalase+ bacteria |
| Chronic granulomatous disease Cytochrome b-negative | CYBA | p22-Phagocyte oxidase | AR | |
| Chronic granulomatous disease Cytochrome b-positive type 1 | NCF1 | p47-Phagocyte oxidase | AR | |
| Chronic granulomatous disease Cytochrome b-positive type 2 | NCF2 | p67-Phagocyte oxidase | AR | |
| Cleft lip-Palate with ectodermal dysplasia | PVRL1 | Poliovirus receptor-like 1 | AR | Cell adhesion molecule/herpes virus receptor; Margarita Island ED, Rosselli–Giulienetti, Zlotogora–Ogur |

continued p. 112

| Disease | Gene | Protein | Comment |
|---------|------|---------|---------|
| Cockayne | ERCC6 ERCC8 | Excision repair cross-complementing group 6 or 8 | AR |
| Congenital adrenal hyperplasia | CYP21A2 CYP11B1 CYP17A1 STAR | 21-hydroxylase 11-β-hydroxylase 17-α-hydroxylase Steroidogenic acute regulatory protein | AR | 21-hydroxylase = most common; STAR = lipoid variant, most severe |
| Congenital contractural arachnodactyly (Beals) | FBN2 | Fibrillin 2 | AD | Similar to Marfan syndrome |
| Congenital generalized lipodystrophy (Berardinelli–Seip) | AGPAT2 BSCL2 | 1-acylglycerol-3-phosphate O-acyltransferase-2 (lysophosphatidic acid cyltransferase) Seipin | AR |
| Congenital ichthyosiform erythroderma (nonbullous) | TGM1 ALOXE3 ALOX12B CGI58/ABHD5 | Transglutaminase-1 Lipoxygenase-3 12R-Lipoxygenase Abhydrolase domain-containing 5 (Dorfman–Chanarin) | AR | Allelic variants of TGM1 include lamellar ichthyosis and self-healing collodion baby |
| Corneal dystrophy of Meesmann | KRT3 KRT12 | Keratin 3 Keratin 12 | AD |
| Cornelia de Lange | NIPBL SMC1A (X-linked) SMC3 | Nipped-β-like structural maintenance of chromosomes 1A and 3 | Sp > AD | Components of cohesin complex |

| Costello | HRAS<br>KRAS | Harvey and Kirsten rat sarcoma virus oncogene homolog | Unk | |
|---|---|---|---|---|
| Cowden | PTEN | Phosphatase and tensin homolog | AD | Tumor suppressor; Allelic to Bannayan–Riley–Ruvalcaba and Lhermitte–Duclos |
| Crohn's disease susceptibility | CARD15/NOD2 | Caspase recruitment domain-containing protein 15<br>Nucleotide-binding oliogmerization domain protein 2 | Cplx | CED4/APAF family of apoptosis regulators<br>Allelic to Blau syndrome and early-onset sarcoidosis |
| Crouzon | FGFR2 | Fibroblast growth factor 2 | AD | Allelic to Apert and Beare–Stevenson |
| Crouzon with acanthosis nigricans | FGFR3 | Fibroblast growth factor 3 | AD | Allelic to severe achondroplasia with developmental delay and acanthosis nigricans (SADDAN) |
| Cutaneomucosal venous malformation | TIE2/TEK, VMCM1 | Tyrosine kinase, endothelial | AD | Endothelial cell-specific receptor tyrosine kinase |
| Cutis Laxa (X-linked variant = Ehlers–Danlos 9, Occipital Horn Syndrome) | FBLN5<br>FBLN4<br>ELN<br>ATP7A | Fibulin 5<br>Fibulin 4<br>Elastin<br>ATP7A | AR,AD<br>AR<br>AD<br>XLR | Copper ion-binding ATPase<br>ATP7A allelic to Menkes |
| Darier | ATP2A2 | SERCA2 – Sarcoendoplasmic reticulum Ca$^{2+}$ ATPase isoform 2 | AD | Ca$^{2+}$ ATPase; allelic to acrokeratosis verruciformis |
| Dowling–Degos–Kitamura | KRT5 | Keratin 5 | AD | Allelic to EBS |

continued p. 114

| Disease | Gene | Protein | Comment |
|---|---|---|---|
| Drug hypersensitivity (anticonvulsant hypersensitivity syndrome) | EPHX | Epoxide hydrolase | ? |
| Dyschromatosis symmetrica hereditaria | DSRAD | Double-stranded RNA-specific adenosine deaminase | AD |
| Dyskeratosis congenita | DKC1 TERC | Dyskerin telomerase RNA candidate 3 | XLRAD Ribosomal assembly chaperone |
| Ectodermal dysplasia, skin fragility | PKP1 | Plakophilin 1 | AD Desmosomal component |
| Epidermolysis Bullosa (EB), dominant dystrophic (Cockayne–Touraine) | COL7A1 | Collagen 7 | AD 290 kDa, Anchoring fibrils |
| EB, recessive dystrophic (Hallopeau–Siemens) | COL7A1 | Collagen 7 | AR 290 kDa, Anchoring fibrils |
| EB simplex | KRT5, 14 | Keratin 5, 14 | AD Intermediate filaments |
| EB simplex, Koebner type | KRT5 | Keratin 5 | AD Allelic to Dowling–Degos–Kitamura |
| EBS with muscular dystrophy, Also EBS ogna variant | PLEC1 | Plectin | AR In hemidesmosomes, intermediate filament binding protein |
| GABEB (generalized atrophic benign epidermolysis bullosa) – junctional | COL17A1 LAMA3 LAMB3 LAMC2 | Collagen 17 Laminin A3 Laminin B3 Laminin C2 | AR Structural protein – BP Ag 2 Laminin subunits |
| Junctional EB – Herlitz type | LAMA3 LAMB3 LAMC2 | Laminin 5 subunits | AR In lamina lucida, anchoring filaments |

| | | | | |
|---|---|---|---|---|
| Junctional EB – Non-Herlitz | LAM5, COL17A1 | Laminin 5, Collagen 17 | AR | Laminin 5 or type 17 collagen |
| Junctional EB with pyloric atresia | ITGA6, ITGB4 | Alpha 6 Beta 4 Integrin | AR | Hemidesmosome transmembrane protein complex |
| Junctional EB with nephropathy and deafness | CD151 | RBC antigen MER2 | AR | Resembles Alport (nephropathy + deafness) |
| Ectodermal dysplasia, skin fragility | PKP1 | Plakophilin 1 | AR | Desmosomal plaque protein |
| Ehlers–Danlos, severe classic/Gravis 1 | COL5A1, COL5A2, COL1A1 | Collagen 5α1, Collagen 5α2, Collagen 1α1 | AD | Allelic to Ehlers–Danlos 2 (COL5A1/2), Allelic to Ehlers–Danlos 7 and osteogenesis imperfecta (COL1A1) |
| Ehlers–Danlos, mild classic/Mitis 2 | COL5A1, COL5A2 | Collagen 5α1, Collagen 5α2 | AD | Allelic to Ehlers–Danlos 1 |
| Ehlers–Danlos, hypermobility 3 | COL3A1, TNXB | Collagen 3α1, Tenascin XB | AD | Allelic to Ehlers–Danlos 4, TNXB = extracellular membrane protein |
| Ehlers–Danlos, vascular 4 | COL3A1 | Collagen 3A1 | AD, AR | Allelic to Ehlers–Danlos 3 |
| Ehlers–Danlos, X-linked 5 | Unknown | | XLR | |
| Ehlers–Danlos, kyphoscoliosis/Ocular 6 | PLOD | Lysyl hydroxylase | AR | |
| Ehlers–Danlos arthrochalasis 7a, 7b | COL1A1, COL1A2 | Collagen 1α1, Collagen 1α2 | AD | Defective conversion of procollagen into type I collagen |
| Ehlers–Danlos dermatosparaxis 7c | ADAMTS-2 | Procollagen N-peptidase | AR | |

continued p. 116

| Disease | Gene | Protein | Comment |
|---|---|---|---|
| Ehlers–Danlos, periodontosis 8 | Unknown | | AD |
| Ehlers–Danlos, occipital horn 9 | ATP7A | ATP7A | XLR — X-linked cutis laxa; Allelic to Menkes; copper transporter |
| Ehlers–Danlos, Fibronectin-deficient 10 | Fibronectin | | AR |
| Ellis–Van Creveld–Weyers acrodental dysostosis complex (chondroectodermal dysplasia) | EVC1 EVC2 | Ellis–Van Creveld 1, 2 | EVC = AR WAD = AD — EVC2 = Limbin |
| Epidermodysplasia verruciformis | EVER1 EVER2 | Epidermodysplasia verruciformis 1, 2 | AR — Susceptible to HPV 3, 5, 8 |
| Erythrokeratoderma variabilis (Mendes de Costa) | GJB3 GJB4 | Connexin 31 Connexin 30.3 | AD — GAP junction protein |
| Erythromelalgia | SCN9A/Nav1.7 | Sodium channel, voltage-gated, type 9, subunit α | AD |
| Fabry | GLA | α-galactosidase A | XLR — Lysosomal hydrolase; build up of glycosphingolipids in the body – ceramide trihexose |
| Familial dysautonomia (Riley-Day) | IKBKAP | Inhibitor of kappa light polypeptide gene enhancer in B cells, kinase complex-associated protein | AR — Ashkenazi Jews |
| Familial GIST with hyperpigmentation | C-KIT | = Mast cell growth/stem cell factor | AD — ± mastocytosis; Activating mutations unlike piebaldism |
| Familial mediterranean fever | MEFV | Pyrin | AR — PMN inhibitor |

| | | | | |
|---|---|---|---|---|
| Familial partial lipodystrophy 1 (Kobberling) | Unknown | | | |
| Familial partial lipodystrophy 2 (Dunnigan) | LMNA | Nuclear lamins A/C | AD | |
| Familial partial lipodystrophy 3 | PPARC | Peroxisome proliferator-activated receptor-gamma | | |
| Farber lipogranulomatosis | AC/ASAH | Acid ceramidase/N-acylsphingosine amidohydrolase | AR | Ceramide accumulates |
| Gardner | APC | Adenomatous polyposis coli | AD | Tumor suppressor, cleaves β-catenin |
| Gaucher | GBA | Acid-β-glucosidase | AR | Decreased glucocerebrosidase activity |
| Giant axonal neuropathy with curly hair | GAN1 | Gigaxonin | AR | Protein degradation, neuronal survival |
| Glomuvenous malformations | GLMN | Glomulin | AD | |
| Griscelli 1 | MYO5A | Myosin 5A | AR | Melanosome transport to keratinocytes |
| Griscelli 2 | RAB27A | RAB27A | AR | Ras-related GTP-binding protein |
| Griscelli 3 | MLPH MYO5A | Melanophilin Myosin 5A | AR | |
| Hailey–Hailey | ATP2C | ATPase, Ca$^{2+}$ transporting | AD | Calcium ATPase |
| Haim–Munk | CTSC | Cathepsin C | AR | Allelic to Papillon–Lefèvre |
| Harlequin ichthyosis | ABCA12 | ATP-binding cassette, subfamily A, member 12 | AR | ABC transporter superfamily; Allelic to lamellar ichthyosis 2 |

continued p. 118

| Disease | Gene | Protein | | Comment |
|---------|------|---------|---|---------|
| Hartnup | SLC6A19 | System B(0) neutral amino acid transporter-1 | AR | Failure to transport tryptophan; Pellagra-like photosensitive rash, cerebellar ataxia, emotional instability, and aminoaciduria |
| Hemochromatosis 1 | HFE | Hemochromatosis | AR | Increased intestinal Fe absorption |
| Hemochromatosis 2A | HJV | Hemojuvelin | AR | Juvenile type |
| Hemochromatosis 2B | HAMP | Hepcidin antimicrobial peptide | AR | Juvenile type |
| Hemochromatosis 3 | TFR2 | Transferrin receptor 2 | AR | |
| Hemochromatosis 4 | SLC40A1 | Ferroportin | AD | |
| Hereditary angioedema 1, 2 | C1INH | C1 esterase inhibitor | AD | |
| Hereditary angioedema 3 | F12 | Coagulation factor 12 | AD | |
| Hereditary hemorrhagic telangiectasia 1 (Osler–Weber–Rendu) | ENG | Endoglin | AD | TGF β-binding protein |
| Hereditary hemorrhagic telangiectasia 2 | ALK1/ACVRL1 | Activin receptor-like kinase | AD | TGF β receptor-like |
| Hereditary hemorrhagic telangiectasia with juvenile polyposis | SMAD4 | Mothers against decapentaplegic, drosophila, homolog of, 4 | AD | Tumor suppressor; intracellular TGFb receptor signal transducer |
| Hereditary lymphedema 1 (Nonne-Milroy) | FLT4 | Vascular endothelial growth factor receptor 3 (VEGFR–3) | AD | Gene is FMS-like tyrosine kinase |
| Hereditary lymphedema 2 (Meige, late-onset, praecox) | MFH1/FOXC2 | Forkhead box C2 | AD | Transcription factor; allelic to lymphedema-distichiasis, lymphedema and ptosis, and lymphedema and yellow nail syndrome |

| | | | | |
|---|---|---|---|---|
| Hermansky–Pudlak syndrome 1 | HPS1, 3–8 | Hermansky–Pudlak | AR | Lysosome, melanosome, and platelet dense body formation; HPS7 = DTNBP1, HPS8 = BLOC1S3 |
| Hermansky–Pudlak syndrome 2 | AP3B1 | Adaptin β-3a subunit | AR | Type 2 has immunodeficiency |
| Hidrotic ectodermal dysplasia (Clouston) | GJB6 | Connexin 30 | AD | |
| Holt–Oram Syndrome (Heart–Hand) | TBX5 | T-box 5 | AD | Thumb anomaly and atrial septal defect |
| Homocystinuria | CBS | Cystathionine β-synthetase | AR | Condensation of homocystine and serine; homocystine builds up |
| Howel–evans syndrome (tylosis with esophageal cancer) | TOC | Tylosis with esophageal cancer | AD | |
| Hypereosinophilic syndrome | FIP1L1-PDGFRA fusion | Fusion of FIP1-like-1 and PDGF receptor-α | | 4q12 deletion; constitutively activated tyrosine kinase |
| Hyper-IgD | MVK | Mevalonate kinase | AR | Allelic to mevalonic aciduria |
| Hyper-IgE | STAT3 TYK2 | Signal transducer and activator of transcription 3 Tyrcsin kinase 2 | AD | Downstream target of IL-6 |
| Hyperlipoproteinemia Type 1A | LPL | Lipcprotein lipase | AR | Increased chylomicrons |
| Hyperlipoproteinemia Type 1B | APOC2 | Apolipoprotein C2 | AR | Increased chylomicrons |
| Hyperlipoproteinemia Type 2A | LDLR | Low-density lipoprotein receptor | AD | Familial hypercholesterolemia High LDL and cholesterol |

continued p. 120

119

| Disease | Gene | Protein | | Comment |
|---|---|---|---|---|
| Hyperlipoproteinemia Type 2B | APOB | Apolipoprotein B-100 | AD | Mutation in LDL receptor binding domain of this apolipoprotein |
| Hyperlipoproteinemia Type 3 (dysbetalipoproteinemia) | APOE | Apolipoprotein E2 | AR | Defective clearing of intermediate density lipoproteins and chylomicrons |
| Hypotrichosis with juvenile macular dystrophy | PCAD/CDH3 | P-cadherin | AR | Membrane glycoprotein, calcium-dependent cell–cell adhesion; Allelic to ectodermal dysplasia, ectrodactyly, macular dystrophy, monilethrix-like |
| Hypotrichosis, localized, AR | DSG4 LIPH | Desmoglein 4 Lipase H | AR | Overlap with AR monilethrix |
| Hypotrichosis–lymphedema–telangiectasia | SOX18 | SRY-box 18 | AD, AR | HMG box-containing transcription factor |
| Hypotrichosis simplex | CDSN | Corneodesmosin | AD | Corneodesmosome component (desquamation of corneocytes), psoriasis susceptibility gene |
| Ichthyosis bullosa of Siemens | KRT2A | Keratin 2A (2e) | AD | Expressed in upper spinous layer with keratin 9 |
| Ichthyosis hystrix Curth–Macklin | KRT1 | Keratin 1 | AD | Tonofibril defect, resembles EHK |
| Ichthyosis, lamellar 1 | TGM1 | Transglutaminase 1 | AR | Abnormal epidermal cross-linking; Allelic to NCIE and self-healing collodion baby |
| Ichthyosis, lamellar 2 | ABCA12 | ATP-binding cassette, subfamily A, member 12 | AR | ABC transporter superfamily; Allelic to harlequin ichthyosis |

| | | | |
|---|---|---|---|
| Ichthyosis vulgaris | FLG | Filaggrin | AD | |
| Ichthyosis, X-linked | STS | Aryl sulfatase C | XLR | Steroid sulfatase |
| Incontinentia pigmenti | NEMO | NF-κB essential modulator/IKK-gamma | XLD | Allelic to AED with immune deficiency ± osteoporosis and lymphedema |
| Immunodysregulation, polyendocrinopathy, and enteropathy, X-linked | FOXP3 | Forkhead box P3 | XLR | Forkhead family transcription factor |
| Insensitivity to pain, congenital, with anhidrosis | NTRK1 | Neurotrophic tyrosine kinase receptor 1 | AR | Signal transduction of nerve growth factor |
| Juvenile hyaline fibromatosis (systemic juvenile hyalinosis) | CMG2/ANTXR2 | Capillary morphogenesis protein-2/anthrax toxin receptor 2 | AR | |
| Kallman 1 | KAL1 | Anosmin | XLR | |
| Kallman 2 | KAL2 (FGFR1) | Fibroblast growth factor receptor 1 | AD | |
| Keratosis palmoplantaris striata type 1 (Brunauer–Fohs–Siemens) | DSG1 | Desmoglein 1 | AD | Calcium-binding transmembrane cesmosomal glycoprotein; PF antigen |
| Keratosis palmoplantaris striata type 2 | DSP | Desmoplakin | AD | Desmosomal plaque protein, allelic to Carvajal, skin fragility–woolly hair, and lethal a-antholytic EB |
| Keratosis palmoplantaris striata type 3 | KRT1 | Keratin 1 | AD | Suprabasal expression |

continued p. 122

| Disease | Gene | Protein | | Comment |
|---------|------|---------|---|---------|
| KID syndrome (Keratitis–Ichthyosis–Deafness) | GJB2 | Connexin 26 | AD or AR | Allelic to Bart–Pumphrey and Classic Vohwinkel |
| Kindler | KIND1 | Kindlin-1 | AR | Focal contact for keratinocyte |
| Klippel–Trenaunay–Weber | VG5Q (AGGF1) | Angiogenic factor with G patch and FHA domains 1 | Sp | This defect in some cases only |
| Leiomyomata, multiple cutaneous and uterine | FH | Fumarate hydratase | AD | Enzyme in Krebs cycle Defect also causes hereditary leiomyomatosis and renal cell ca |
| LEOPARD-1 | PTPN11 | Protein–tyrosine phosphatase, nonreceptor | AD | Same gene as Noonan-1 |
| Leprechaunism | INSR | Insulin receptor | AR | Allelic to Rabson–Mendenhall |
| Lesch–Nyhan | HGPRT | Hypoxanthine guanine phosphoribosyltransferase | XLR | Purine salvage pathway |
| Lhermitte–Duclos | PTEN | Phosphatase and tensin homolog gene | AR | Allelic to Bannayan–Riley–Ruvalcaba and Cowden |
| Lipoid proteinosis | ECM1 | Extracellular matrix protein 1 | AR | Anti-ECM1 antibodies in lichen sclerosis |
| Loeys–Dietz | TGFβ R1,2 | TGFβ receptors 1 and 2 | AD | Marfan-like but short-arterial aneurysms and tortuosity, hypertelorism, bifid uvula, cleft palate |
| Lymphedema and ptosis, lymphedema-distichiasis, hereditary lymphedema 2 | FOXC2 (MSH1) | Forkhead box C2 | AD | Transcription factor |

| | | | |
|---|---|---|---|
| Mal de Meleda | SLURP1 | Ly6/uPar-related protein 1 | AR | Keratoderma palmoplantaris transgrediens |
| Marfan | FBN1 | Fibrillin 1 | AD | Elastic fibers fragmented |
| Marinesco–Sjögren | SIL1 | BIP-associated protein (BAP) | AR, AD | Endoplasmic reticulum glycoprotein, interacts with BIP, involved in nucleotide exchange |
| McCune–Albright | GNAS1 | Guanine nucleotide-binding protein alpha subunit | Som | Stimulates G protein, increases cAMP by regulating adenylate cyclase |
| Melanoma | CDKN2A CDK4 MC1R | Cyclin-dependent kinase inhibitor 2a Cyclin-dependent kinase 4 Melanocortin 1 receptor | AD | Hereditary melanoma; Defective MC1R cannot convert eumelanin to pheomelanin |
| Menkes Kinky hair syndrome | ATP7A | ATPase, Cu2+ transporting, alpha subunit | XLR | Allelic to occipital horn syndrome and X-linked cutis laxa Wilson disease = ATP7B |
| MIDAS | HCCS | Holocytochrome C synthase | XLD | Mitochondrial |
| Monilethrix | KRTHB1 KRTHB3 KRTHB6 DSG4 | Keratin hair, basic 1, 3, and 6 Desmoglein-4 | AD AR | Intermediate filaments; human hair keratins Hair shaft "blebs" |
| Muckle–Wells | CIAS1 | Cryopyrin | AD | Allelic to chronic infantile neurologic cutaneous and artciular (CINCA) syndrome and familial cold autoinflammatory syndrome |

continued p. 124

| Disease | Gene | Protein | Comment |
|---|---|---|---|
| Mucopolysaccharidosis 1 (Hurler syndrome) | IDUA | α-ι-iduronidase | AR | Build up of glycosaminoglycans due to lack of degradation |
| Mucopolysaccharidosis 2 (Hunter syndrome) | IDS | Iduronate 2-sulfatase | XLR | Build up of glycosaminoglycans due to lack of degradation |
| Muir-Torre | MLH1 | MutL homolog 1, colon cancer, nonpolyposis type 2 | AD | DNA mismatch repair genes; also seen in Lynch cancer family syndrome (hereditary nonpolyposis colorectal cancer) |
| | MSH2 | MutS homolog 2, colon cancer, nonpolyposis type 1 | | |
| Multiple carboxylase deficiency | BTD | Biotinidase | AR | Decreased free serum biotin; metabolic acidosis |
| | HLCS | Holocarboxylase synthetase | | |
| Multiple cutaneous and uterine leiomyomas | FH | Fumarate hydratase | AD | Krebs cycle enzyme |
| Multiple endocrine neoplasia 1 (Werner) | MEN1 | Menin | AD | Binds nuclear GUND |
| Multiple endocrine neoplasia 2a (Sipple), 2b | RET | Receptor tyrosine kinase | AD | Protooncogene, encodes a tyrosine kinase receptor |
| Multiple familial trichoepithelioma | CYLD | Cylindromatosis | AD | Same gene as Brooke–Spiegler tumor suppressor |
| Naegeli–Franceschetti–Jadassohn | K14 | Keratin 14 | AD | Allelic to EBS and dermatopathia pigmentosa reticularis; NF/DPR – mutations in nonhelical head (E1/V1) domain EBS – mutations in central alpha-helical rod domain |
| Nail–Patella | LMX1B | LIM homeobox transcription factor 1β | AD | |

| Disease | Gene | Protein | Inheritance | Notes |
|---|---|---|---|---|
| Naxos | JUP | Junction plakoglobin | AR | PPK with woolly hair and RV cardiomyopathy |
| Netherton | SPINK5 (LEKT1) | Serine protease inhibitor, Kazal-type 5 | AR | Serine protease inhibitor |
| Neurofibromatosis 1 | NF1 | Neurofibromin | AD | Inhibits Ras; Allelic to NF-1-Noonan overlap syndrome, similar to NF1-like syndrome due to SPRED1 defects |
| Neurofibromatosis 2 | NF2 | Neurofibromin 2 (schwannomin, merlin) | AD | |
| Niemann–Pick disease A, B | SMPD–1 | Sphingomyelin phosphodiesterase-1 | AR | Sphingomyelinase deficiency |
| Niemann–Pick disease C 1, D | NPC1 | Niemann–Pick C1 | AR | Cholesterol esterification |
| Niemann–Pick disease C2 | NPC2/-IE1 | Niemann–Pick C2 | Ar | Cholesterol binding |
| Noonan 1 | PTPN11 (SHP2) | Protein tyrosine phosphatase, non-receptor type 11 | AD, Sp | Allelic to LEOPARD-1 |
| Noonan 3 | KRAS | Kirsten rat sarcoma virus oncogene homolog | AD | Allelic to CFC and Costello |
| Noonan 4 | SOS1 | Son of sevenless, drosophila homolog | | Guanine nucleotide exchange factor; Allelic to gingival fibromatosis |
| Noonan 5 | RAF1 | V-RAF-1 murine leukemia viral oncogen homolog 1 | AD | Serine–threonine kinase, activates MEK1/2; Allelic to LEOPARD-2 |
| Oculocutaneous albinism 1 | TYR | Tyrosinase | AR | Melanin pathway |

continued p. 126

125

| Disease | Gene | Protein | | Comment |
|---|---|---|---|---|
| Oculocutaneous albinism 2 | P gene | Mouse pink-eyed dilution gene | AR | Regulation of melanosome pH |
| Oculocutaneous albinism, rufous and OCA 3 | TYRP1 | Tyrosine-related protein 1 | AR | Stabilizes tyrosinase |
| Omenn syndrome | RAG1 RAG2 DCLRE1C | Recombinase activating Artemis | AR | Omenn = SCID with hypereosinophilia; RAG1 and RAG2 mutations may also cause a more severe T-B-NK+ SCID; DCLRE1C mutations may also cause SCID with sensitivity to ionizing radiation |
| Orofaciodigital 1 (Papillon–Léage) | CXORF5 | Chromosome X open reading frame 5 | XLD | |
| Osteogenesis imperfecta I–IV | COL1A1 COL1A2 | Collagen 1α1 Collagen 1α2 | AD or AR | Allelic to Ehlers–Danlos 7 |
| Pachyonychia congenita 1 (Jadassohn–Lewandowsky) | KRT6A KRT16 | Keratin 6a Keratin 16 | AD | Intermediate filaments; KRT16 mutations also associated with non-epidermolytic palmoplantar keratoderma (non-epidermolytic Unna–Thost) |
| Pachyonychia congenita 2 (Jackson–Lawler) | KRT6B KRT17 | Keratin 6b Keratin 17 | AD | Intermediate filaments; KRT17 version allelic to SCM |
| Palmoplantar keratoderma, epidermolytic (Vörner) | KRT9 | Keratin 9 | AD | Expressed in upper spinous layer |
| Palmoplantar keratoderma, non-epidermolytic (Unna–Thost) | KRT1 KRT16 | Keratin 1 Keratin 16 | AD | KRT1 mutations also associated with epidermolytic hyperkeratosis, BCIE, ichthyosis hystrix; KRT16 mutations also associated with PC1 |
| Papillon–Lefèvre | CTSC | Cathepsin C | AR | Lysosomal protease; Allelic to Haim–Munk |

| Disease | Gene | Protein | Inheritance | Notes |
|---|---|---|---|---|
| Peutz–Jeghers | STK11 | Serine threonine kinase 11 | AD | Tumor suppressor |
| Phenylketonuria | PAH | Phenylalanine hydroxylase | AR | Phenylalanine and metabolites build up |
| Piebaldism | KIT<br>SNAI2 | C-KIT<br>Snail, drosophila homolog of, 2 | AD | Inactivating mutations;<br>Protooncogene, tyrosine kinase<br>Neural crest transcription factor |
| Popliteal pterygium | IRF6 | Interferon regulatory factor 6 | AD | Allelic to Van der Woude |
| Porphyria, acute intermittent | PBGD | Porphobilinogen deaminase | AD | PBGD also referred to as hydroxymethylbilane synthase (HMBS) |
| Porphyria, congenital erythropoietic (Gunther) | UROS | Uroporphyrinogen III synthase | AR | UROS also referred to as hydroxymethylbilane hydrolyase |
| Porphyria, hepatoerythropoietic | UROD | Uroporphyrinogen decarboxylase | AD | Cytosolic |
| Hereditary coproporphyria | CPOX | Coproporphyrinogen oxidase | AD | Mitochondrial gene |
| Erythropoietc protoporphyria | FECH | Ferrochelatase | AD/R | Mitochondrial gene |
| Porphyria cutanea tarda | UROD | Uroporphyrinogen decarboxylase | AD | Increased skin uroporphyrin causes photosensitivity to light at 400–410 nm |
| Porphyria, variegate | PPOX | Protoporphyrinogen oxidase | AD | Mitochondrial gene |
| Progeria (Hutchinson–Gilford) | LMNA | Lamin A | AD | Nuclear envelope |

continued p. 128

127

| Disease | Gene | Protein | | Comment |
|---------|------|---------|---|---------|
| Progressive Symmetric Erythrokeratoderma (PSEK) | LOR | Loricrin | AD | Allelic to Vohwinkel and EKV |
| Prolidase deficiency | PEPD | Peptidase D | AR | Splits iminodipeptides |
| Pseudofolliculitis barbae | K6hf | Keratin 6, hair follicle | | Susceptibility gene |
| Pseudoxanthoma elasticum | ABCC6 | ATP-binding cassette subfamily C, member 6 | AR AD | Transmembrane transporter gene |
| Psoriasis | HLA-Cw6, IL-15, SLC12A8, IL-23/IL-23R, HLA-B17 | | | Susceptibility genes |
| PXE-like syndrome | GGCX | Gamma-glutamyl carboxylase | AD/AR | Gamma-carboxylation of gla-proteins; associated with cutis laxa and coagulation defects |
| Pyogenic Arthritis–Pyoderma Gangrenosum–Acne (PAPA) | PSTPIP1 | Protein-serine-threonine phosphatase-interacting protein 1 | AD | |
| Refsum | PAHX PEX7 | Phytanoyl Co-A Hydroxylase peroxin-7 | AR > AD | Phytanic acid builds up Receptor targets enzymes to peroxisomes |
| Refsum, infantile form | PEX1 PEX2 PEX6 | Peroxin-1, 2, and 6 | AR | Deficient and impaired peroxisomes, severe defects cause Zellweger syndrome |
| Restrictive dermopathy | ZMPSTE24 (FACE-1) LMNA | Zinc metalloproteinase STE24, Lamin A | AR | |
| Richner–Hanhart (Tyrosinemia II) | TAT | Tyrosine aminotransferase | AR | Tyrosine accumulates in all tissues |

| | | | | |
|---|---|---|---|---|
| Rothmund–Thomson (poikiloderma congenita) | RECQL4 | RecQ protein-like 4 | AR | DNA helicase |
| Rubinstein–Taybi | CREBBP EP300 | CREB-binding protein E1A-binding protein, 300 kd | AD | CREB = cAMP response element-binding protein Transcriptional coactivators |
| SCID, X-linked | IL2Rγ | IL-2 receptor γ chain | XLR | T-B+NK- |
| SCID, autosomal recessive | ADA | Adenosine deaminase | AR | T-B-NK- |
| | JAK3 | Janus kinase 3 | | T-B+NK- |
| | IL7Rα | | | T-B+NK+ |
| | CD3δ | | | T-B+NK+ |
| | CD3ε | | | T-B+NK+ |
| | CD3ζ | | | T-B+NK+ |
| | CD45 | | | T-B+NK+ |
| | ZAP-70 | | | T-B+NK+ |
| SCID with sensitivity to ionizing radiation | DCLRE1C | DNA cross-link repair 1C (Artemis) | AR | T-B-NK+ Allelic to Omenn |
| SCID, T-B-NK + | RAG1 RAG2 | Recombinase-activating gene | AR | Allelic to Omenn |
| Self-healing collodion baby | TGM1 | Transglutaminase | AR | Allelic to lamellar ichthyosis 1 and NBCIE |
| Sjögren–Larssen | ALDH3A2 | Fatty aldehyde dehydrogenase | AR | |
| Steatocystoma multiplex | KRT17 | Keratin 17 | AD | In pachyonychia congenita 2 |
| Systemic sclerosis | CTGF | Connective tissue growth factor | AR | Polymorphism in promoter region |

continued p. 130

| Disease | Gene | Protein | | Comment |
|---------|------|---------|---|---------|
| T-cell immunodeficiency, congenital alopecia, and nail dystrophy | FOXN1 (WHN) | Forkhead box N1 | AR | Transcription factor |
| Takahara (Acatalasemia) | CAT | Catalase | AR | |
| Tangier | ABCA1/CERP | ATP-binding cassette A1/Cholesterol efflux regulatory protein | AR | Allelic to familial HDL deficiency (which may also result from apolipoprotein A-1 mutations) |
| Thrombotic thrombocytopenic purpura, congenital (Schulman–Upshaw) | ADAMTS13/VWFCP | von Willebrand factor-cleaving protease | AR | |
| Tietz (Albinism–Deafness) | MITF | Microphthalmia-associated transcription factor | AD | Allelic to Waardenberg 2A |
| TNF Receptor-Associated Periodic fever (TRAPS) | TNFRSF1A | TNF receptor 1 | AD | |
| Trichodentoosseous | DLX3 | Distal-less homeobox 3 | AD | |
| Trichorhinophalangeal 1 and 3 | TRPS1 | Trichorhinophalangeal syndrome 1 | AD | Putative transcription factor |
| Trichorhinophalangeal 2 | Continuous TRPS1 and EXT1 deletion | TRP1 and Exostosin | AD | TRP1 with multiple exostoses |
| Trichothiodystrophy (PIBIDS) | ERCC2 (XPD) ERCC3 (XPB) | Excision repair cross-complementing rodent repair deficiency, complementation groups 2 and 4 | AR | ERCC2 same as XP group D; DNA helicase; most cases caused by mutations in XPD, a subunit of transcription factor IIH |
| TTD, non-photosensitive 1 (TTDN1/BIDS) | TTDN1/C7ORF11 | Chromosome 7 open reading frame 11 | AR | |

| Ullrich, congenital scleroatonic muscular dystrophy | COL6A1/2/3 | Collagen VI | AR | |
|---|---|---|---|---|
| Tuberous sclerosis | TSC1<br>TSC2 | Hamartin<br>Tuberin | AD | GTPase-activating protein domain |
| Van de Woude | IRF6 | Interferon regulatory factor 6 | AD | Allelic to popliteal pterygium |
| Vitiligo, associated autoimmune/inflammatory conditions | NALP1 | NACHT leucine-rich-repeat protein 1 | AD | Regulator of the innate immune system; SNPs related to susceptibility |
| Vohwinkel syndrome, variant form (mutilating keratoderma with ichthyosis) | LOR | Loricrin | AD | Cornified cell envelope component; Allelic to PSEK |
| Vohwinkel syndrome, classic, with deafness | GJB2 | Connexin 26 | AD | Allelic to Bart–Pumphrey and KID |
| Von–Hippel Lindau Syndrome | VHL | von Hippel–Lindau | AD | Tumor suppressor gene |
| Waardenburg 1 | PAX3 | Paired box gene 3 | AD | Transcription factor, activates MITF promoter; dystopia |
| Waardenburg 2A | MITF | Microphthalmia-associated transcription factor | AD | Transactivates tyrosinase gene, no dystopia; Allelic to Tietz (Waardenburg 2D is due to SNAI2) |
| Waardenburg 3 (Klein–Waardenburg) | PAX3 | Paired box gene 3 | AD, AR | |
| Waardenburg 4 (Waardenburg–Shah) | EDNRB<br>EDN3<br>SOX10 | Endothelin receptor B<br>Endothelin 3<br>SOX10 | AD | Involved in neural crest cell migration; Endothelin 3 is a ligand for endothelin B receptor; SOX 10 is a transcription factor, activates MITF promoter |

continued p. 132

| Disease | Gene | Protein | | Comment |
|---|---|---|---|---|
| Watson | NF-1 | Neurofibromin | AD | Café-au-lait macules with pulmonic stenosis, ~ to NF-1 |
| Werner | RECQL2 | RecQ protein-like 2 | AR | DNA helicase enzyme |
| | LMNA | Nuclear lamin A/C | | Lamin defect – severe phenotype |
| White sponge nevus (Cannon) | KRT4 | Keratin 4 | AD | |
| | KRT13 | Keratin 13 | | |
| Wilson | ATP7B | ATPase, Cu2+ transporting, beta subunit | AR | Defect in copper transport and biliary excretion of copper |
| Wiskott-Aldrich | WAS | Wiskott Aldrich syndrome protein | XLR | Binds GTPase and actin |
| Witkop | MSX1 | Muscle segment, homeobox, drosophila, homolog of, 1 | AD | |
| Xeroderma pigmentosum | | XPA-DDB1 (DNA damage binding protein) | AR | |
| | | XPB-ERCC3 (excision repair cross-complementing) | | |
| | | XPC-Endonuclease | | |
| | | XPD-ERCC2 | | |
| | | XPE-DDB2 | | |
| | | XPF-ERCC4 | | |
| | | XPG-Endonuclease | | |
| | | XPV-Polymerase | | |

**X-linked dominant:** Incontinentia Pigmenti, Goltz, CHILD, MIDAS, OFD–1, Conradi-Hunermann, Bazex

**X-linked recessive: Chad's Kinky Wife**

CGD, Hunter, Anhidrotic Ectodermal Dysplasia, Dyskeratosis Congenita, SCID, Kinky (Menkes, Cutis Laxa, Occipital Horn), Wiskott-Aldrich, Ichythosis X-linked, Fabry, Ehlers–Danlos 5,9; Also: Bruton's Agammaglobulinemia, Chondrodysplasia Punctata 1, Kallman 1, Lesch-Nyhan, X-linked SCID (IL2R⌐).

## Chromosome abnormalities

| Syndrome | Chromosome |
|---|---|
| Cri du Chat | 5p- |
| Down | Trisomy 21 |
| Edwards | Trisomy 18 |
| Hypomelanosis of Ito | Various |
| Klinefelter | X aneuploidy – i.e., XXY |
| Pallister–Killian | Mosaic tetrasomy 12p |
| Patau | Trisomy 13 (Phyloid pigmentation = mosaic trisomy 13) |
| Turner | XO monosomy |
| Warkany | Mosaic Trisomy 8 (nail/patella dysplasia) |

## Tumors

| Tumor | Gene | Protein | Comment |
|---|---|---|---|
| Anaplastic large cell lymphoma, primary systemic | NPM-ALK fustion | Nucleophosmin-anaplastic lymphoma kinase fusion protein | T(2:5)[p23:q35]; ALK+ systemic anaplastic large cell lymphomas have better prognosis than ALK neg systemic large cell lymphomas (primary cutaneous cases are ALK neg) |
| Basal cell carcinoma | PTCH2 | Patched | Somatic and BCNS |
| Clear cell sarcoma | EWS-ATF1 | Fusion of Ewing sarcoma and activating transcription factor 1 | a.k.a. "malignant melanoma of the soft parts" |
| Dermatofibrosarcoma protuberans | COL1A PDGF | Collagen 1A Platelet-derived growth factor | t(17:22)(q22:q13), may have supernumerary ring chromosome |
| Hypereosinophilia syndrome | FIP1L1-PDGFRA | F/P fusion | ~chronic eosinophilic leukemia |
| Mantle cell lymphoma | T(11;14) | Fusion of Bcl-1/Cyclin D1 and immunoglobulin heavy chain | |
| Mastocytosis | KIT | C-kit | Adult but not childhood forms |
| Melanoma* | CDKN2A/p16-INK4A/p14-ARF, BRAF, KIT, NRAS, MITF, PTEN, AKT, MC1R, APAF-1 | | BRAF often mutated in melanoma and benign melanocytic nevi but unusual in Spitz nevi (similar to NRAS but reverse w/ HRAS); BRAF and NRAS mutations are reciprocal; BRAF phosphorylates ERKs/MAPKs; MC1R mutations impair cAMP synthesis; p16-INK4A inhibits Rb; p14-ARF inhibits p53 degradation |

| | | |
|---|---|---|
| Merkel cell carcinoma | Trisomy 6 | |
| Mycosis fungoides | CDKN2A, TNFRSF6 (Fas), JUNB | |
| Pilomatricoma | CTNNB1 | Activating mutation; wnt signaling pathway |
| Seborrheic keratosis | FGFR3, PIK3CA | FGF receptor 3, phosphatidylinositol kinase 3, catalytic, alpha | Same genes as epidermal nevi |
| Spitz nevi | 11p amplifications | HRAS | Minority of Spitz have HRAS mutations, but much more often than in melanoma |

* Melanomas from skin *without* chronic photodamage – **BRAF** and NRAS mutations but nl CDK4 and CCND1 vs. melanomas from skin *with* chronic photodamage – increase in number of CDK4 and CCND1 but nl BRAF and NRAS vs. melanomas from *non-sun-exposed* skin (acral, mucosal) – KIT mutations but nl BRAF and NRAS; Acral MMs have higher degrees of chromosomal aberrations; p53 mutations uncommon in MM except LMM or MM associated with XP-C or Li-Fraumeni.

# Genodermatoses

## Disorders of cornification
### Ichthyosis
**Ichthyosis vulgaris:** Onset: infancy, gray-brown, erythematous scales, may spare flexures and face, atopy, KP, hyperlinear palms, decreased stratum granulosum. AD, Filaggrin defects. (Mutated filaggrin is also a risk factor for atopic dermatitis and associated with disease severity. Among patients with atopic dermatitis, mutated filaggrin is associated with asthma, allergic rhinitis, and allergic sensitization. However, mutated filaggrin is not independently associated with asthma. Mutated filaggrin is not associated with psoriasis or KP. Among patients with alopecia areata, filaggrin mutations predict more severe courses.)

**X-linked ichthyosis:** Onset: third to sixth month (never collodion baby!), widespread, dirty, brown scales, dirty face, may spare flexures, delayed parturition, comma-shaped/flower-like (pre-Descemet) corneal opacities in posterior capsule, cryptorchidism, if broad deletion → hypogonadotropic hypogonadism with anosmia (Kallman) or chondrodysplasia punctata, neither hyperlinear palms nor KP, low maternal serum unconjugated estriol during pregnancy screening. XLR, steroid sulfatase defects.

**Lamellar ichthyosis:** Collodion baby, ectropion, eclabion, everted ears, plate-like scale, PPK, erythroderma, phalangeal reabsorption, rickets in severe cases. AR, TGM1, ABCA12, FLJ39501/CYP4F2 defects.

**Congenital ichthyosiform erythroderma/nonbullous CIE:** Subtype of lamellar ichthyosis. AR, TGM1, ALOXE3, ALOX12B, CGI58/ABHD5, Ichthyin defects.

**Bullous CIE/epidermolytic hyperkeratosis:** Rapidly resolving collodion baby → diffuse erythema, scale, bullae, erosions, acantholysis, "gothic church" hyperkeratosis. AD, KRT1 or 10 defects.

**Icthyosis bullosa of Seimens:** Collodion-like → superficial, rippled hyperkeratosis, erosions, bullae in early childhood, PPK, mauserung = oval desquamation, minimal erythema. AD, KRT2e defects.

**Harlequin fetus:** Massive hyperkeratosis, deep fissures, ectropion, eclabium, necrotic phalanges, absent lamellar granules, fatal without high-dose retinoids. AR, ABCA12 defects.

**Netherton:** Collodion baby, erythroderma, ichthyosis linearis circumflexa (serpiginous, double-edged, migratory erythema), atopy, trichorrhexis invaginata, asthenia. AR, SPINK5/LEKT1 defects.

**Refsum:** IV-like ichthyosis, retinitis pigmentosa, peripheral neuropathy, cerebellar ataxia, nerve deafness, ECG abnormalities/arrhythmias, yellow nevi, increased tissue and plasma phytanic acid, Tx: eliminate dietary chlorophyll (animal fat/phytol, green vegetables/phytanic acid) and avoid rapid loss of weight (releases phytanic acid). AR, PAHX or PEX7 defects.

**Rud:** Ichthyosis, hypogonadism, short stature, MR, epilepsy, retinitis pigmentosa.

**Sjögren–Larsson:** Onset: birth or early infancy, generalized, pruritic ichthyosis, spastic paralysis, MR, szs, degenerative retinitis, maculopathy (white macular dots), AR, FALDH defects.

**CHILD:** Congenital hemidysplasia, icthyosiform erythroderma, Limb Defects, >2/3 in females, cardiovascular (main cause of death), CNS and renal defects, 2/3 right-sided involvement. XLD, NSDHL defects.

**Conradi–Hunerman/XLD chondrodysplasia punctata:** Collodion-like presentation, large scale, ichthyosiform erythroderma in Blaschko lines → follicular atrophoderma ± hypo/hyperpigmentation, flat face, linear alopecia, stippled epiphyses, asymmetric limb shortening, scoliosis, hip dysplasia, eye abnormalities. XLD, EBP defects.

**KID:** Keratitis, ichthyosis, deafness, spiny hyperkeratosis, sparse hair, absent eyelashes, follicular plugging, onychodystrophy, hypohidrosis, limbal stem cell deficiency, SCC. AD, GJB2/Connexin 26 defects.

**Erythrokeratoderma variabilis/Mendes de Costa:** Erythematous, hyperkeratotic, well-demarcated plaques in bizarre geographic, figurate distributions with daily variations. AD, defects: GJB3/Connexin 31 and GJB4/Connexin 30.3.

**Icthyosis follicularis with atrichia and photophobia:** Alopecia, non-erythematous, follicular keratoses, atopy, epilepsy, recurrent respiratory infections, corneal vascularization, blindness, retinal vascular tortuosity.

**Lipoid proteinosis:** Skin and mucous membrane infiltrated with hyaline-like material, weak cry/hoarseness as infant, bullae, pustules, crusts, pitted scars, verrucous plaques on elbows and knees, sickle/bean-shaped calcification of temporal lobes, szs. AR, ECM1 defects.

**Dorfman–Chanarin/neutral lipid storage disease with ichthyosis:** Lamellar ichthyosis, MR, cataracts, lipid vacuoles in circulating leukocytes (Jordans' anomaly). AR, CGI58/ABHD5 defects.

**Acquired ichthyosis:** Neoplastic (Hodgkins, multiple myeloma, MF), autoimmune (sarcoid, dermatomyositis, GVHD, SLE), drugs (nicotinic acid, corticosteroids), infections (HIV, leprosy), endocrine (hypothyroidism, hyperparathyroidism), metabolic (chronic liver or kidney disease).

**Ichthyosis hystrix – Curth Macklin:** AD, KRT1 defects.

**Epidermal nevus syndrome:** Sporadic, linear whorled verrucous plaques, MR, szs, hemiparesis, deafness, ocular defects (lipodermoids, colobomas, corneal opacities), scoliosis, rickets, syringocystadenoma papilliferum, Wilm's tumor, astrocytoma.

**Pityriasis rotunda:** Circular, hypopigmented, hyperkeratotic plaques, confluent and geometric, AD, South Africa, Sardinia, Japan, Type 1: Asians, Blacks, hyperpigmented, older, malignancies (hepatic), Type 2: Whites, hypopigmented, younger.

**Multiple minute digitate hyperkeratosis:** Minute keratotic spikes on extremities and trunk.

**Ulerythema ophryogenes/KP atrophicans facei:** Erythematous, follicular papules with scarring alopecia, KP, atopy, woolly hair, AD, loss of lateral 1/3 eyebrows, seen in: Noonan, CFC, IFAP.

**Atrophoderma vermiculatum:** Reticular atrophy on cheeks, AD, may be seen in: Rombo, Nicolau–Balus (+ eruptive syringoma and milia) (atrophoderma vermiculatum is similar to atrophia maculosa varioliformis cutis of Tuzun).

**Self-healing collodion baby:** AR, TGM1 defects.

**Collodion baby:** Most often: lamellar or NBCIE; others: Sjögren–Larsson, Dorfman–Chanarin, EHK, self-healing, TTD, Netherton, ectodermal dysplasias.

## Keratodermas
### Inherited Keratoderma

| | |
|---|---|
| Transgrediens | Clouston, Mal de Meleda, Olmsted, Papillon–LeFevre, Greither |
| Non-transgrediens | Unna–Thost, Vorner, Howel-Evans |

**Unna–Thost/non-epidermolytic PPK:** Thick, yellow, well-demarcated PPK, non-transgrediens, hyperhidrosis. AD, KRT1 or 16 defects.

**Vorner/epidermolytic PPK:** Resembles Unna–Thost, non-transgrediens, may blister, EH on histopath. AD, KRT9 defects.

**Olmsted:** Periorificial plaques, thick, transgrediens PPK, mutilating, pseudoainhum, leukokeratosis.

**Papillon-LeFevre:** Transgrediens PPK, periodontitis, can involve knees/elbows, calcified dura mater and falx cerebri, pyogenic liver abscesses. AR, Cathepsin C defects.

**Haim–Munk:** PPK, periodontitis, onychogryphosis, arachnodactyly. AR, Cathepsin C defects.

**Vohwinkel:** Honeycomb hyperkeratosis, pseudoainhum, starfish keratoses, scarring alopecia. AD, GJB2/Connexin 26 (Classic with Deafness) or Loricrin (Mutilating Variant with Ichthyosis) defects.

**Bart–Pumphrey:** Knuckle pads, leukonychia, deafness. AD, GJB2/Connexin 26.

**Mal de Meleda:** Glove and sock PPK, transgradiens, hyperhidrosis, pseudoainhum, onychodystrophy, high-arched palate. AR, SLURP1 defect.

**Acrokeratoelastoidosis of Costa:** Asymptomatic, firm, translucent papules on lateral acral margins, starts at puberty, uncommon and controversial association with scleroderma, AD but F>M, if elastorrhexis is absent on biopsy then dx = focal acral hyperkeratosis, DDx includes keratoelastoidosis marginalis (due to chronic sun exposure and trauma).

**Howel–Evans:** Tylosis, blotchy PPK, non-transgrediens, esophageal CA, soles>palms. AD, TOC defects.

**Carvajal:** PPK, woolly hair, LV cardiomyopathy. AR, Desmoplakin defects.

**Naxos:** PPK, woolly hair, RV cardiomyopathy. AR, Plakogobin defects.

**Richner–Hanhart:** Tyrosinemia Type 2, painful PPK, weight bearing surfaces, plaques on elbows/knees, leukokeratosis, MR, corneal ulceration. AR, tyrosine aminotransferase defects.

**Symmetric progressive erythrokeratoderma/Gottron:** Non-migratory, hyperkeratotic, erythematous plaques, favors extremities and buttocks, PPK, pseudoainhum. AD, Loricrin defects.

**Huriez:** Scleroatrophy, sclerodactyly, PPK, nail hypoplasia, nasal poikiloderma, lip telangiectasia, hypohidrosis, fifth finger contractures, SCC, bowel cancer, AD.

**Punctate palmoplantar keratoderma/Buschke–Fischer–Brauer:** Keratotic plugs, may be limited to palmar creases, AD.

**Disseminated superficial actinic porokeratosis (DSAP):** 3rd–4th decade, F>M, lowest risk of malignant transformation among the porokeratosis syndromes (except punctate variety which has no risk; linear and long-standing lesions have the greatest risks). AD, SART3 defects.

## Acquired Keratoderma

**Keratoderma climactericum:** Pressure bearing acral area, peri-menopausal, may represent psoriasis.

**Porokeratosis plantaris discreta:** Painful, sharply marginated, rubbery nodules on weight bearing surface, adult females, SCC.

## Acantholytic Disorders

**Darier:** Dirty, malodorous papules on face, trunk, flexural, punctate keratosis on palms/soles, V-shaped nicking, red/white nail bands, mucosal cobblestoning, guttate leukoderma, schizophrenia, MR. AD, ATP2A2/SERCA2 defects.

**Acrokeratosis verruciformis of Hopf:** Verrucous papules on dorsal hands/feet, punctate pits on palms/soles, onychodystrophy. AD, ATP2A2 defects.

**Hailey–Hailey/benign familial chronic pemphigus:** Vesicles, crust, erosions in intertriginous areas, begins in adolescence. AD, ATP2C1 defects.

**Peeling skin syndrome/keratolysis exfoliativa congenita:** Exfoliation and scale ± erythema and pruritus, esp. palms/soles, AR.

# Disorder of hair, nail, ectoderm
## Hair

**Trichothiodystrophy:** Sulfur (cystine, cysteine)-deficient brittle hair, tiger-tail polarizing, trichoschisis, absent cuticle, immunodeficiency, osteosclerosis; PIBIDS: Photosensitivity, ichthyosis, brittle hair, decreased intellect, decreased fertility, short. AR, defects in ERCC2/XPD, ERCC3/XPB, TFB5 – all TFIIH subunits – and TTDN1/C7ORF11 (non-photosensitive TTD).

**Marinesco–Sjögren:** TTD + neonatal hypotonia, cerebellar ataxia, congenital cataracts, MR, thin brittle nails, short, hypogonadism, myopathy, chewing difficulties. AR, SIL1 defects.

**Hallermann–Streiff:** Beaked nose, microphthalmia, micrognathia, mandibular hypoplasia, dental abnormalities, congenital cataracts, hypotrichosis (following cranial sutures), dwarfism.

**Klippel–Feil:** Low posterior hairline, short webbed neck, fused cervical vertebra, scoliosis, renal anomalies, hearing impairment, torticollis, cardiac septal defects, cleft palate, increased in females, AD or AR.

**Pili Torti:** Twisting, brittle hair, AD, syndromes: Menkes, Bjornstad, Crandall, TTD, hypohidrotic ED, Bazex, anorexia nervosa, Laron.

**Bjornstad:** Deafness, pili torti. AD, BCS1L defects.

**Crandall:** Deafness, hypogonadism, pili torti.

**Citrullinemia:** Pili torti, periorificial dermatitis. AR, defects: Argininosuccinate synthetase or SLC25A13.

**Menkes:** Steel wool-like hair, pili torti, monilethrix, trichorrexis nodosa, epilepsy, hypothermia, decreased copper and ceruloplasmin. XLR, ATP7A defects.

**Uncombable hair:** AR, spun glass hair, longitudinal groove, pili canaliculati et trianguli.

**Monilethrix:** Beaded hairs, dry, fragile, sparse, KP, brittle nails. AD or AR: type 2 hair keratins KRTHB1, 3, or 6 defects (AD), Desmoglein-4 (AR).

**Trichorrexis nodosa:** Arginosuccinic aciduria (red fluorescence of hair), citrullinemia, Menkes, TTD, Netherton, isotretinoin, hypothyroidism, physical/chemical trauma, proximal in Blacks and genetic forms vs. distal in Whites and Asians.

**Trichorrexis invaginata:** Bamboo hair, Netherton.

**Pili annulati:** Ringed hair, spangled, alternating bands (light bands to the naked eye = dark bands on light microscopy = air-filled cavities within the cortex of the hair shaft), associated with alopecia areata, AD.

**Woolly hair:** Onset: birth, "Afro in a non-African," Associations: KP, PPK, facial dysmorphism, skin fragility, neuropathy, osteoma cutis, diarrhea, ulerythema ophryogenes; DDx: Noonan, CFC, Trichodento-osseous, CHANDS, woolly hair nevus, Carvajal, Naxos.

**Acquired progressive kinking of the hair (APKH):** Rapid, adolescent onset, curly, lusterless, frizzy hair, frontotemporal and vertex, may evolve into androgenetic alopecia.

**Localized hypertrichosis:** Becker nevi, casts, POEMS, pretibial myxedema, cubiti, auricle.

**Generalized congenital hypertrichosis/hypertrichosis lanuginosa:** "Werewolf," curly hairs, sparing palms/soles and mucosa, X-linked.

**Congenital temporal triangular alopecia:** Onset: birth to 6 years old, uni- or bilateral, nl number of follicles but all vellus AD.

**Kinky hair:** Menkes, woolly hair syndromes, woolly hair nevus, pili torti syndromes, pseudomonilethrix, uncombable hair, APKH, Tricho-Dento-Osseous, oral retinoids.

**GAPO:** Growth retardation, alopecia, pseudoanodontia, optic atrophy, cranial defects, frontal bossing, umbilical hernia, muscular appearance, renal abnormalities.

**Cantu:** Congenital hypertrichosis, osteochondrodysplasia, cardiomegaly, MR, short stature, macrocranium, hypertelorism, cutis laxa, wrinkled palms and soles, joint hyperextensibility, AD.

**Keratosis Follicularis Spinulosa Decalvans:** Corneal dystrophy, photophobia, KP (becomes atrophicans), cicatricial alopecia (scalp, eyebrows), PPK, atopy, aminoaciduria, XLR.

**Atrichia with Papular Lesions:** Atrichia, milia, hypopigmented scalp streaks. AR, Hairless defects (Hereditary Vitamin D-dependent Rickets may be identical + hypocalcemia, hyperparathyroidism, osteomalacia, rickets).

## Hair color

**PKU:** Blonde hair.

**Homocystinuria:** Bleached hair.

**Menkes:** Light hair.

**Chediak–Higashi, Griscelli, Elajalde:** Silvery hair.

**Fe deficiency:** Segmental heterochromia (Canities segmentata sideropaenica).

**Early graying:** Familial, Hutchinson–Gilford, Werner, Book syndrome (premolar aplasia, hyperhidrosis, and canities premature).

**Gray patches:** Piebaldism, Vitiligo, Vogt–Koyanagi–Harada, NF1, Tietze, Alezzandrini, TS.

## Nail and oral disorders

**Pachyonychia congenita:** Type 1 (Jadassohn–Lewandowsky): Thickened nails, yellow, pincer nails, PPK, follicular keratosis on elbows/knees, oral leukokeratosis, Type 2 (Jackson–Sertoli): 1 + steatocystoma multiplex, PPK may blister, hyperhidrosis, natal teeth, Type 3: 1 + 2 + ocular lesions, cheilosis, Type 4: 1 + 2 + 3 + thin, sparse hair, MR, laryngeal involvement. AD, Defects: KRT6A and 16 (Type 1), KRT6B and 17 (Type 2).

**Dyskeratosis congenita/Zinsser–Cole–Engman:** Nail thinning, longitudinal ridging, oral leukokeratosis (premalignant), neck – poikiloderma vasculare atrophicans, thin hair, hands/feet: dorsal atrophy/ventral hyperkeratosis, epiphora, aplastic anemia, caries, defects: DKC1 (XLR), TERC (AD) **(Hoyeraal–Hreidarsson** – DC + cerebellar hypoplasia)

**Nail-patella:** Hypo- or anonychia, triangular lunula, absent/hypoplastic patella, luxation, posterior iliac horns, renal dysplasia, GU anomalies, Lester iris. AD, LMX1B defects.

**Iso–Kikuchi/COIF:** Congenital Onychodysplasia of the Index Finger, brachydactyly, short hands, inguinal hernia, digital artery stenosis, AD.

**Yellow nail:** Yellow nails, lymphedema, pleural effusions, bronchiectasis. AD, FOXC2/MFH1 defects.

**Naegeli–Franceschetti–Jadassohn:** Hyperkeratotic nails with congenital malalignment, reticulate pigmentation (axillae, neck), punctate PPK, enamel hypoplasia, hypohidrosis abnormal dermatoglyphics. AD, KRT14 defects.

**Cannon:** White sponge nevus, not premalignant. AD, KRT4 and 13 defects.

**Oral–facial–digital-1/Papillon–League:** Bifid tongue, accessory frenulae, cleft palate/lip, lip nodules, milia, alopecia, dystopia canthorum, syndactyly, brachydactyly, CNS anomalies, polycystic kidneys. XLD, CXORF5/OFD1 defects.
**Rubinstein–Taybi:** MR, broad thumbs/great toes, hypertrichosis, high-arched palate, crowded teeth, beak nose, heavy eyebrows, capillary malformations, keloids, pilomatricomas (multiple pilomatricomas also reported with Steinert myotonic dystrophy, Turner, sarcoidosis), cardiac abnormalities. AD or AR, CREBBP or EP300 defects.
**Cooks:** Anoncyhia-onychodystrophy (fingers and toes) absent or hypoplastic distal phalanges, AD.

## Ectodermal dysplasia

**Hidrotic ectodermal dysplasia/Clouston:** Hypotrichosis, nail dystrophy, keratoderma, normal teeth, normal sweating. AD, GJB6/Connexin 30 defects.
**Hypohidrotic/anhidrotic ectodermal dysplasia/Christ–Siemens–Touraine:** Heat intolerance 2/2 decreased or absent sweating, hypodontia, fine sparse hair, brittle nails, thick lips, saddle nose, sunken cheeks, frontal bossing, depressed cell mediated immunity, elevated IgE, rhinitis, no smell or taste, salivary abnormalities, decreased pulmonary/GI secretions, xerosis, eczema. XLR: EDA, AD: EDAR, AR: EDAR, EDARADD.
**Hypohidrotic ectodermal dysplasia with immunodeficiency ± osteoporosis and lymphedema:** AR, NEMO defects.
**Witkop/tooth-and-nail:** Onychodystrophy, toenails > fingernails, retained primary dentition. AD, MSX1 defects.
**Tricho-Dento-Osseous:** Whitish, curly hair, brittle nails, xerosis, dental pitting, taurodontism, tall. AD, DLX3 defects.
**Ellis–Van Creveld–Weyers/acrodental dysostosis:** Hypoplastic nails, sparse hair, dwarfism (short distal extremities), cone-shaped epiphyses (hand), natal teeth, septal heart defects.
**P63 complex:** EEC, AEC, Rapp-Hodgkin, Limb-Mammary type 4, ADULT, all are AR.
**Ectrodactyly–ectodermal dysplasia–clefting/EEC:** Lobster claw deformity, ectodermal dysplasia, sparse wiry blond hair, peg-shaped teeth, dystrophic nails, cleft lip, lacrimal duct defects.
**Ankyloblepharon–ectodermal dysplasia–clefting/AEC:** Ankyloblepharon, ectodermal dysplasia, clefting, chronic erosive dermatitis – esp. scalp, patchy alopecia, hypotrichosis, lacrimal duct defects, hypospadias, includes CHAND syndrome.
**Rapp–Hodgkin:** Ectodermal dysplasia, clefting, onychodysplasia, dry wiry hair, hypodontia, hypospadias.
**Limb–Mammary Type 4:** Aplastic nipples/mammary glands, limb defects, onychodysplasia, MR, hair defects.
**Acral–dermato–ungual–lacrimal–tooth/ADULT:** Ectrodactyly, freckling, onychodysplasia, lacrimal duct defects, hypodontia.

### Ectomesodermal dysplasia

**Goltz:** Cribiform fat herniations in Blaschko lines, perinasal red papules, papillomas in genital and folds, mosaic hypohidrosis, onychodysplasia, scarring alopecia, syndactyly, eye defects, delayed dentition, osteopathia striata, coloboma. XLD, PORCN defects.

**MIDAS:** Microphthalmia, dermal aplasia, sclerocornea, linear atrophic Blaschkonian plaques, MR, coloboma, strabismus, CNS lesions, cardiac defects. XLD, Holocytochrome C Synthase/HCCS defects.

### Phakomatosis

**TS:** Angiofibromas, angiomyolipomas, shagreen patch, Koenen tumors, ash leaf macules, CALM, lymphangioleiomyomatosis, dental pitting, cardiac rhabdomyomas, phalangeal cysts, retinal gliomas, szs, gingival fibromas, brain calcifications, molluscum pendulum. AD, TSC-1 (Hamartin) and TSC-2 (Tuberin) defects.

**NF1:** Diagnosis – At least 2 of: >6 CALM, >2 neurofibromas or 1 plexiform neurofibroma, axillary/inguinal freckling, optic glioma, first degree relative, Lisch nodules, winged sphenoid, pheochromocytoma (1% of pts). AD, Neurofibromin defects.

**NF2:** Neurofibromas, bilateral acoustic neuromas, schwannomas, posterior supcapsular lenticular opacity. AD, Merlin defects.

**NF-Noonan overlap:** AD, Neurofibromin defects.

**SPRED1 NF-1-like syndrome:** Axillary freckling, CALM, macrocephaly, Noonan-like appearance. AD, SPRED1 defects.

### Craniofacial abnormalities

**Treacher Collins:** Mandibulofacial dysostosis, downward eyes, lid coloboma, ear anomalies, NL intelligence. AD, TCOF1 defects.

**Beare–Stevenson cutis gyrata:** Craniosynostosis, cutis gyrata, AN, ear anomalies, anogenital anomalies, acrochordons, prominent umbilical stump. AD, FGFR2 defects.

**Apert:** Craniosynostosis, craniofacial anomalies, severe syndactyly, acneiform lesions, hyperhidrosis, 10% cardiac defects, 10% GU anomalies. Sporadic, FGFR2 defects.

**Crouzon:** Craniosynostosis, hypertelorism, parrot nose, exophthalmos. AD, FGFR2 defects.

**Crouzon with acanthosis nigricans:** AD, FGFR3 defects.

**Cornelia/Brachmann de Lange:** Synophrys, hirsutism, low hairline, MR, heart defects, thin lips, small nose, low-set ears, livedo reticularis/cutis marmorata, small hands and feet, cryptorchidism/hypospadias. Defects: NIPBL (AD), SMC1L1 (XL), or SMC3 (mild, AD) – all in cohesin complex.

**Costello:** Cutis laxa-like skin, verruca-like papillomas (face, anus, axillae), acrochordons, AN, PPK, coarse facies, macroglossia, hypertelorism, broad nasal root, thick lips, onychodystrophy, hyperextensible fingers, short stature, malignancies (bladder, neuroblastoma, rhabdomyosarcoma), nevi, must distinguish from Noonan and CFC. AR, HRAS or KRAS defects.

**Trichorhinophalangeal:** Sparse brittle hair, pear-shaped nose, long philtrum, brachyphalangia, cone-shaped digital epiphysis, crooked fingers, short, brittle nails, short, loose skin, cartilaginous exostoses. AD, defects: Types 1 and 3: TRPS1; Type 2: continuous TRPS1 and EXT1 deletion.

**Goldenhar/oculoauriculovertebral dysplasia/hemifacial microsomia:** Extraauricular appendage, choristoma, eyelid coloboma, cervical vertebral abnormalities, cardiac defects.

**Nevus sebaceous syndrome:** Linear NS, szs, CNS abnormalities, coloboma, skeletal defects.

**Noonan:** Mimics Turner, acral lymphedema, nevi, hypertelorism, low-set ears, coarse curly hair, low posterior hairline, broad/webbed neck, KP atrophicans, ulerythema ophryogenes, short stature, chest deformities, heart defects, bleeding diathesis. AD, PTPN11/SHP2, KRAS, SOS1 defects.

**Cardio-facio-cutaneous:** Sparse/absent eyelashes, KP, low posterior hairline, ichthyosis, palmoplantar hyperkeratosis, sparse curly hair, short neck, pulmonary stenosis, AV septal defects, short stature, similar to Noonan. AD, KRAS, BRAF, MEK1, MEK2 defects.

**Fanconi anemia:** Pancytopenia, diffuse hypo/hyperpigmentation, CALMs, absent thumbs and radius (~40%), retinal hemorrhage, strabismus, short stature, GU anomalies. AR, defects in Fanconi anemia complementation group genes A–N.

## Tumor syndromes

**Cowden:** Tricholemmomas, oral mucosal papillomatosis/cobblestoning, acral keratoses, lipomas, sclerotic fibromas, thyroid gland lesions (2/3) (esp. adenomatous goiter or follicular adenomas), fibrocystic breast lesions, breast cancer (3/4 of F), GI polyposis, GU lesions (1/2 of F, endometrial cancer), adenoid facies, high-arched palate, lingua plicata, acral papular neuromatosis, inverted follicular keratoses. AD, PTEN defects.

**Gardner:** Epidermal cysts (pilomatricoma-like), desmoid tumors, fibromas (esp. back/paraspinal/nuchal), osteomas, lipomas, leiomyomas, neurofibromas, supernumerary teeth, GI polyps (frequent malignant transformation), CHRPE, dental anomalies, adrenal adenomas, hepatoblastoma, CNS tumors (Turcot), thyroid carcinoma. AD, APC defects.

**MEN I:** Parathyroid, pituitary, pancreas, adrenal, thyroid tumors, lipomas, inclusion cysts, angiofibromas, collagenomas, CALMs, gingival macules. AD, Menin defects.

**MEN IIa:** Medullary thyroid CA, phaeochromocytoma, parathyroid adenomas, macular and lichen amyloidosis. AD, RET defects.

**MEN IIb:** Medullary thyroid CA, pheochromocytoma, mucosal neuromas, large lips, lordosis, genu valgum, kyphosis, CALMs, lentigines, marfanoid habitus, synophrys, megacolon/ganglioneuromatosis. AD, RET defects.

**Von Hippel–Lindau:** Retinal angioma, cerebellar medullary angioblastic tumor, pancreatic cysts, RCC, pheochromocytoma, polycythemia, AD.

**Brooke–Spiegler:** Trichoepitheliomas, cylindromas, spiradenomas, milia. AD, CYLD defects.

**Multiple familial trichoepithelioma/epithelioma adenoides cysticum of Brooke:** Trichoepitheliomas, milia. AD, maps to 9p21 (distinct from Brooke–Spiegler).

**Birt–Hogg–Dube:** Fibrofolliculomas, trichodiscomas, acrochordons, lipomas, collagenomas, RCC (50% chromophobe/oncocytic hybrid), PTX/lung cysts, hypercalcemia, colon polyps. AD, FLCN defects.

**Schopf–Schulz–Passarge:** Eyelid hydrocytomas, hypodontia, hypotrichosis, nail defects, PPK, eccrine syringofibroadenoma, AR.

**Multiple cutaneous and uterine leiomyomata (fibromas):** 15–60% develop renal duct or papillary renal type II cancer, rarely cerebral cavernomas. AD, Fumarate Hydratase defects (homozygous mutations cause severe mitochondrial encephalopathy, fumaric aciduria).

**Li–Fraumeni:** Diverse malignancies – breast, leukemia, brain, soft tissue/ bone sarcomas, adrenal, melanoma.

## KA syndromes

**Muir–Torre:** KA, sebaceous carcinoma, sebaceous adenomas, colorectal cancer (50%), GU neoplasms (25%), breast/lung neoplasms. AD, MSH2, MLH1, or MSH6 defects.

**Ferguson–Smith:** Multiple self-healing KAs, onset: 2nd decade, usually sun-exposed areas, scar, singly or in crops. AD, 9q31 (near PTCH1).

**Grzybowski:** Numerous small eruptive (2–3 mm), adult onset, oral mucosa and larynx may be involved, pruritus.

**Witten and Zak:** Combo of Ferguson–Smith and Grzybowski.

**Keratoacanthoma centrifugum marginatum:** Large with peripheral growth and central healing, non involuting, dorsal hand or leg.

**Others:** Subungual, KA dyskeratoticum and segregans, and KAs occurring post-UV, post-surgery, post-aldara, or post-laser resurfacing.

## BCC syndromes

**Rombo:** BCC, trichoepitheliomas, hypotrichosis, atrophoderma vermiculata, milia, cyanosis of lips/hands/feet, telangiectasia, AD.

**Bazex–Dupre–Christol:** BCC, follicular atrophoderma, pili torti, milia, ulerythema ophryogenes, scrotal tongue, spiny hyperkeratoses, neuropsychiatric, XLD.

**Gorlin/basal cell nevus/nevoid BCC:** BCC, palmoplantar pits, odontogenic jaw cysts, hypertelorism, frontal bossing, ovarian CA/ fibroma, medulloblastomas, milia, lipomas, epidermal cysts, calcification of falx, fused/bifid ribs, eye anomalies, hypogonadism. AD, PTCH1 defects.

## Disorders of connective tissue

**Pachydermoperiostosis/Touraine–Solente–Gole:** Thickening of skin, folds and creases on face, scalp, and extremities, clubbing, AD.

**Aplasia cutis congenita (ACC):** Group 1: solitary scalp ACC, Group 2: scalp ACC + limb defects, Group 3: scalp ACC + epidermal/sebaceous nevus, Group 4: scalp ACC overlying embryologic defect, Group 5: ACC + fetus papyraceous (linear/stellate, trunk or limb), Group 6: ACC + EB, Group 7: localized ACC on extremities, Group 8: ACC due to HSV, VZV, methimazole (imperforate anus), Group 9: ACC in trisomy 13 (Patau, large membranous scalp defects), 4p- (Wolf-Hirschhorn), Setleis, Johanson-Blizzard, Goltz, amniotic band, Delleman, Xp22 (Reticulolinear).

**Adams–Oliver:** Aplasia cutis, cutis marmorata, heart defects, limb hypoplasia, AD.

**Bart:** Aplasia cutis (esp. legs), DDEB>JEB.

**Setleis:** Bitemporal forcep-like lesions, leonine facies, absent eyelashes, low frontal hairline, periorbital swelling, flat nasal bridge, upslanting eyebrows, large lips, bulbous nose (Brauer syndrome – isolated temporal lesions), AD or AR.

**Pseudoxanthoma elasticum/PXE/Gronblad–Strandberg:** Calcification/clumping/fragmentation of elastic fibers, "plucked chicken" skin, angoid streaks, tears in Bruch's membrane, ocular hemorrhage, retinal pigmentary changes, claudication, CAD/MI, GI hemorrhage, HTN, EPS. AR, ABCC6 defects.

**PXE-like:** PXE-like phenotype + cutis laxa, vitamin K-dependent clotting factor deficiency, cerebral aneurysms, minimal ocular sxs. AR, GGCX defects (PXE-like syndrome can be seen in sickle cell or beta-thalassemia).

**Goltz/focal dermal hypoplasia:** Cribiform fat herniations in Blaschko lines, papillomas (genital, anal, face), osteopathia striata, syndactyly, oligodactyly, colobomas. XLD, PORCN defects.

**Buschke–Ollendorff:** Osteopoikilosis, disseminated lenticular CT nevus, sclerotic bone foci. AD, LEMD3 defects.

**Marfan:** Hyperextensible joints, arachnodactyly, aortic aneurysms, dissection/insufficiency, MVP, downward ectopia lentis, PTX, striae, xerosis, EPS, tall stature, long facies, pectus excavatum. AD, Fibrillin-1 defects (Fibrillin-2 defects = Beals, Congenital Contractural Arachnodactyly – "crumpled ears").

**Osteogenesis imperfecta:** Brittle bones, thin translucent skin, EPS, bruising, hyperextensible joints, wormian bones, hearing loss, normal teeth, ~normal stature, hernias, arcus senilis, respiratory failure 2/2 kyphoscoliosis, Tx: bisphosphonates, Type 1: blue sclerae, Type 2: perinatal lethal/congenital, Type 3: progressively deforming with normal sclerae, Type 4: normal sclerae, Genetic basis – Type 1, 2A, 3, 4: AD defects in COL1A1 or COL1A2; Type 2B, 7: AR defects in CRTAP.

**Cutis laxa:** Elastolysis, sagging skin, hound dog appearance, deep voice, emphysema, diverticuli, hernia, hook nose, oligohydramnios, CV anomalies. AR (FBLN4 or 5, or ATP6V0A2), AD (Elastin or FBLN5), XL (ATP7A – EDS9 and Menkes).

## Ehlers–Danlos

| | Type | Inhr | Defect | Characteristics |
|---|---|---|---|---|
| I | Gravis | AD | COL 5A1,2 | Skin fragility, joint/skin hyperextensibility, bruising, "cigarette paper" scars, prematurity of newborn, molluscoid pseudotumors (at scars), SQ spheroids |
| II | Mitis | AD | COL 5A1 | Similar to Gravis but less severe |
| III | Hypermobile | AD | COL 3A1, Tenascin-XB | Marked small and large joint hypermobility and dislocation, *minimal* skin changes, MSK pain |
| IV | Vascular/ecchymotic/sack | AD | COL 3A1 | *Arterial, bowel, and uterine rupture,* bruising, thin, translucent skin with visible/*varicose* veins, only mild small joint hyperextensibility, tendon/muscle rupture, EPS, facies – thin nose, hollow cheeks, staring eyes |
| V | X-linked | XLR | | Similar to Mitis, bruising/skin hyperextensibility > skin fragility |
| VI | Kyphoscoliotic/ocular-scoliotic | AR | Lysyl hydroxylase, PLOD1 | Skin/joint laxity, *corneal/scleral fragility,* keratoconus, ocular hemorrhage, *muscle hypotonia* (neonatal), kyphoscoliosis, arterial rupture, reduced urinary pyridinium cross-links |
| VII A,B | Arthrochalasia multiplex | AD | COL 1A1,2 | *Congenital hip dislocation,* severe joint hypermobility, soft skin, abnormal scars, short, micrognathia |
| VII C | Dermatosparaxis | AR | ProCOL I N-proteinase/ ADAMST2 | Skin fragility (dermatosparaxis = "*skin tearing*"), *sagging and redundant skin,* joint/skin hyperextensibility, bruising, short, micrognathia |
| VIII | Periodontal | AD | | Similar to types I/II + prominent *periodontal* disease, pretibial hyperpigmented (NLD-like) scars |
| IX | Occipital horn/cutis laxa | XLR | ATP7A | Occipital exostoses, abnormal clavicles, abnormal copper transport, joint hypermobility, GU abnormalities, malabsorption, allelic to Menkes |
| X | Fibronectin | AR | Fibronectin | Bruising, abnormal clotting, defective platelet aggregation, skin laxity, joint hypermobility |
| XI | Large joint hypermobile | AD | | |

**Progeria/Hutchinson–Gilford:** Atrophic, sclerodermoid, poikilodermatous skin, prominent veins, alopecia, bird facies, failure to thrive, premature graying, short stature, coax valga, flexural contractures, abnormal dentition, early death from atherosclerotic heart disease. AR, LMNA defects.

**Acrogeria:** May be a spectrum of Vascular EDS, atrophic acral skin, mottled pigmentation, nail dystrophy, micrognathia, atrophic tip of nose.

**Werner/adult progeria:** Short, high-pitched voice, beaked nose, cataracts, DM2, muscle atrophy, osteoporosis, sclerodermoid changes, painful callosities, severe atherosclerosis, progressive alopecia, canities, hyperkeratosis at elbows/knees/palms/soles, ischemic ulcers, reduced fertility, sarcomas, thyroid carcinoma. AR, RECQL2 defects.

**Rothmund–Thomson/hereditary congenital poikiloderma:** Photosensitivity, poikiloderma, dorsal hand keratoses (25% SCC transformation), sparse hair, loss of eyebrows/eyelashes, short, bone defects (radius and hands), juvenile zonular cataracts (50% blind), MR, hypodontia, EPS, osteosarcomas, hypogonadism. AR, RECQL4 defects.

**Cockayne:** Premature graying, cachetic dwarfism, retinal atrophy, deafness, sunken eyes, beaked nose, large ears, photosensitivity, telangiectasia, dementia, premature aging, loss of subcutaneous fat, thin hair, flexion contractures, severe MR, salt and pepper retina. AR, CSA – ERCC8 defects, CSB – ERCC6 defects.

**Juvenile systemic fibromatosis/infantile systemic hyalinosis:** Nodules on H/N (ears/nose/scalp) and fingers, gingival hypertrophy, joint contractures, osteopenia, short stature, myopathy. AR, Capillary Morphogenesis Protein-2 (CMG2/ANTXR2) defects.

**Francois/dermochondrocorneal dystrophy:** Papulonodules on dorsal hands, nose, ears, gingival hyperplasia, osteochondrodystrophy, corneal dystrophy, AR.

**Restrictive dermopathy:** Taut, translucent skin, open mouth, joint contractures, arthrogryposis, pulmonary insufficiency. AR, LMNA or ZMPSTE24 defects.

**Whistling face/Freeman-Sheldon:** Contractures (hands, feet, neck), microstomia, deep-set eyes, strabismus, colobomas, scoliosis, cryptochordism.

## Collagen types

| Type | Distribution | Diseases |
|---|---|---|
| I | Skin (85% of adult dermis), bone, tendon, ECMs | Arthrochalasia multiplex, Osteogenesis imperfecta |
| II | Vitreous humor, cartilage | Stickler arthro-ophthalmopathy, Kneist dysplasia, Spondyloepiphysela dysplasia, Achondrogenesis, Avascular necrosis of femoral head, Antibodies: Relapsing polychondritis |

| III | Skin (10% of adult dermis), fetal skin, GI/lung, vasculature | Vascular > Hypermobile |
|---|---|---|
| IV | Basement membranes | Goodpasture, Alport, Benign familial hematuria, Porencephaly, Diffuse leiomyomatosis |
| V | Ubiquitous | Gravis/Mitis |
| VI | Cartilage, skin, aorta, placenta, others | Ullrich muscular dystrophy, Bethlem myopathy |
| VII | Anchoring fibrils, skin, cornea, mucous membranes, amnion | DEB, Isolated toenail dystrophy, Transient bullous disease of the newborn, EB pruriginosa, Antibodies: CP and BLE |
| VIII | Endothelial cells, skin, Descemet's membrane | Fuchs corneal dystrophy |
| IX | Cartilage | Stickler arthro-ophthalmopathy, Multiple epiphyseal dysplasia ± myopathy, Intervertebral disc disease susceptibility |
| X | Cartilage (hypertrophic) | Metaphyseal chondrodysplasia |
| XI | Hyaline cartilage | Stickler arthro-ophthalmopathy, Marshall skeletal dysplasia, Familial deafness, Otospondylomegaepiphyseal dysplasia |
| XVII | Skin hemidesmosomes | JEB, Generalized atrophic EB, Antibodies: BP |

Fibril-forming: I, II, III, IV, V, XI.
Fibril-associated collagens with interrupted triple helices: IX, XII, XIV, XVI, XIX, XX, XXI.
Microfibrillar: VI.
Network-forming: VIII, X.
Transmembrane domains: XIII, XVII.
Lysyl oxidase – cross-linking of collagen; cofactors – vitamin C, B6, copper.
Cystathionine synthase – cross-linking of collagen; homocytinuria.
Tenascin-XB – EDS3 and EDS-like syndrome.

## Disorders of metabolism
### Enzymatic deficiencies
**PKU:** MR, szs, pigmentary dilution, atopic dermatitis. AR, phenylalanine hydroxylase or dihydropteridine reductase defects.

**Homocystinuria:** Marfanoid, premature heart disease, low IQ, szs, osteoporosis, codfish vertebrae with collapse, livedo on legs, fine sparse hair, pigmentary dilution, upward ectopia lentis. AR, cystathione β-synthase or MTHFR defects.

**Alkaptonuria:** Dark urine/sweat, arthritis, discolored cartilage, kyphoscoliosis, joint destruction, tendon rupture, deafness, vs. exogenous ochronosis due to hydroxyquinone, phenol, or picric acid. AR, homogentisic acid oxidase/homogentisate 1,2-dioxygenase defects.

**Lesch–Nyhan:** HGPRT deficiency, hyperuricemia, self-mutilation, MR, spastic CP, tophi. XLR, HPRT defects.

**Niemann–Pick:** Classical infantile form (A, Ashkenazi), visceral form (B, adults, non-neuropathic), subacute/juvenile form (C), Nova Scotia form (D), adult form (E), HSM, lymphadenopathy, MR, cherry red macula, yellow skin, dark macules in mouth. AR, Sphingomyelinase or NPC1 defects.

**Gaucher:** Glucosylceramide/GlcCer/glucosylcerebroside accumulates in the brain, liver, spleen, marrow, Type 1: "nonneuronopathic," HSM, bronze skin, pinguecula of sclera, adults; Type 2: "acute neuronopathic," infant, may be preceded by ichthyosis; Type 3: "subacute neuronopathic," juvenile, chronic neuro sxs; Type 3C: with CV calcifications. AR, acid β-glucosidase defects (except atypical Gaucher – PSAP/Saposin C defect).

**Fabry:** Angiokeratoma corporis diffusum, whorl-like corneal opacities, "maltese cross" in urine, painful paresthesias, ceramide accumulates in heart, autonomic nervous system, and kidneys (main cause of mortality), CVA/MI (second most cause of mortality), autoantibodies (esp. LAC and antiphospholipid), thrombosis. XLR, α-Galactosidase A.

## Angiokeratoma

**Solitary Papular:** usu extremity, preceding trauma
**Circumscriptum:** large single Blaschkonian plaque, extremity
**Corporis Diffusum:** Fabry, Fucosidosis
**Mibelli:** Fingers and toes, adolescence, cold-provoked
**Fordyce:** Scrotum, vulva, middle-aged
**Caviar Spot:** Tongue

**Fucosidosis:** Angiokeratoma corporis diffusum, coarse thick skin, MR, szs, spasticity, dysostosis multiplex, visceromegaly, growth retardation, respiratory infections. AR, α-L-Fucosidase.

**Hartnup:** Error in tryptophan secretion, pellagra-like rash, psychiatric changes. AR, SLC6A19 defects.

**Hurler:** HSM, BM failure, thick lips, large tongue, MR, corneal opacities, broad hands with claw-like fingers, dried urine with toluidine blue turns purple, dermatan sulfate and heparan sulfate in urine. AR, α-L-Iduronidase defects.

**Hunter:** Like Hurler but milder, pebbly lesions. XLR, iduronate sulfatase defects.

**Oxalosis:** Livedo, nephrocalcinosis, cardiomyopathy. AR, Type 1 – alanine-glyoxylate aminotransferase (AGXT) defects, glyoxylate reductase/hydroxypyruvate reductase (GRHPR) defects.

**Tangier:** Alpha lipoprotein deficiency, orange-yellow striations on large tonsils, splenomegaly, neuropathy, decreased cholesterol. AR, ATP-binding cassette-1 (ABC1) defects.

**Lipogranulomatosis/Farber:** SQ masses over wrists/ankles, arthritis, hoarse, involves larynx, liver, spleen, kidneys, CNS. AR, Acid Ceramidase (also called N-acylsphingosine amidohydrolase – ASAH) defects.

## Lipomatosis

**Madelung/Launois–Bensaude/familial symmetrical lipomatosis:** Alcoholism, liver disease, DM2, gout, hyperlipidemia, massive symmetrical lipomas around neck and upper trunk, "body-builder" appearance.

**Dercum/Adiposa dolorosa:** Psychiatric issues, obese women, multiple painful lipomas, asthenia, AD.

**Familial multiple lipomatosis:** AD, spares shoulders and neck.

## Total lipodystrophies

**Bernadelli–Seip:** Congenital total/generalized lipodystrophy, increased appetite, increased height velocity, AN, hyperpigmentation, thick curly hair, mild MR, DM2, CAD, hypertriglyceridemia, hepatic steatosis. AR, Type 1 – 1-acylglycerol-3-phosphate $O$-acyltransferase-2 (AGPAT2) defects, Type 2 – Seipin (BSCL2) defects.

**Seip–Lawrence:** Acquired total lipodystrophy, begins before age 15, preceded by infxn or CTD, DM2, AN, liver involvement is worse and commonly fatal, muscle wasting, growth retardation.

## Partial lipodystrophies

**Kobberling–Dunnigan:** At puberty, loss of SQ fat from extremities, buttocks, and lower trunk, gain fat on face, neck, back, and axilla, AN, hirsutism, PCOS, DM2, increased TG. AD or XLD, Type 1 – unknown genetic defect, Type 2 – LMNA defects, Type 3 – PPARG defects.

**Barraquer–Simons:** Acquired progressive lipodystrophy, first and second decade onset after viral illness, begins in face and progresses downward to iliac crests/buttocks, increased C3 nephritic factor, glomerulonephritis, third trimester abortions, DM2, LMNB2 defects.

**Insulinopenic partial lipodystrophy w/Rieger anomaly/SHORT:** In infancy, loss of fat on face and buttocks, retarded growth, bone age, and dentition, DM2 with low insulin, NO AN, Rieger anomaly = eye and tooth anomalies, S = stature; H = hyperextensibility of joints or hernia; O = ocular depression; R = Rieger anomaly; T = teething delay.

## Porphyria

| | | |
|---|---|---|
| Pseudoporphyria | – | 2/2 NSAIDS, tetracycline, hemodialysis, tanning booths, thiazide, furosemide | Normal urine, blood, feces<br>PCT-like, photosensitive blistering and skin fragility; no hypertrichosis/hyperpigmentation/ sclerodermoid changes |
| PCT | AD | Uroporphyrinogen decarboxylase | U/B: uroporphyrin 3× > coproporphyrin<br>Stool: Isocoproporphyrin<br>Photosensitive blistering, skin fragility, hypertrichosis, sclerodermoid changes<br>Tx: phlebotomy, anti-malarials. Check Fe, HCV, hemochromatosis |
| Hepatoerythropoietic porphyria (Homozygous PCT) | AR | Uroporphyrinogen decarboxylase | Similar U/B/Stool as PCT, plus elevated protoporphyrins in RBCs<br>Similar to CEP – p-notosensitive blistering in infancy, hypertrichosis, hyperpigmentation, neurologic changes, anemia, dark urine, erythrodontia |
| Variegate porphyria | AD | Protoporphyrinogen oxidase | U: dALA, PBG (during attack); coproporphyrin > uroporphyrin (unlike PCT)<br>B: 626 nm fluorescence<br>Stool: elevated coproporphyrins > protoporphyrins<br>Most often asx; may have PCT-like skin, AIP-like neurologic and GI sx<br>Avoid precipitating factors |
| Acute intermittent porphyria | AD | Porphobilinogen deaminase | U: PBG, dALA   B: dALA<br>Abdominal pain, muscle weakness, psychiatric sx, no skin findings/photosensitivity, risk of liver cancer |

| | | | |
|---|---|---|---|
| Hereditary coproporphyria | AD | Coproporphyrinogen oxidase | U: coproporphyrin, dALA, PBG (during attack)<br>Stool: coproporphyrin (always)<br>PCT-like skin, AIP-like neurologic and GI sx neuron |
| Congenital erythropoietic porphyria (Gunther) | AR | Uroporphyrinogen-III synthase | U/Stool/RBC: uroporphyrin and coproporphyrin<br>Severe photosensitivity, erythrodontia, mutilating scars, hypertrichosis, madarosis, scleromalacia perforans, red urine, anemia, gallstones<br>Tx: Transfuse to keep Hct 33% (turn off porphyrin production) |
| Erythropoietic protoporphyria | AD AR | Ferrochelatase | U: nl  B/RBC/stool: protoporphyrin<br>Severe photosensitivity (elevated protoporphyrin IX), purpura, erosions/scars, waxy/"weather beate" thickening (nose, knuckles), gallstones, anemia, liver dysfunction<br>Tx: β-carotene, antihistamine, NBUVB to induce UV tolerance |

U: Urine    B: Blood

153

## Disorders of pigmentation

**Carney complex: NAME** (Nevi, Atrial myxoma, Myxomatous neurofibromata, Ephelids), **LAMB** (Lentigines, Atrial myxoma, Myxoid tumors, Blue nevi), Sertoli cell tumors, psammomatous melanotic schwannomas, mammary neoplasia, CVA from cardiac emboli, pigmentary nodular adrenal tumors, pituitary adenomas. AD, PRKAR1A defects.

**LEOPARD/Moynahan:** Lentigines, EKG abnormalities, Ocular hypertelorism, Pulmonary stenosis, Abnormal genitalia, growth Retardation, Deafness. AD, PTPN11 defects.

**Peutz–Jeghers:** 90% small bowel involved, colic pain, bleeding, intussusception, rectal prolapse, 20–40% malignant transformation of GI polyps, cancer (breast, ovary, testes, uterus, pancreas, lungs), sertoli cell tumors, oral lentigines (also facial, hands/soles, genital, perianal), longitudinal melanonychia, presents before or in early puberty. AD, STK11 defects (vs. **Laugier–Hunziker:** Non-familial orolabial pigmented macules similar to P–J without GI involvement, Caucasians presenting between ages 20 and 40 years).

**Familial GI stromal tumors (GISTs) with hyperpigmentation:** GISTs, perineal hyperpigmentation, hyperpigmented macules (perioral, axillae, hands, perineal – not oral/lips), + urticaria pigmentosum. AD, C-KIT defects (activating mutations).

**Bannayan–Riley–Revalcaba/Bannayan–Zonana:** Macrocephaly, genital lentigines, MR, hamartomas (GI polyps), lipomas, hemangiomas. AD, PTEN defects.

**Russell–Silver:** Growth retardation, feeding difficulties, triangular facies, downturned lips, blue sclerae, limb asymmetries, clinodactyly of fifth digit, CALM, urologic abnormalities, 10% demonstrate maternal uniparental disomy of chromosome 7.

**McCune–Albright:** "Coast of Maine" CALM, precocious puberty, polyostotic fibrous dysplasia (fractures, asymmetry, pseudocystic radiographic lesions), endocrinopathies (hyperthyroidism, Cushing, hypersomatotropism, hyperprolactinemia, hyperparathyroidism). Mosaic activating GNAS1 defects.

**Albright hereditary osteodystrophy:** Pseudo or pseudopseudo-hyperparathyroidism, short fourth and fifth digits, osteoma cutis, short stature, dimpling over knuckles, MR. Maternally inherited GNAS1 mutations.

**Pallister–Killian:** Hyperpigmentation in Blaschko lines, coarse facies, temporal hypotrichosis, CV anomalies, MR. Mosaic tetrasomy 12p.

**OCA1A, 1B/tyrosine negative albinism (OCA = oculocutaneous albinism):** 1A: No Tyrosinase activity, strabismus, photophobia, reduced acuity, 1B: Slightly more tyrosinase activity. AR, Tyrosinase defects (if temperature sensitive mutation → "Siamese cat" pattern).

**OCA2:** Tyrosinase +, increased in Blacks/South Africa, 1% of Prader-Willi and Angelman patients have OCA2. AR, P gene defects.

**OCA3:** Blacks, copper/ginger hair, light tan skin, ± eye involvement. AR, TYRP1 defects.

**Rufous oculocutaneous albinism/ROCA:** Copper-red skin/hair, iris color diluted, South Africa. AR, TYRP1 defects.

**OCA4:** AR, MATP/SLC45A2 defects.

**Cross–McKusick/oculocerebral syndrome with hypopigmentation:** Albinism, MR, szs, spastic di/quadriplegia, silvery-gray hair.

**Hermansky–Pudlak:** Tyrosinase +, hemorrhagic diathesis, absent dense bodies in platelets, nystagmus, blue eyes, granulomatous colitis, pulmonary involvement, progressive pigment recovery, Puerto Ricans, Jews, Muslims. AR, HPS1–8 defects (includes DTNBP1 and BLOC1S3).

**Piebaldism:** White forelock, depigmented patch ("diamond-patches"). AD, C-KIT defects (inactivating mutations).

**Waardenberg:** Depigmented patches, sensorineural defects, white forelock, dystopia canthorum, iris heterochromia, broad nasal root, white eyelashes, cleft lip, scrotal tongue, megacolon (Type 4), limb defects (Type 3) AD>AR, Type 1: PAX3, Type 2A: MITF, Type 2D: SNAI2, Type 3: PAX3, Type 4: SOX10, endothelin-B receptor, or endothelin-3 defects.

**IP/Bloch–Sulberger:** Four stages: (1) Blistering, (2) Verrucous, (3) Hyperpigmented, (4) Hypopigmented/Atrophic; Eosinophilia/leukocytosis, pegged teeth, szs, MR, strabismus, scarring alopecia, onychodystrophy, ocular sxs. XLD, NEMO defects.

**IP Acromians/hypomelanosis of Ito:** Hypopigmented nevi (linear/whorled) + CNS anomalies, strabismus, szs, MR, mosaic chromosomal anomalies.

**Linear and whorled/figurated nevoid hypo/hypermelanosis:** No bullae, Blaschko distribution, often with MR, PDA, ASD.

**Kindler–Weary:** Acral, traumatic bullae during childhood, sclerotic poikiloderma, photosensitivity, periodontosis, pseudosyndactyly, scleroderma/XP-like facies, esophageal strictures, oral leukokeratoses, SCC. AR, KIND1 defects.

**Dermatopathia pigmentosa reticularis:** Generalized reticulate pigmentation, sweating disregulation, decreased dermatoglyphics, noncicatricial alopecia, onychodystrophy, PPK. AD, KRT14 defects.

**Acromelanosis progressiva:** Rare, black pigment of hands/feet, spread by age ~5 years.

**Acropigmentation of Dohi/dyschromatosis symmetrica hereditaria:** Hypo- and hyperpigmented macules on extremeties in a reticulated pattern, esp. dorsal hands/feets. AD, DSRAD defects.

**Dowling–Degos:** Postpubertal, progressive, brown, reticulate hyperpigmentation of the flexures, no hypopigmented macules, soft fibromas, pitted perioral scars, rarely hidradenitis suppurativa, path = elongated pigmented rete ridges, thinned suprapapillary plates, dermal melanosis. AD, KRT5 defects (**Galli–Galli** – acantholytic Dowling–Degos; Dowling–Degos shares features with **Haber** – early rosacea, trunkal keratoses (esp. axillae SK/VV-like), pitted scars, PPK).

**Reticulate pigmentation of Kitamura:** Linear palmar pits, reticulate, hyperpigmented macules, 1–4 mm on volar and dorsal hands, no hypopigmented macules. AD, KRT5 defects.

**Familial progressive hyperpigmentation:** Hyperpigmented patches at birth, spread, involve conjunctivae and buccal mucosa, AD.

**Phakomatosis pigmentokeratotica:** Speckled lentiginous nevus (usu checkerboard) + organoid nevus with sebaceous differentiation ± musculoskeletal, neuro, and ophtho abnormalities.

**Hemochromatosis:** Onset: 40–60 years old, Classic Tetrad: bronze skin (esp. face), hepatomegaly, DM2, cardiomyopathy; pigmentation due to (basilar) melanin and hemosiderin, cardiac dysrhythmia, arthropathy, black stasis dermatitis, Tx: phlebotomy and chelating agents. AR, HFE defects.

## Non-hereditary syndromic disorders of pigmentation

**Vogt–Koyanagi–Harada:** Depigmented skin/eyelashes, chronic granulomatous iridocyclitis, retinal detachment, aseptic meningoencephalitis.

**Alezzandrini:** Unilateral degenerative pigmentary retinitis, ipsilateral vitiligo, poliosis.

**Cronkhite–Canada:** Melanotic macules on fingers, more diffuse hyperpigmentation than Peutz–Jeghers, alopecia, onychodystrophy, protein losing enteropathy, GI polyposis.

**Riehl melanosis:** Pigmented contact dermatitis on face, esp. brown-gray discolored forehead/temples, often due to cosmetics, interface reaction on path.

**Gray baby syndrome:** Chloramphenicol.

**Bronze baby syndrome:** Complication of phototherapy for bilirubinemia, elevated direct bili, hepatic dysfunction, induced by photoproducts of bilirubin and biliverdin.

## Disorders of vascularization

**Proteus syndrome:** Partial gigantism of the hands/feet, lipomas, linear verrucous nevi, macrocephaly, hyperostosis, PWS, body hemihypertrophy, ocular anomalies, scoliosis.

**Cutis marmorata telangiectatica congenita/Van Lohuizen:** Persistant livedo, atrophy/ulceration, CNS defects, MR, craniofacial anomalies, glaucoma, syndromes with cutis marmorata: Adams–Oliver, Cornelia de Lange, Coffin–Siris (related condition: Macrocephaly-CMTC syndrome – macrocephaly + cutis marmorata + several additional features among the following: hypotonia, toe syndactyly, segmental overgrowth, hydrocephalus, midline facial nevus flammeus, frontal bossing).

**Maffucci:** Enchondromas, increased osteosarcomas, vascular malformations. AD, PTHR1 defects not confirmed (Ollier – no vascular malformations).

**Gorham–Stout/disappearing (aka vanishing or phantom) bone:** Onset: childhood or young adulthood, progressive osteolysis of one or more bones, vascular malformations (bone and skin), pathologic fractures, limb tenderness and weakness, thoracic duct occlusion, chylothorax, Tx: radiation.

**Beckwith–Wiedemann:** Facial PWS, macroglossia, omphalocoele, hemihypertrophy, adrenocortical carcinomas, pancreatoblastomas, hepatoblastomas. Defects: p57/KIP2/CDKN1C or NSD1.

**Cobb:** Cutaneomeningospinal angiomatosis, hemangioma or vascular malformation of a spinal segment and its corresponding dermatome.

**Blue rubber bleb nevus/Bean:** Painful blue nodules with hyperhidrosis, GI bleeds.

**Roberts/SC phocomelia/SC pseudothalidomide:** Facial PWS, hypomelia, hypotrichosis, growth retardation, cleft lip/palate, limb defects. AR, ESCO2 defects.

**Thrombocytopenia-absent radius/TAR:** Absent radius, decreased platelets, PWS.

**Alagille:** Arteriohepatic dysplasia, nevus comedonicus, xanthomas, retinal pigment anomalies, peripheral arterial stenosis, pulmonic valvular stenosis, "butterfly" vertebrae, absent deep tendon reflexes, broad forehead, bulbous nasal tip, foreshortened fingers. AD, JAG1 or NOTCH2 defects.

**PHACES:** Posterior fossa abnormalities, Hemangiomas, Arterial anomalies (including intracranial aneurysms), Cardiac anomalies (often aortic coarctation), Eye anomalies, Sternal defects, usually females, most often left-sided hemangioma, Dandy–Walker malformation, cleft palate.

**Sturge–Weber:** V1 PWS, V2 and V3 may be involved but must be in conjunction with V1, full V1 involvement has greater risk than partial V1 involvement, glaucoma, szs, ipsilateral vascular malformation of meninges and train track calcifications, MR.

**Klippel–Trenaunay:** Capillary malformation with limb hypertrophy, venous/lymphatic malformations, angiokeratomas, lymphangiomas, AV fistula, phlebitis, thrombosis, ulcerations.

**Von Hippel–Lindau:** Capillary malformation of head/neck, retinal/cerebellar hemangioblastoma, renal cell CA, renal cysts, pheochromocytoma, adrenal CA, pancreatic cysts. AD, VHL defects.

**Multiple cutaneous and mucosal venous malformations/VMCM:** AD, TIE2 defects.

**Capillary malformation–arteriovenous malformation/CM-AVM:**
Atypical capillary malformations + AVM, AV fistula, or Parkes Weber
syndrome. AD, RASA1 defects.

**Ataxia telangiectasia/Louis–Bar:** Cerebellar ataxia starts first (at ~1
year old), wheelchair-bound by ~12 years old, oculocutaneous
telangiectasias develop by 3–6 years old, sinopulm infxn, IgA & IgG
are diminished, IgE and IgM may be diminished, premature aging,
poikilodermatous and sclerodermatous skin, MR, insulin-resistant DM2,
increased AFP (makes it difficult to screen for hepatic tumors) and CEA,
radiosensitivity, lymphoid/solid (stomach, breast) malignancies, cutaneous
granulomas. AR but cancer risk in heterozygotes, ATM defects.

**Bloom:** Short stature, telangiectatic facial erythema, malar hypoplasia,
photosensitivity, hypogonadism/decreased fertility, high-pitched voice,
leukemia, lymphoma, low IgM and IgA, recurrent pneumonia, CALM,
crusted/blistered lips, narrow face, DM2 (and acanthosis nigricans), MR,
loss of eyelashes. AR, RECQL3=RECQ2 defects.

**Osler–Weber–Rendu/hereditary hemorrhagic telangiectasia:**
Telangiectasia of mucosa/ face/palms/soles, epistaxis, GI bleed, pulmonary
AVMs. AD, Endoglin (HHT1), ALK-1 (HHT2), HHT3, or HHT4 defects.

**Xeroderma pigmentosa:** Types A–G, Type A most severe, A is most
common in Japan, (30%) and D (20%) are most common overall, defective
UV damage repair, ectropion, blepharitis, keratitis, low intelligence,
dementia, ataxia, lentigines, premature aging, NMSC, melanoma, KA, AR.

**De Sanctis–Cacchione:** Type A XP, mental deficiency, dwarfism,
hypogonadism. AR, ERCC6 defects.

**Nonne–Milroy:** Congenital lymphedema, unilateral or bilateral, pleural
effusions, chylous ascites, scrotal swelling, protein-losing enteropathy, risk
for lymphangiosarcoma and angiosarcoma, right > left leg. AD but F>M,
FLT4/VEGFR3 defects.

**Meige/lymphedema praecox:** Most common form of primary
lymphedema AD, FOXC2/MFH1 defects (also causes Yellow Nail,
Lymphedema–Distichiasis, and Lymphedema and Ptosis syndromes).

**Yellow nail:** Lymphedema, pleural effusions, bronchiectasis, yellow nails.
AD, FOXC2/MFH1 defects.

### Non-hereditary syndromic vascular disorders

**APACHE:** Acral Pseudolymphomatous Angiokeratoma of CHildrEn.

**Kasabach–Merritt:** Consumptive coagulopathy associated with large
vascular lesion esp. kaposiform hemangioendothelioma or tufted angioma.

**Mondor:** Thrombophlebitis of the veins in the thoracogastric area, often
breast, sometimes strain/trauma.

**POEMS/Crow–Fukase:** Glomeruloid hemangiomas, Polyneuropathy,
Organomegaly (liver, lymph nodes, spleen), Endocrinopathy, Monoclonal
protein (IgA or G)/Myeloma (15% Castleman disease), Skin changes

(hyperpigmentation, skin thickening, hypertrichosis, sclerodermoid changes), sclerotic bone lesions, edema, papilledema.

**Secretan:** Acral factitial lymphedema.

**Stewart–Treves:** Mastectomy → angiosarcoma.

**Stewart-Bluefarb:** Pseudo-KS, leg AVM.

**Wyburn-Mason:** Facial PWS, ipsilateral AVM of retinal/optic pathway.

**Hennekam:** Congenital lymphedema, intestinal lymphangiectasia, MR.

**Coats:** Retinal telangiectasia, ipsilateral PWS.

**Syndromes with photosensitivity:** XP, Bloom, Rothmund–Thomson, Cockayne, Hartnup, porphyrias, TTD, Cockayne, Kindler, Prolidase deficiency, Hailey-Hailey, Darier.

## Immunodeficiency syndromes

**X-linked agammaglobulinemia/Bruton:** Males, onset: infancy, recurrent infxns (Gram+ sinopulmonary, meningoencephalitis, arthritis), reduced or undetectable Ig levels, atopy, vasculitis, urticaria, no germinal centers or plasma cells, RA-like sxs, neutropenia, chronic lung disease, defect in PreB to B cell differentiation, tx: IVIG. XL, BTK defects.

**Isolated IgA deficiency:** 50% with recurrent infxns, 25% with autoimmune disease, Celiac, UC, AD, asthma, IVIG infusion may cause allergic rxn 2/2 IgA Ab, hard to confirm dx before 4 years old because IgA develops late in children.

**CVID:** Typical sx onset and diagnosis in late 20s, increased HLA-B8, DR3, recurrent sinopulmonary infxns, increased autoimmune disease, lymphoreticular and GI malignancies, arthritis, noncaseating granulomas (may be confused with sarcoidosis), some T-cell dysfxn, reduced Ig levels (esp. IgG and IgA, also IgM in ½ of patients), tx: IVIG.

**Isolated IgM deficiency:** 1/5 with eczematous dermatitis, VV, patients with MF and celiac disease may have secondary IgM deficiency, thyroiditis, splenomegaly, hemolytic anemia.

**Hyper–IgM:** Recurrent infxns, low IgG, E, A, respiratory infxn, diarrhea, otitis, oral ulcers, VV, recurrent neutropenia, tx: with IVIG, BMT. XL (CD40L), AR (CD40, AICD, HIGM3).

**DiGeorge:** Notched, low-set ears, micrognathia, shortened philtrum, hypertelorism, absent parathyroids → neonatal hypocalcemia, thymic hypoplasia, cardiac anomlies (truncus arteriosis, interrupted aortic arch), psychiatric sxs cleft lip/palate, CHARGE overlap, 1/3 with Complete DiGeorge have eczematous dermatitis. AD, deletion in proximal long arm of chromosome 22 (TBX1 is esp. important).

**Thymic dysplasia with normal immunoglobulins/Nezelof:** T-cell deficit, severe candidiasis, varicella, diarrhea, pulm infxns, nl Ig, AR.

**Omenn/familial reticuloendotheliosis with eosinophilia:** Exfoliative erythroderma, alopecia, eosinophilia, HSM, LAN, infections, diarrhea, hypogammaglobulinemia, hyper-IgE, decreased B cells, increased T cells. AR, RAG1, RAG2 defects.

**SCID:** Absent cellular and humoral immunity, monilithiasis, diarrhea, pneumonia. AR, Adenosine Deaminase, RAG1, RAG2 defects.

**Wiskott–Aldrich:** Young boys, triad (atopic, recurrent infxn – esp. encapsulated organisms, thrombocytopenia), small platelets, lymphoid malignancies, cellular and humoral immunodeficiency, autoimmune disorders, often present with bleeding (from circumcision or diarrhea), defects in cellular and humoral immunity: IgM deficiency with IgA and IgE often elevated and IgM often normal, HSM, Tx: BMT. XLR, WASP defects.

**Chronic Granulomatous Disease/CGD:** Recurrent purulent and granulomatous infxns of the long bones, lymphatic tissue, liver, skin, lungs, 2/3 in boys, eczema, defect in NADPH oxidase complex, autoimmunity, lupus-like sxs in XL carriers (rash, arthralgias, oral ulcers, fatigue, but usu ANA-), gene for XLR (60%): CYBB, AR forms: NCF1, NCF2, CYBA (p22–, p47–, p67–, and p91-phox).

**Myeloperoxidase deficiency:** Most asymptomatic. AR, MPO defects.

**Hyper–IgE:** AD-like lesions, recurrent pyogenic infxns/cold abscesses, eosinophilia, may have PPK, asthma, chronic candidiasis, urticaria, coarse facies with wide nose, deep-set eyes, hyperextensible joints, fractures, lymphomas, pneumatoceles, retained primary teeth, scoliosis, pathologic fractures. AD: STAT3 defects, AR: TYK2 defects (AR form has severe viral infections, HSV, extreme eosinophilia, neurologic complications, no skeletal/dental defects), subset with **Job:** Girls with red hair, freckles, blue eyes, hyperextensible joints.

**APECED:** Autoimmune Polyendocrinopathy, (chronic mucocutaneous) Candidiasis, Ectodermal Dystrophy, frequent Addison and/or hypoparathyroidism, selective T-cell anergy for candida, alopecia, vitiligo, oral SCC. AR, AIRE defects.

**Leukocyte Adhesion Molecule deficiency:** Delayed umbilical separation, periodontitis, gingivitis, poor wound healing, Tx: BMT. AR, CD18 β2 integrin (can't bind CD11, C3b).

|  | Chediak–Higashi | Elejalde | Griscelli |
|---|---|---|---|
| Neurologic | Normal (rarely defects in adult form) | Severe defects, mental and motor, regressive | Defects in Type 1, normal in Types 2 and 3 |
| Immunologic | PMN, NK, and lymph cell defects, fatal accelerated phase (uncontrolled macrophage and lymphocyte activation) | Normal | Normal in Types 1 and 3, Defects in Type 2 (lymphs and NK cells), no fatal accelerated phase |
| Hair | Silvery, regular melanin clumps in small granules (6× smaller than granules of Elejalde or Griscelli) | Silvery, irregular melanin clumps in large and small granules | Silvery, irregular melanin clumps in large and small granules |

| Skin | Pigment dilution | Pigment dilution | Pigment dilution |
| --- | --- | --- | --- |
| Platelet | Dense granule defects | Dense granule defects | Dense granule defects |
| Ophtho | Defects | Defects | Defects |
| Inheritance | AR, LYST | AR, MYO5A | AR, MYO5A (Type 1), RAB27A (Type 2), MLPH or MYO5A (Type 3) |

## Hereditary periodic fever syndromes

**Familial mediterranean fever/FMF:** Recurrent fever (few hours to several days), recurrent polyserositis (peritoneum, synovium, pleura), AA amyloidosis, renal failure, erysipelas-like erythema esp. BLE, rare associations: HSP and PAN. AR or AD, MEFV/Pyrin defects.

**TNF receptor-associated periodic/TRAPS/Hibernian fever:** Recurrent fever (usu > 5 days, often 1–3 weeks), myalgia (w/ overlying migratory erythema), pleurisy, abdominal pain, conjunctivitis/periorbital edema, serpiginous, edematous, purpuric, or reticulated lesions esp. at extremities, AA amyloidosis, renal failure, leukocytosis, elevated ESR. AD, TNF-Receptor 1 defects.

**Hyper-IgD with periodic fever/HIDS:** Recurrent fever (3–7 days, 1–2 months apart), abdominal pain, diarrhea, headache, arthralgias, cervical lymphadenopathy, erythematous macules > papules and nodules, elevated IgD and IgA, rare associations: HSP and EED, mevalonic aciduria. AR, MVK defects.

## Cryopyrin-associated periodic syndromes

**Histo:** Lots of PMNs, no mast cells.

**Familial cold autoinflammatory/urticaria/FCAS:** Urticaria-like eruption, limb pain, recurrent fever, flare with generalized cold exposure, normal hearing, AA amyloidosis. AD, CIAS1 defects.

**Muckle–Wells:** Urticaria-like eruption, limb pain, recurrent fever, AA amyloidosis (more common than FCAS), deafness. AD, CIAS1 defects.

**Neonatal–onset multisystemic inflammatory disease/NOMID/ CINCA:** Triad of CNS disorder, arthropathy, and rash (edematous, urticarial-like papules and plaques, neutrophilic eccrine hidradenitis); also deafness and visual disturbance, recurrent fever, AA amyloidosis. AD, CIAS1 defects.

## Pyogenic sterile arthritis, pyoderma gangrenosum and acne/

**PAPA:** Periodic Fever with Aphthous Stomatitis, Pharyngitis, and Cervical Adenopathy (PFAPA), attacks last ~5 days. AD, PSTPIP1 defects (vs. SAPHO: synovitis, acne, pustulosis, hyperostosis, osteitis).

**Blau:** Arthritis, uveitis, granulomatous dermatitis – early onset sarcoidosis. AD, NOD2/CARD15 defects.

**Majeed:** Subacute or chronic multifocal osteomyelitis with neutrophilic dermatosis or Sweet syndrome. AR, LPIN2 defects.

## Miscellaneous

**Melkersson–Rosenthal:** Scrotal tongue, orofacial swelling, facial nerve palsy.

**Ascher:** Blepharochalasis, double upper lip, endocrine abnormalities (goiter).

**Epidermodysplasia verruciformis:** HPV types 3, 5, 8, SCC. AR, EVER1 or EVER2 defects.

**Prader–Willi:** Obesity after 12 months of age, MR, skin picking, chromosome 15 deletion in 60% (paternal imprinting), downslanting corners of mouth, almond-shaped eyes, hypopigmentation.

**Angelman:** Happy puppet syndrome, MR, szs, pale blue eyes, tongue protrusion, unprovoked laughter, hypopigmentation, maternal chromosome 15 deletion or (1/4) Ubiquitin-protein Ligase E3A (UBE3A) defects.

**Donahue:** Leprechaunism, lipodystrophy, AN, hypertrichosis. AR, INSR defects.

**CADASIL:** Cerebral Arteriopathy, Autosomal Dominant, with Subcortical Infarcts and Leukoencephalopathy, recurrent ischemic strokes, early dementia, granular osmiophilic deposits around vascular smooth muscles cells and under the basement membrane on EM. AD, NOTCH3 defects.

**Lafora:** Onset: late adolescence with death within a decade, progressive myoclonic epilepsy, ataxia, cerebellar atrophy, PAS±cytoplasmic eccrine duct inclusions. AR, EPM2A/Laforin defects.

**Heck/focal epithelial hyperplasia:** Occurs in American Indians, Eskimos, Latin Americans, oral mucosa infections with HPV 13, 32.

**Lhermitte–Duclos:** Dysplastic gangliocytoma, isolated or associated with Cowden. AD, PTEN defects.

**Branchio-oculofacial/BOF:** Laterocervical psoriasiform lesions, similar to aplasia cutis congenital, abnormal nasolacrimal ducts → infections, sebaceous scalp cysts, low pinnae, accessory tragus, broad nose, hypertelorism, loss of punctae, premature aging, AD.

**Barber–Say:** Hypertrichosis, lax skin, abnormal fingerprints, ectropion, macrostomia, MR.

**CHIME:** Migratory ichthyosiform dermatosis, Coloboma, Heart defects, migratory Ichthyosiform dermatitis, Mental retardation, Ear defects (deafness); also szs, abnormal gait.

**Van der Woude:** Congenital lower lip pits, cleft palate, hypodontia. AD, IRF6 defects.

**Fibrodysplasia Ossificans Progressiva:** Malformed great toes, osteoma cutis (endochondral). AD, ACVR1 defects.

**Riley-Day/Familial dysautonomia:** Feeding difficulties, lack of emotional tears, absent fungiform papillae (vs. absent filiform papillae in geographic tongue), diminished reflexes/pain/taste, no flare with intraepidermal histamine, drooling, labile BP, blotchy erythema while eating, pulmonary infxn, Ashkenazi. AR, IKBKAP defects.

## Miscellaneous non-genetic syndromes

**Schnitzler:** Urticarial vasculitis, bone pain, fever, hyperostosis, IgM monoclonal gammopathy, arthralgia, LAN, HSM, elev ESR.

**Frey:** Gustatory hyperhidrosis, usually following trauma/surgery to the parotid gland (auriculotemporal nerve).

# Dermoscopy

### Polarized (PD) vs. nonpolarized (NPD)
- NPD requires liquid interface, direct skin contact (using a gel rather than alcohol leads to less distortion from pressure)
- NPD better for milia-like cysts, comedo-like openings, peppering/regression, blue-white areas, lighter colors
- PD better for vessels, red areas, shiny-white streaks/fibrosis

### Algorithms
- **Two-step algorithm** – (1) Melanocytic or non-melanocytic (2) If melanocytic, then use global pattern and local features to distinguish melanoma
- **CASH algorithm** – Color, architecture, symmetry, homogeneity

### Pigment network
- Pigment network – either typical (brown, narrow, regular mesh) or atypical (thick black, brown, or gray lines, irregular meshes, suggestive of melanoma)
- Pseudopigmented network – on face
- Pigment network but not melanocytic – SK, DF, accessory nipple

### Features suggestive of melanoma
Streaks – melanoma
Blue-white veil – melanoma, Spitz, angiokeratoma
Black blotches – if irregular, suggestive of melanoma (if uniform, consider Reed)
Regression structures – melanoma (esp. with melanin peppering)
Radial streaming/pseudopods/branched streaks/broken network – melanoma
Milky-red areas – early melanoma
Dots/globules – if irregular, suggestive of melanoma

### Acral melanocytic lesions
- Parallel–furrow, fibrillar, lattice-like or homogeneous patterns – acral melanocytic nevi
- Parallel–ridge pattern – acral melanoma (acrosyringia open onto ridges, ridges are wider than furrows)

### Features suggestive of SK
Milia-like cysts – SK, papillomatous IDN
Comedo-like openings – SK, papillomatous IDN

Exophytic papillary structures – SK
Fat fingers – SK
Cerebriform surface – SK, BCC

## Features suggestive of BCC
(Maple) leaf-like areas – BCC
Blue-gray blotches/ovoid nests/globules – pigmented BCC
Pink-white shiny areas – BCC
Spoke wheels – BCC

## Dermoscopic vessels
Comma-like vessels – benign melanocytic lesion
Arborizing vessels – BCC
Hairpin vessels – SK, melanoma (if irregular), KA, SCC
Dotted/Irregular vessels – melanoma
Polymorphous vessels – melanoma
Corkscrew vessels – amelanotic melanoma metastases
Corona/wreath/crown vessels – surround sebaceous hyperplasia (central yellow globular structure)
Glomerular vessels – SCC, SCCIS
Point vessels – melanocytic neoplasms, superficial epithelial neoplasms (AK, SCCIS)

## Features suggestive of other lesions
Red-blue/black lacunae/saccules – hemangioma, angiokeratoma (dark lacuna), subcorneal/subungual hematoma
Central white patch – DF (star-like white area surrounded by delicate pigment network)
Reddish homogeneous region surrounded by white collarette – PG
Moth–eaten border and fingerprint pattern – solar lentigo
Steel blue areas – blue nevi
EB nevi – often demonstrate certain specific features associated with melanoma (atypical pigment network, irregular dots/globules, atypical vascular pattern), but not other features (blue-white veil, regression structures/blue-white areas, irregular streaks, black dots)
LPLK – depends on involution stage, localized (early) or diffuse (late) pigmented granular pattern, regressive features (blue-white scar-like depigmented or vascular structures)
Facial lentigo maligna – asymmetric pigmented follicular openings, dark rhomboidal structures, slate-gray dots and globules
Scabies – triangular shape (delta glider) resembling circumflex accent (corresponds to head and front legs) dihydroxyacetone may cause changes in nevi (increased globules and comedolike pseudofollicular openings)

**Patterns of melanocytic nevi/Lesions** – Reticular, globular, homogeneous (blue), starburst (complete starburst – reed, spitz; incomplete starburst – melanoma), parallel (acral), multicomponent (melanoma), cobblestone (papillomatous IDN and congenital nevi), non-specific

### Histopathologic correlates of dermoscopic features:

- Color according to Melanin location:
  - Black – upper epidermis
  - Brown – DEJ
  - Slate Blue – papillary dermis
  - Steel Blue – reticular dermis
- Pigment network – lines = rete ridges; spaces = superpapillary plates
- Pseudopigmented network on face – adnexal structures = holes (face has minimal rete ridges)
- Dots and globules – nests of melanocytic cells at different depths
- Black blotches – pigment everywhere (radially, epidermal, dermal)
- Cerebriform surface – gyrus = fat fingers; sulcus = pigmented keratin
- Leaf-like areas – islands of pigmented BCC (large islands = blue-gray ovoid nests)
- Blue-white veil – white = orthokeratotic hyperkeratosis; blue = dermal melanin.

## Pathology

### Histochemical staining

| Stain | Purpose |
|---|---|
| Hematoxylin–eosin | Routine |
| Masson trichrome | Collagen (green), Muscle (red), Nuclei (black). Helps to distinguishing leiomyoma (red) from dermatofibroma (green) |
| Verhoeff von Gieson | Elastic fibers |
| Pinkus acid orcein | Elastic fibers |
| Gomori's aldehyde fuchsin | Elastic fibers (blue); collagen (red) |
| Movat's pentachrome | Connective tissue |
| Silver nitrate | Melanin, reticulin fibers |
| Fontana Masson | Melanin |
| Schmorl's | Melanin |
| DOPA-oxidase | Melanin |
| Gram | Gram+: blue-purple; Gram−: red |

continued p. 166

| Stain | Purpose |
|---|---|
| Methenamine silver (Gomori, GMS) | Fungi, Donovan bodies, Frisch bacilli, BM, sodium urate |
| Grocott | Fungi |
| Periodic acid-Schiff (PAS) | Glycogen, fungi, neutral MPS (diastase removes glycogen) |
| Alcian blue pH 0.5 | Sulfated MPS |
| Alcian blue pH 2.5 | Acid MPS |
| Toluidine blue | Acid MPS |
| Colloidal iron | Acid MPS |
| Hyaluronidase | Hyaluronic acid |
| Mucicarmine | Epithelial mucin |
| Leder | Mast cells (chloroacetate esterase) |
| Giemsa | Mast cell granules, acid MPS, myeloid granules, leishmania |
| Fite | Acid-fast bacilli |
| Ziehl–Neelson | Acid-fast bacilli |
| Kinyoun's | Acid-fast bacilli |
| Auramine O | Acid-fast bacilli (fluorescence) |
| Perls potassium ferrocyanide | Hemosiderin/Iron |
| Prussian blue | Hemosiderin/Iron |
| Turnbull blue | Hemosiderin/Iron |
| Alkaline Congo red | Amyloid (the Congo red variant pagoda red No. 9/Dylon is more specific for amyloid) |
| Thioflavin T | Amyloid |
| Acid orcein Giemsa | Amyloid |
| Cresyl violet | Amyloid, ochronosis |
| Von Kossa | Calcium |
| Alizarin red | Calcium |
| Pentahydroxy flavanol | Calcium |
| Scarlet red | Lipids |
| Oil red O | Lipids |
| Sudan black | Lipids, lipofuscin |
| Osmium tetroxide | Lipids |
| Dopa | Tyrosinase |
| Warthin Starry | Spirochetes, Donovan bodies |
| Dieterle silver | Spirochetes |

| Stain | Purpose |
|---|---|
| Steiner | Spirochetes |
| Bodian | Nerve fibers |
| PGP 9.5 | Nerve fibers |
| GFAP | Glial, astrocytes, schwann cells |
| Feulgen | DNA |
| Methyl-green pyronin | DNA |
| Foote's, Snook's | Reticulin fibers |
| PTAH | Fibrin, infantile digital fibromatosis<br>Inclusions (also stained by trichrome),<br>  granules of granular cell tumor, amoeba |
| Methylene blue | Ochronosis |
| Brown–Hopps | Bacteria |
| Brown–Brenn | Bacteria |
| McCallum–Goodpasture | Bacteria |
| DeGalantha | Urate crystals (20% silver nitrate also stains<br>  Gout; Gout preserved with etoh) |
| Ulex europaeus lectin | Endothelial cells |
| Peanut agglutinin | Histiocytes |
| Neuron-specific enolase | Neural, neuroendocrine, Merkel, granular<br>  cell tumor |
| Gross cystic disease fluid protein | Apocrine, Paget's, met breast CA |

## Immunohistochemical staining

### EPIDERMAL

| | |
|---|---|
| Cytokeratin 20 | Merkel cell (perinuclear dot) |
| Cytokeratin 7 | Paget's |
| EMA | Eccrine, apocrine, sebaceous (also plasma cells, LyP,<br>  anaplastic CTCL – primary systemic not primary<br>  cutaneous) |
| CEA | Met adenoca, Paget's, eccrine, apocrine |
| BerEP4 | BCC+, Merkel cell+, SCC- |

### MESENCHYMAL

| | |
|---|---|
| Desmin | Muscle |
| Vimentin | Mesenchymal cells (AFX, melanoma, sarcomas) |
| Actin | Muscle, glomus cell tumors |
| Factor VIII-related Ag (VWF) | Endothelial cells, megakaryocytes, platelets |

continued p. 168

| Stain | Purpose |
|-------|---------|
| Ulex europasus agglutinin I | Endothelial cells, angiosarcoma, Kaposi, keratinocytes |
| CD31 | Endothelial cells, vascular tumor, angiosarcoma, NSF, scleromyxedema |
| CD34 | DFSP‡: CD34+, Factor XIIIa- |
| | DF: CD34−, Factor XIIIa+ |
| | Endothelial cells, NSF, scleromyxedema |
| | Morphea: CD34+ spindle cells selectively depleted |
| | Focal CD34+ spindle cells around trichoepithelioma but not BCC |
| Procollagen I | Scleromyxedema > NFD/NSF |
| GLUT1 | Positive in infantile hemangiomas and placenta, negative in vascular malformations, RICH, NICH, PG, tufted angiomas, kaposiform hemangioendotheliomas (reduced or negative in subglottic infantile hemangiomas) |
| WT1 and LeY | Positive in infantile hemangiomas, negative in vascular malformations |
| D2-40* and LYVE-1 | Lymphatics and kaposiform hemangioendothelioma |

**NEUROECTODERMAL**

| | |
|-------|---------|
| S100 | Melanocytes, nerve, Langerhans, eccrine, apocrine, chondrocytes, sebocytes |
| HMB-45 | Melanocytes |
| MART-1 | Melanocytes |
| Mel-5 | Melanocytes |
| CD1A | Langerhans cells |
| Synatophysin | Merkel cells |
| Chromogranin | Merkel cells |

**HEMATOPOIETIC**

| | |
|-------|---------|
| Factor XIIIa | PLTs, macrophages, megakaryocytes, dendritics (NSF**, scleromyxedema), DF but not DFSP |
| HAM-56 | Macrophages |
| Alpha-1-antitrypsin | Macrophages |
| κ & λ | Mature B cells & plasma cells |
| BCL1 | Mantle cell lymphoma |
| BCL2 | Follicular center lymphoma (except primary cutaneous follicle center lymphoma), BCC, trichoepithelioma (bcl2- except outer layer) |
| BCL6 | Follicular center lymphoma |
| CD2 | T-cell |

| Stain | Purpose |
| --- | --- |
| CD3 | Pan T-cell marker, NK cells |
| CD4 | T helper cell, Langerhans |
| CD5 | T cells, some B cells in mantle zone, depleted in MF[†] |
| CD7 | T cells, depleted in MF |
| CD8 | T cytotoxic cells |
| CD10 | B cell in BL, follicular center lymphoma, lymphoblastic lymphoma, AFX |
| CD14 | Monocytes |
| CD15 | Granulocytes, Hodgkin's |
| CD16 | NK cells |
| CD20 | B cells |
| CD22 | B cells |
| CD23 | B cells, marginal zone lymphoma, CLL |
| CD25 (IL-2R) | Activated B/T/Macs, evaluate before denileukin diftitox |
| CD30 (Ki-1) | Anaplastic CTCL, LyP, anaplastic large cell lymphoma, activated T and B cells, RS cells, (Hodgkin's) |
| CD43 (Leu-22) | Pan T-cell marker, mast cells, myeloid cells |
| CD45 (LCA) | CD45RO: memory T cells<br>CD45RA: B cells, naive T cells |
| CD56 | NK cells, angiocentric T-cell lymphoma, Merkel cell |
| CD68 | Histiocytes, AFX, NSF, scleromyxedema, mast cells, myeloid cells |
| CD75 | Folicular center cells |
| CD79d | B cells, plasma cells (plasmacytoma) |
| CD99 | Precursor B-lymphoblastic leukemia/lymphoma, Ewing's, PNET |
| CD117 (c-kit) | Mast cells |
| CD138 | Plasma cells |

‡ DFSP — CD34+ XIIIa- Stromelysin-3- CD68- CD163- HMGA1/2- vs. DF: CD34- XIIIa+ Stromelysin-3+ CD68+ CD163+ HMGA1/2+; Increased hyaluronate in the stroma of DFSP vs. DF; Tenascin positivity at DEJ overlying DF but not DFSP.

* D2-40 — Often negative, but may have focal positivity in congenital hemangioma and tufted angioma.

** "circulating fibrocyte" — procollagen I+ C11b+ CD13+ CD34+ CD45RO+ MHCII+ CD68+.

† MF — usually CD3+ CD4+ CD5- CD7- CD8- Leu-8- CD45RO+ with $\alpha\beta$ TCR; MF is also usually CD30— but not all CD30+ cases undergo anaplastic large cell transformation (anaplastic large cell transformation from MF, Hodgkin's, or LyP is usually ALK- and EMA- similar to primary systemic anaplastic large T-cell lymphoma but unlike primary cutaneous anaplastic large T-cell lymphoma).

## Pathologic bodies

| Body/sign/clue | Features | Diagnosis |
|---|---|---|
| Antoni A tissue | Densely cellular areas with palisaded nuclei, fascicles and verocay bodies | Schwannoma |
| Antoni B tissue | Loose, gelatinous stroma, fewer cells, microcystic changes | Schwannoma |
| Arao-Perkins Bodies | Elastin bodies in connective tissue streamers below vellus follicles | Androgenic alopecia |
| Asteroid bodies | Star-like cytoplasmic inclusions in giant cells | Sarcoidosis and other granulomatous diseases (TB, botryomycosis, sporotrichosis, actinomycosis, leprosy, foreign body granuloma, berylliosis) |
| Azzopardi effect | Basophilic vascular streaking (encrusted nuclear material/DNA around vessels) | Tumor necrosis, crush |
| Banana bodies | 1. Curvilinear, membrane bround bodies in Schwann cells on EM | 1. Farber disease |
| | 2. Crescentic, ocher bodies in the dermis | 2. Ochronosis |
| Beanbag cells | Large macrophages demonstrating cytophagocytosis | Subcutaneous panniculitis-like T-cell lymphoma/cytophagic histiocytic panniculitis |
| Birbeck granules | Tennis racket structures on EM | Langerhans cells |
| Busy dermis | | GA, interstitial granulomatous dermatitis, resolving vasculitis, folliculitis, early KS, desmoplastic MM, chronic photodermatosis, breast CA mets |

| | | |
|---|---|---|
| Caspary–Joseph spaces | Clefts at DEJ associated with basal layer injury, a.k.a. Max-Joseph cleft | LP, lichen nitidus |
| Caterpillar bodies | Eosinophilic, segmented, elongated (epidermal) bodies on roof of blisters (Col IV) | Porphyrias |
| Cholesterol clefts | Needle-like crystals | Sclerema neonatorum, subcutaneous fat necrosis of the newborn (may have more inflammation and calcification than sclerema), post-steroid panniculitis, NXG, cholesterol emboli, NLD, trichilemmal cyst |
| Chunks of coal | Large atypical lymphoid cells with hyperchromatic nuclei | Lymphomatoid papulosis |
| Cigar bodies | Oval, elongated yeast cells | Sporotrichosis |
| Colloid/Civatte bodies | Apoptotic bodies in epidermis (civatte) or extruded into papillary dermis (colloid) | Lichen planus and variants |
| Comma-shaped bodies | Cytoplasmic worm-like bodies on EM | Benign cephalic histiocytosis |
| Conchoidal bodies (Schaumann Bodies) | Shell-like, lamellated, basophilic, calcified protein complexes in giant cells | Sarcoidosis and other granulomatous diseases |
| Corps grains | Small, dyskeratotic, acantholytic keratinocytes with elongated grain-shaped nuclei seen in stratum corneum | Darier, Grover, warty dyskeratoma, Hailey–Hailey (rare) |
| Corps ronds | Enlarged, dyskeratotic, acantholytic keratinocytes with round nuclei and perinuclear halo seen in Malpighian layer and surrounding basophilic dyskeratotic material | Darier, Grover, warty dyskeratoma, Hailey–Hailey (rare) |
| Councilman bodies | Cytoplasmic inclusion | BCC |

continued p. 172

171

| Body/sign/clue | Features | Diagnosis |
|---|---|---|
| Cowdry Type A & B | Eosinophilic, intranuclear inclusions surrounded by clear halo | A – HSV, CMV (+ "owl's eye cells" – viral inclusions in endothelial cells), VZV; B – Polio |
| Cytoid bodies | Heterogeneous round, oval, or polygonal deposits, usually in dermis | Collective term for colloid bodies, Russell bodies, amyloid, elastic globes |
| Donovan bodies | Single or clustered rod safety pin-like bacteria in macrophages | Granuloma inguinale |
| Dutcher bodies | Intranuclear pseudoinclusions in malignant plasma cells, Ig | B-cell lymphoma, multiple myeloma |
| Farber bodies | Comma-shaped tubular structures in cytoplasm of fibroblasts and endothelial cells on EM | Farber disease |
| Flame figures | Poorly circumscribed, small areas of amorphous eosinophilic material adherent to dermal collagen | Eosinophilic cellulitis + flame figures = Well's syndrome > arthropod bites, parasites, BP, DH, eosinophilic panniculitis |
| Floret cells | Multinucleated giant cells with marginally placed nuclei | Pleomorphic (spindle cell) lipoma |
| Flower cells | Atypical CD4+ T cells, prominent nuclear lobation | HTLV-1, ATL |
| Ghost cells | Calcified necrotic anucleate adipocytes with thickened membrane | Pancreatic panniculitis (+ saponification) (vs. shadow/ghost cells in pilomatricomas) |
| Giant granules in neutrophils | Large granules | Chédiak–Higashi |
| Globi | Globular clumps of AFB in macrophages (foam/lepra/virchow cells) | Lepromatous leprosy |
| Guarnieri bodies | Cytoplasmic, eosinophilic inclusions in epidermal cells | Smallpox, vaccinia |
| Henderson–Patterson bodies | Large, cytoplasmic, eosinophilic inclusions in keratinocytes | Molluscum contagiosum |

| | |
|---|---|
| Homer–Wright Rosettes | Central nerve fibrils, peripheral small tumor cells | Cutaneous neuroblastoma |
| Jordans' anomaly | Vacuolated leukocytes on peripheral smear | Dorfman–Chanarin |
| Kamino bodies | Eosinophilic globules at DEJ made of BMZ components | Spitz nevus |
| Lafora bodies | Concentric amyloid deposits (= polyglucosan bodies) | Lafora disease |
| Lipofuscin-like granules | Yellow-brown granules in dermal macrophages | Amiodarone hyperpigmentation |
| Macromelanosomes | Large melanosomes | Café au lait macules, Chédiak-Higashi, XP macules, Hermansky–Pudlak |
| Marquee sign | Organisms at the periphery of macrophages | Leishmania |
| Medlar/sclerotic bodies | Muriform cells, "copper pennies," round thick-walled brown fungi | Chromoblastomycosis |
| Michaelis–Gutman bodies | Calcified, degraded bacteria in macrophages, lamellated | Malakoplakia |
| Mikulicz cells | Large macrophages containing Klebsiella rhinoscleromatis | Rhinoscleroma |
| Morulae | Leukocyte intracytoplasmic inclusions, Ehrlichia multiplying in cell vacuoles | Ehrlichiosis |
| Mulberry bodies | Dermal mulberry-like endosporulation/sporangia | Protothecosis (vs. "mulberry-like figures" on EM in Fabry eccrine glands) |
| Mulberry cells | Moruloid, granular, eosinophilic adipocytes – "ping pong balls" | Hibernoma |
| Negri bodies | Eosinophilic, cytoplasmic inclusions in neurons | Rabies |

continued p. 174

173

| Body/sign/clue | Features | Diagnosis |
|---|---|---|
| Odland bodies | Small, lamellated granules rich in lipids in granular layer, membrane-coating granules on EM | Important for permeability barrier, absent in harlequin fetus |
| Onion skinning | Perivascular, hyaline material | Lipoid proteinosis (onion skin fibrosis in GF, angiofibroma) |
| Papillary mesenchymal bodies | Germinal hair bulb | Tricholastoma, trichoepithelioma |
| Pautrier microabscesses | Three or more atypical lymphocytes within epidermis | Mycosis fungoides |
| Pericapillary fibrin caps | | Venous leg ulcers, venous stasis, venous hypertension, non-venous leg ulcers |
| Pohl–Pinkus Marks | Isolated hair shaft narrowing (severe = bayonet hair) | Surgery, trauma |
| Psammoma bodies | Concentrically laminated, round, calcified bodies | Cutaneous meningioma, ovarian and thyroid neoplasms, papillary kidney carcinoma, mesothelioma |
| Pustulo-ovoid bodies of Milian | Large eosinophilic granules with clear halo | Granular cell tumor |
| Russell bodies | Immunoglobulin deposits in plasma cells | Rhinoscleroma, plasmacystosis |
| Spiderweb cells | Globular, striated, vacuolated cells | Adult rhabdomyoma |
| Splendore–Hoeppli deposits | Flame figure-like eosinophilic deposits around organisms | Parasites, fungus, bacteria |
| Verocay bodies | Palisading nuclei in rows around eosinophilic cytoplasm | Schwannoma |
| Weibel–Palade bodies | Dense rod or oval organelles on EM | Endothelial cells |

Adapted from Solky BA, Jones JL, Pipkin CA. *Boards' Fodder – Histologic Bodies* (http://www.aad.org/members/residents/fodder.html)

## Other derm path buzzwords, patterns, DDx

| Findings | Association(s) |
|---|---|
| **BUZZWORDS** | |
| "Sawtoothing" | Lichen planus |
| "Ball and claw" | Lichen nitidus (also see histiocytes) |
| "Swarm of bees" | Alopecia areata |
| "Toy soldiers," "strings of pearls," "fettucine collagen" | Mycosis fungoides |
| "Coat-sleeve" perivascular lymphocytosis | Gyrate erythema (consider lymphocytic vasculitis) |
| "Tea cup" scale/Tea cup sign (oblique, upwardly angulated parakeratosis) | Pityriasis rosea |
| "Dirty feet" | Solar lentigo (vs. "dirty fingers" – lentigo simplex), Becker's nevus |
| "Bubblegum stroma" | Neurofibroma |
| "Glassy collagen" | Keloid |
| "Tadpoles/sperm in the dermis" | Syringoma (if clear cell variant, think diabetes) |
| "Corn flakes" | Keratin granuloma |
| "Red crayons" (blood vessels) | Atrophie blanche |
| Eyeliner sign ("the thin brown line" – basal layer preventing invasion), "windblown" | Bowen |
| "Caput medusa" (radially streaming follicles/sebaceous glands) | Trichofolliculoma |
| "Crazy pavement" | Colloid milium > nodular amyloidosis |
| Collagen trapping | DF, DFSP (+ fat entrapment) |
| Squamous eddies | Irritated seborrheic keratosis, inverted follicular keratosis, incontinentia pigmenti |
| Checkerboard alternating para/ortho-keratosis | Pityriasis rubra pilaris |
| Mounding parakeratosis | Pityriasis rosea (+spongiosis, RBC extravasation), guttate psoriasis (+PMNs), PL (interface, lymphocytic vasculitis), nummular eczema |
| Layered dermal infiltrate | Necrobiosis lipoidica diabeticorum (+ necrobiosis, plasma cells) |
| Sandwich sign (PMNs between ortho and parakeratosis) | Tinea |

continued p. 176

| Findings | Association(s) |
|---|---|
| Cysts with arabesques lining | Lipodermatosclerosis |
| Nuclear molding | Merkel cell carcinoma ("bunch of grapes"), metastatic neuroendocrine carcinoma |
| Comedonecrosis ("comedo" pattern with central necrosis) | Sebaceous carcinoma |
| Wiry collagen (fibroplasias of papillary dermis) | Mycosis fungoides |

## GROWTH PATTERNS

| | |
|---|---|
| Storiform/cartwheel pattern | Storiform/sclerotic/plywood collagenoma, DF, DFSP, fibromyxoid sarcoma, schwannoma, solitary fibrous tumor, perineurioma, primary cutaneous meningioma |
| Herringbone pattern | Fibrosarcoma |
| Jigsaw puzzle pattern (+ "pink cuticle") | Cylindroma |
| Tissue culture pattern (+ microcysts) | Nodular fasciitis ("myxoid scar") |
| Chicken-wire vascular pattern | Myxoid liposarcoma (collapsed linear blood vessels) |
| Swiss cheese pattern ("oil cysts") | Sclerosing lipogranuloma |
| Reticulated pattern | Fibroepithelioma of pinkus, reticulated seborrheic keratosis, tumor of the follicular infundibulum |
| Peripheral palisading | Tumors: BCC, trichoepithelioma, basaloid follicular hamartoma, trichilemmoma (thick BM), tumor of the follicular infundibulum, sebaceoma, pilar tumor, schwannoma, epitheliod sarcoma (necrobiosis); Rashes: GA (mucin), RA/RF nodule (fibrinoid necrosis), gout (urate crystals), NLD (necrobiosis), NXG (degenerated collagen), palisaded neutrophilic and granulomatous dermatitis, eruptive xanthoma |

## DIFFERENTIAL DIAGNOSES

| | |
|---|---|
| Eosinophilic spongiosis | Arthropod bite, incontinentia pigmenti (First stage) (look for necrotic keratinocytes), pemphigus (esp. vegetans), BP, CP, herpes gestationis, PUPPP, ACD, eosinophilic folliculitis, id, drug |

| Findings | Association(s) |
|----------|----------------|
| Grenz zone | GF, EED, leprosy, lymphocytoma cutis, B-cell lymphoma/leukemia, acrodermatitis chronica atrophicans, DFSP/DF |
| Bland dermal spindle cell proliferations | DF, DFSP, neurofibroma, dermatomyofibroma, leiomyoma (perinuclear halo), solitary fibrous tumor |
| Atypical dermal spindle cell proliferations | AFX, melanoma, SCC, leiomyosarcoma, angiosarcoma ("falling apart" appearance), Kaposi (+ eosinophilic globules, promontory sign, plasma cells) |
| Small blue cell dermal proliferations | Glomus tumor, Merkel cell carcinoma, lymphoma, eccrine spiradenoma, metastatic carcinoma |
| Small red deep well-circumscribed tumor | Angioleiomyoma |
| Busy dermis | GA, interstitial granulomatous dermatitis, resolving vasculitis, folliculitis, early KS, desmoplastic MM, chronic photodermatosis, breast CA |
| Boxcar/square biopsy | Scleroderma, scleredema, scleromyxedema, NLD, nl back skin, radiation (prominent telangiectasia) |
| ~Normal appearance | TMEP, amyloidosis (lichen/macular-look for pigment incontinence), connective tissue nevus, myxedema, ichthyosis, cutis laxa, anetoderma, tinea versicolor, GVHD, argyria |
| Single filing of cells | Leukemia, (pseudo)lymphoma, metastatic carcinoma (breast), glomus cell tumor, GA, congenital melanocytic nevus, microcystic adnexal carcinoma |
| Pseudobullae (massive superficial dermal edema) | PMLE, sweet, erysipelas, erysipeloid, arthropod bite reaction, chilblains/perniosis |
| Pale epidermis | Pellagra, acrodermatitis enteropathica, necrolytic migratory erythema, Hartnup, clear cell acanthoma/papulosis |
| Basement membrane thickening (with rash) | Lupus, lichen sclerosis, dermatomysositis |
| Accessory polypoid lesion | Accessory tragus (vellus hairs), accessory nipple (smooth muscle, traumatic/amputation neuroma), accessory digit (nerves – vs. prominent often vertical collagen in acquired digital fibrokeratoma) |

*continued p. 178*

| Findings | Association(s) |
| --- | --- |
| Pagetoid spread | Paget's (spares basal layer), melanoma, SCC, Bowen, sebaceous carcinoma, MF, neuroendocrine tumor, rectal carcinoma |
| Wedge-shaped | Lymphomatoid papulosis (infiltrate), tick bite reaction (infiltrate), Degos (infarct), PLEVA (infiltrate) (EM-like with parakeratosis), lichen planus (wedge-shape hypergranulosis), melanocytic nevi (esp. with halo) |
| Peripheral collarette | Lobulated capillary hemangioma, cherry angioma, myxoid cyst, angiokeratoma, AFX, sebaceous adenoma, clear cell acanthoma |
| Lymphoid follicles | ALHE, pseudolymphoma (top heavy, well-formed, tingible body macs), B-cell lymphoma (bottom heavy, poorly-formed) |

**ARTIFACTS**

| | |
| --- | --- |
| Vacuolated keratinocytes | Freeze artifact |
| Ribbon-like blue material | Gel foam artifact |
| "Chafs of wheat" (spindled epidermal cells) | Electrodessication artifact |

**MINOCYCLINE PIGMENTATION**

| | |
| --- | --- |
| Type I: Facial, blue-black, scars | Iron stains +, melanin stains − (unlike types II and III, type I is not related to prolonged exposure to MCN) |
| Type II: Extremities, blue-gray | Iron stains +, Fontana reaction + but not melanin |
| Type III: Photodistributed or generalized, muddy brown | Epidermal hypermelanosis, melanin stains +, iron stains − |

**GIANT CELLS**

| | |
| --- | --- |
| Touton | Circumferential arrangement of nuclei ('wreath'), central glassy and foamy peripheral cytoplasm |
| Langhans | Horseshoe arrangement of nuclei |
| Foreign body | Haphazard nuclei |

| Cysts | Lining, contents | Clinical, hints |
|---|---|---|
| Keratinous, infundibular type (epidermoid) | Epidermis-like, includes granular layer, loose orthokeratin | Punctum, foreign body giant cell reaction |
| Milia | Like KCIT but thin wall and small | |
| Keratinous, trichilemmal type (pilar) | Stratified squamous, no granular layer, cholesterol clefts, compact keratin | Scalp, may calcify |
| Steatocystoma | Ruggated, thin stratified squamous, glassy pink surface, sebaceous glands | Pachyonychia congenital type II, KCIT-like keratin, trunk |
| Vellus hair cyst | Thin epidermal-like lining, laminated keratin, vellus hairs | Small, trunk, AD, numerous, ± pigment |
| Pigmented follicular | Stratified squamous, many pigmented hairs | M>F, pigmented, face |
| Apocrine hidrocystoma | Apocrine cells | Solitary, small, H/N, Schopf-Schulz-Passarge, focal dermal hypoplasia |
| Dermoid | Stratified squamous, adnexal structures | Lateral eyebrow, periocular, midline, newborn/infant |
| HPV-related | Epideral-like + inclusions, vacuolar changes, hypergranulosis, verrucous lining | HPV-60 related version on soles |
| Thyroglossal duct | Stratified squamous, may have cilia, columnar/ cuboidal elements | Thyroid follicles, midline neck |
| Branchial cleft | Stratified squamous, may have cilia, pseudostatified columnar elements | Lymph tissue, lateral neck, jaw, preauricular |
| Bronchogenic | Goblet cells, cilia, respiratory epithelial lining | Suprasternal, precordial, smooth muscle, cartilage, often neck |
| Cutaneous ciliated | Cilia, columnar/cuboidal | F>M, thighs/buttocks |
| Median raphe | Pseudostratified columnar, mucinous cells | Ventral penis/scrotum |
| Thymic | Stratified squamous or cuboidal, ± cilia | Thymic tissue, neck, mediastinum |

*continued p. 180*

| Pseudocyst of auricle | Within cartilage, no lining | Often asx, upper pinna |
| Digital mucous | No true lining, stellate fibroblasts, myxoid, thin overlying epidermis | Dorsal digit |
| Mucocele | No true lining, mucin, fibrous tissue, macs | Lower lip, buccal, salivary glands |
| Pilonidal | Sinus tract, inflammation, hair shafts | Sacrococcygeal |

# Part 2
# Surgery

*Handbook of Dermatology: A Practical Manual.* By Margaret W. Mann,
David R. Berk, Daniel L. Popkin, and Susan J. Bayliss. Published 2009 by Blackwell Publishing,
ISBN: 978-1-4051-8110-5.

# Surgical Margins Guidelines

| Tumor type | Tumor characteristic | Excision margin |
|---|---|---|
| Melanoma | *In situ* | 0.5 cm |
| | ≤1 mm in depth | 1 cm |
| | 1.01–2 mm in depth | 1–2 cm + SLN |
| | >2 mm | 2 cm + SLN |
| | (see melanoma guide pg. ) | |
| BCC | <2 cm in diameter | 3–4 mm |
| | >2 cm in diameter | 6 mm or Mohs |
| SCC | low risk* | 4 mm |
| | high risk** | 6 mm or Mohs |

*Low-risk SCC: well-defined margins, well differentiated, low-risk area, primary tumor.
**High-risk SCC: poorly defined margins, large size (>2 cm), poorly differentiated histologically, high-risk tumor location, recurrent tumor, invasion to subcutaneous fat, perineural invasion, organ transplant, or immunosuppressed patient. Adapted from *Huang* C and *Boyce SM.* Surgical margins of excision for basal cell carcinoma and squamous cell carcinoma. *Semin Cutan Med Surg.* 2004; 23:167–73.

## Indications for Mohs micrographic surgery

Location
- *Near functional/cosmetic structure*: eyes, nose, lips, fingers, hand, foot, genitals
- *High-risk locations*: H-zone of the face and skin overlying cartilage and bony structures: periorbital (inner canthus, eyelids); periauricular (ear, preauricular area, retroauricular sulcus); nose, temple; perioral (nasolabial folds, philtrum, upper lip, vermillion border).

Tumor features
- *Large size* (>2 cm any location; >1 cm on face, neck, scalp; >0.6 cm in H-zone)
- *Poorly defined* tumor
- *Recurrence/incomplete* prior excision
- *Aggressive histology*:
  - BCC with morpheaform, micronodular, basosquamous, or sclerosing type
  - SCC with poorly differentiated, acantholytic, adenosquamous, desmoplastic, infiltrative type
  - Perivascular/perineural invasion
  - Other tumors: microcystic adnexal carcinoma, DFSP, merkel cell carcinoma, malignant fibrous histiocytoma
- Location in scar, chronic ulcer (Marjolin's ulcer)
- Tumor arising in sites of *prior radiation Tx.*

SURGERY

Patient features

- *Immunosuppression*, transplant recipient, chronic lymphocytic leukemia, HIV
- History of multiple skin cancers
- Basal cell nevus, XP, Bazex syndromes.

# Guideline for Prophylactic Antibiotics

Use of antibiotic prophylaxis for endocarditis indicated for surgical procedure on infected tissue in patients with high-risk cardiac lesion or as detailed below

| Antibiotic (trade size) | Adults | Children |
|---|---|---|
| Cephalexin (500 mg, 250 mg/5 ml) | 2 g | 50 mg/kg |
| Dicloxacillin (500 mg, 250 mg/5 ml) | 2 g | 50 mg/kg |
| *If penicillin allergic* | | |
| Azithromycin (250, 500 mg) | 500 mg | 15 mg/kg |
| Clarithromycin (500 mg, 250 mg/5 ml) | 500 mg | 15 mg/kg |
| Clindamycin (300 mg) | 600 mg | 20 mg/kg |
| **Oral site:** | | |
| Amoxicillin (500 mg, 250 mg/5 ml) | 2 g | 50 mg/kg |
| *If penicillin allergic* | | |
| Azithromycin (250, 500 mg) | 500 mg | 15 mg/kg |
| Clarithromycin (500 mg, 250 mg/5 ml) | 500 mg | 15 mg/kg |
| Clindamycin (300 mg) | 600 mg | 20 mg/kg |
| **Groin and lower extremity site** | | |
| Cephalexin (500 mg, 250 mg/5 ml) | 2 g | 50 mg/kg |
| *If penicillin allergic* | | |
| Trimethoprim-Sulfamethoxazole, double strength 1 tab Levofloxacin | 500 mg | |

One hour prior to surgery: (all p.o. doses).

## Algorithm for antibiotic prophylaxis

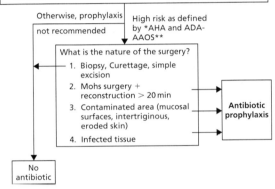

High risk cardiac conditions:*
- Prosthetic cardiac valve or prosthetic material used for valve repair
- Prior infective endocarditis
- Cardiac transplant recipients who develop valvulopathy
- Congenital heart disease (CHD), specifically, unrepaired cyanotic CHD, 1st 6 months after completely repaired CHD with prosthetic material or device, repaired CHD with residual defects which inhibit endothelialization (at or adjacent to prosthetic patch or device)

High risk for prosthetic joint infection:**
- First 2 years post joint replacement
- History of joint infections
- Immunocompromised/immunosuppressed patients
- Patients with malignancy, malnourish, hemophilia, or Type I diabetes

Otherwise, prophylaxis not recommended

High risk as defined by *AHA and ADA-AAOS**

What is the nature of the surgery?
1. Biopsy, Curettage, simple excision
2. Mohs surgery + reconstruction > 20 min
3. Contaminated area (mucosal surfaces, intertriginous, eroded skin)
4. Infected tissue

Antibiotic prophylaxis

No antibiotic

Adapted from *Wilson W. et al. Prevention of Infective Endocarditis. *Circulation* 2007; 116:1736–54; Messingham MJ and Arpey CJ. Update on the Use of Antibiotics in Cutaneous Surgery. *Derm Surg* 2005; 31:1068–78; **Wright TI, et al. Antibiotic prophylaxis in dermatologic surgery: advisory statement 2008. *J Am Acad Dermatol* 2008; 59:464–73.

SURGERY

# Guideline for Prophylactic Antivirals

History of HSV infection of the orofacial area is an indication for prophylaxis for facial resurfacing or orofacial surgery. Treat for 7–14 days with acyclovir, valacyclovir, or famciclovir to suppress viral reactivation during reepithelialization

| | |
|---|---|
| Acyclovir (Zovirax) | 400 mg tid x 7–14 d |
| Valacyclovir (Valtrex) | 500 mg bid x 7–14 d |
| Famciclovir (Famvir) | 250 mg bid x 7–14 d |

# Anesthetics

**Mechanism of action:** Reversibly inhibit nerve conduction by blocking sodium ion influx into peripheral nerve cells = prevent depolarization of nerves.

### Practical tips to decrease pain with injections

The patient
- Distract, pinch the skin
- Consider topical anesthesia (i.e. LMX) prior to infiltration.

The anesthetic agent
- Warming to 37–42°C
- Buffered lidocaine with bicarb (increase the pH 3.3 → 7.4)
  Add 1 cc 8.4% $NaHCO_3$ to 10 cc Lidocaine.

The injection technique
- Fine needle (27 or 30 gauge)
- Inject slowly
- If possible, through a dilated pore or wound edge
- Deeper injections into SQ area hurts less (go from deep subdermal to tight dermal)
- Minimize needle punctures by moving in a fan shape
- Consider nerve blocks or ring blocks.

---

| **Dose calculation** | $1\% = 1\,g/100\,ml = 10\,mg/cc$ |
|---|---|
| | $0.1\% = 0.1\,g/100\,ml = 1\,mg/cc$ |

---

## Tumescent anesthesia
Lidocaine 0.05–0.1% + epinephrine 1:1,000,000
Max tumescent is 35–50 mg/kg
Peak lidocaine level at 12–14 h

| Ingredient | Quantity (ml) |
|---|---|
| Normal saline 0.9% | 1000 |
| Lidocaine 1% | 50–100 |
| Sodium bicarbonate 8.4% | 10 |
| Epinephrine 1:1000 | 1 |

## Topical anesthetic (see drug section p. 253)

| | |
|---|---|
| LMX4 | Lidocaine 4% |
| EMLA cream* | 2.5% Lidocaine + 2.5% prilocaine |

*Risk of methemoglobinemia. Also, may create artefactual vacuolization/swelling of the upper epidermis and basal layer damage/clefting.
Cavef A et al. Histologic Cutaneous Modifications After the Use of EMLA Cream. *Arch Derm*. 2007; 143:1074–76.

SURGERY

## Adverse reaction to local anesthetics

| Condition | Pulse | BP | Signs and symptoms | Management |
|---|---|---|---|---|
| Vasovagal Rxn | ▼ | ▼ | Diaphoresis, hyperventilation, nausea | Trendelenburg, cool compress |
| Epinephrine Rxn | ▲ | ▲ | Sweating, tachypnea, HA, palpitation | Reassurance, beta-blocker |
| Anaphylaxis | ▲ | ▼ | Tachycardia, bronchospasm | Epinephrine 1:1000 × 0.3 ml SQ. Antihistamine, airway maintenance |
| **Lidocaine Toxicity** | | | | |
| 1–6 µg/ml | Nl | Nl | Circumoral paresthesia, metallic taste, tinnitus, lightheadedness | Observe |
| 6–9 µg/ml | Nl | Nl | Tremors, nausea, vomiting, hallucination | Diazepam, airway maintenance |
| 9–12 µg/ml | ▼ | ▼ | Seizures, cardiopulmonary depression | Respiratory support |
| >12 µg/ml | – | – | Coma, cardiopulmonary arrest | CPR/ACLS |

Adapted from Snow SN, Mikhail GR. Mohs Micrographic Surgery. Madison: The University of Wisconsin Press, 2004, 2nd Edition. Chapter 14. Table 14-3.

## Local anesthetic

| Generic name | Trade name | Pregnancy category† | Potency | Onset (min) | Without epinephrine | | With epinephrine | |
|---|---|---|---|---|---|---|---|---|
| | | | | | Duration (min) | Max dose (mg/kg) for adults | Duration (min) | Max dose (mg/kg) for adults |
| **AMIDE ("I" before –caine = amide)** | | | | | | | | |
| Lidocaine | Xylocaine | B | Intermed | <2 | 30–120 | 4.5 (30cc for 70kg) | 60–400 | 7 (50cc for 70kg) |
| Bupivacaine | Marcaine, Sensorcaine | C* | High | 2–10 | 120–240 | 2.5 | 240–480 | 3 |
| Mepivacaine | Carbocaine | C* | Intermed | 3–20 | 30–120 | 6 | 60–400 | 8 |
| Prilocaine | Citanest | B | Intermed | 5–6 | 30–120 | 7 | 60–400 | 10 |
| Etidocaine | Duranest | B | High | 3–5 | 200 | 4.5 | 240–360 | 6.5 |
| **ESTER** | | | | | | | | |
| Procaine | Novocain | C | Low | 5 | 15–30 | 10 | 30–90 | 14 |
| Chloroprocaine | Nesacaine | C | Low | 5–6 | 30–60 | 10 | – | – |
| Tetracaine | Pontocaine | C | High | 7 | 120–240 | 2 | 240–480 | 2 |

†Epinephrine is pregnancy category C.

*Bupivacaine and mepivacaine: pregnancy category C due to potential for fetal bradycardia.

| | Metabolized by | Excretion | Allergic reaction |
|---|---|---|---|
| **AMIDE** | Liver dealkylation | Kidney | Rare, due to preservative methylparaben (if allergic: switch to preservative free lidocaine) |
| **ESTER** | Tissue (pseudocholinesterase) | Kidney | More common due to metabolite to PABA (*p*-aminobenzoic acid) (if allergic: switch to amides) |

## Nerve blocks*
See Plates 1–4.

# Surgical Anatomy

## Anatomy of the face
### Cosmetic unit of the central face

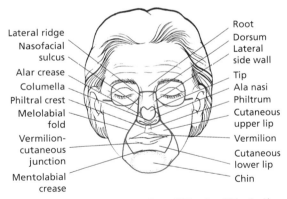

Lateral ridge
Nasofacial sulcus
Alar crease
Columella
Philtral crest
Melolabial fold
Vermilion-cutaneous junction
Mentolabial crease

Root
Dorsum
Lateral side wall
Tip
Ala nasi
Philtrum
Cutaneous upper lip
Vermilion
Cutaneous lower lip
Chin

From Robinson JK (ed.). *Atlas of Cutaneous Surgery.* WB Saunders: 1996, p. 2, with permission from Elsevier.

SURGERY

189

## Cosmetic units of the cheek

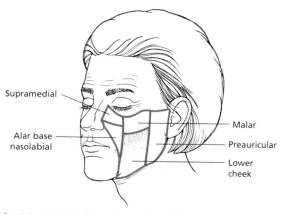

Supramedial

Malar

Alar base nasolabial

Preauricular

Lower cheek

From Robinson JK (ed.). *Atlas of Cutaneous Surgery.* WB Saunders: 1996, p. 2, with permission from Elsevier.

## Cosmetic units of the forehead

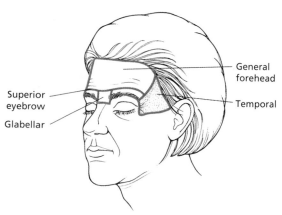

General forehead

Superior eyebrow

Temporal

Glabellar

From Robinson JK (ed.). *Atlas of Cutaneous Surgery.* WB Saunders: 1996, p. 2, with permission from Elsevier.

## Cosmetic units of the nose

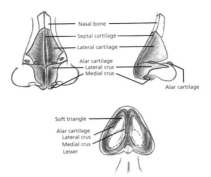

Courtesy of Dr. Quan Vu

## Anatomy of the nasal cartilage

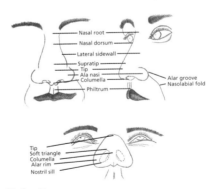

Courtesy of Dr. Quan Vu

## Anatomy of the ear

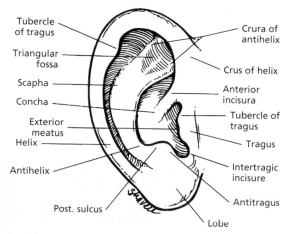

From Robinson JK (ed.). *Atlas of Cutaneous Surgery.* WB Saunders: 1996, p. 186, with permission from Elsevier.

## Cosmetic units of the eye

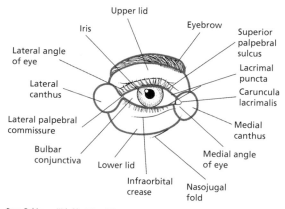

From Robinson JK (ed.). *Atlas of Cutaneous Surgery.* WB Saunders: 1996, p. 3, with permission from Elsevier.

## Anatomy of the eye

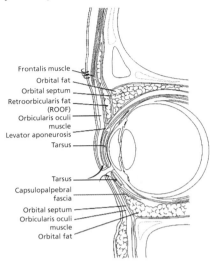

Frontalis muscle
Orbital fat
Orbital septum
Retroorbicularis fat
(ROOF)
Orbicularis oculi
muscle
Levator aponeurosis
Tarsus

Tarsus
Capsulopalpebral
fascia
Orbital septum
Orbicularis oculi
muscle
Orbital fat

From Robinson JK (ed.). *Atlas of Cutaneous Surgery.* WB Saunders: 1996, p. 3, with permission from Elsevier.

## Anatomy of the nail

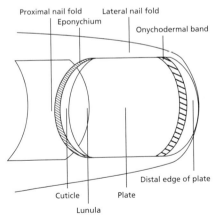

Proximal nail fold    Lateral nail fold
Eponychium
Onychodermal band

Distal edge of plate

Cuticle    Plate
Lunula

From Scher RK and Daniel CR. *Nails: Therapy, Diagnosis, Surgery.* WB Saunders: 1997, pp. 13–14, with permission from Elsevier.

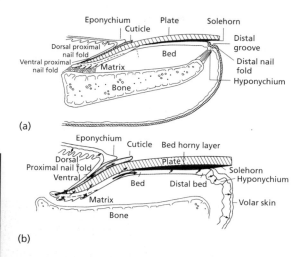

(a)

(b)

## Danger zones in surgery
## Danger zones of the face

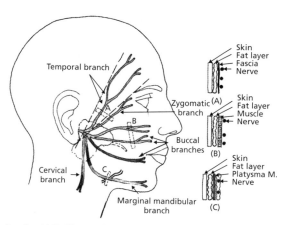

From Bernstein G. *J Dermatol Surg Oncol.* 12; 1986, p. 725, with permission from BC Decker Inc.

## Danger zones: location and innervation

1. Temporal branch of CN VII

   Most vulnerable location: Mid-zygomatic arch.

   Nerve course: Nerve exits the superior–anterior portion of the parotid gland, then courses 0.5 cm below the tragus to 1.5 cm above the lateral eyebrow. Nerve lies just beneath the skin, subcutaneous fat, and SMAS.

   Motor innervation: Frontalis, upper portion of the orbicularis oculi and corrugator supercilii.

   Damage: Inability to raise eyebrow and wrinkle forehead. Results in a flat forehead and droopy eyebrow.

2. Marginal mandibular branch of CN VII

   Most vulnerable location: Mid-mandible 2 cm lateral to the oral commissure.

   Nerve course: Nerve exits the inferior–anterior portion of the parotid gland, then courses along the angle of the mandible across the facial artery and vein. May be 2 cm or more below the inferior edge of the mandible if the head is rotated or hyperextended. Lies beneath the skin, subcutaneous fat and SMAS.

   Motor innervation: Orbicularis oris, risorius, mentalis, and depressor muscles of the mouth.

   Damage: Drooping of the mouth, inability to pull the lip laterally and inferiorly with smiling.

3. Great auricular nerve (C$_2$ and C$_3$)

   Most vulnerable location: 6.5 cm below the external auditory canal along the posterior border of the sternocleidomastoid muscle.

   Nerve course: Nerve courses toward the lobule posterior to the external jugular vein.

   Damage: Sensory innervation, results in numbness of the inferior 2/3 of the ear and adjacent cheek and neck.

4. Spinal accessory nerve (CN XI)

   Most vulnerable location: Erb's point.

   Nerve course: Nerve exits from behind the SCM at Erb's point and courses diagonally and inferiorly across the posterior triangle. Draw a line from the angle of the jaw to the mastoid process – Erb's point is located 6 cm vertically below the midpoint of this line at the posterior border of the sternocleidomastoid (within a 2 cm area). Also may define area by drawing a line horizontally across the neck from the thyroid notch to the posterior border of the sternocleidomastoid (1 cm above and 1 cm below).

   Innervation: Location of the great auricular, less occipital, and spinal accessory nerve. The spinal accessory nerve innerves the trapezius muscle.

   Damage: Winged scapula – inability to shrug the shoulder and abduct the arm.

## Danger zone of the neck: Erb's point

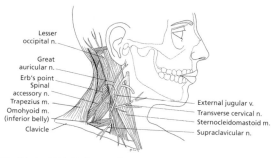

From Wheeland RG (ed.). *Cutaneous Surgery*. WB Saunders: 1994, p. 61, with permission from Elsevier.

## Dermatomal distribution of sensory nerves

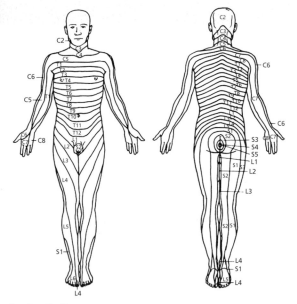

From Leventha. *Fractures, dislocations, and fracture–dislocations of the spine.* In: Canale ST et al. (eds). Campbell's operative orthopaedics, 10th edition. Mosby: 2003, with permission from Elsevier.

## Anatomy of the lower extremity venous system

From Min RJ et al. Duplex ultrasound evaluation of lower extremity venous insufficiency. *J Vasc Interv Radiol* 2003; 14:1233–41, with permission from Elsevier.

### Anatomy of the greater saphenous vein

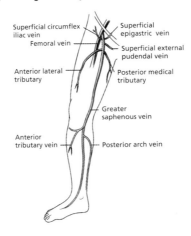

### Anatomy of the perforator veins

### Anatomy of the short saphenous vein

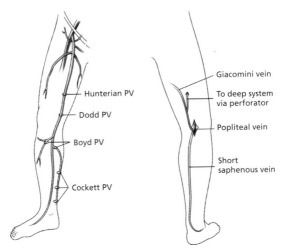

SURGERY

# Cutaneous Reconstruction

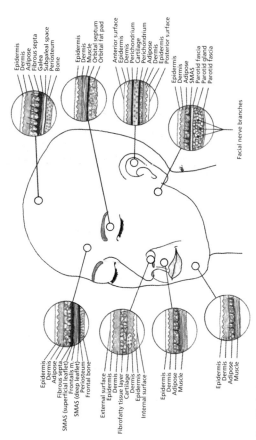

Epidermis
Dermis
Adipose
Fibrous septa
Galea
Subgaleal space
Periosteum
Bone

Epidermis
Dermis
Muscle
Orbital septum
Orbital fat pad

Anterior surface
Epidermis
Dermis
Perichondrium
Cartilage
Perichondrium
Adipose
Dermis
Epidermis
Posterior surface

Epidermis
Dermis
Adipose
SMAS
Parotid fascia
Parotid gland
Parotid fascia

Facial nerve branches

Epidermis
Dermis
Adipose
Fibrous septa
Frontalis m.
SMAS (superficial leaflet)
SMAS (deep leaflet)
Periosteum
Frontal bone

External surface
Epidermis
Dermis
Fibrofatty tissue layer
Cartilage
Dermis
Epidermis
Internal surface

Epidermis
Dermis
Adipose
Muscle

Epidermis
Dermis
Adipose
Muscle

From Wheeland RG (ed.). *Cutaneous Surgery*. WB Saunders; 1994, p. 51, with permission from Elsevier.

## Undermining depths in reconstruction

| Scalp | Subgaleal |
|---|---|
| Forehead | Subgaleal or subcutaneous fat above frontalis fascia |
| Temple/zygomatic arch | Superficial subcutaneous fat above temporal branch of facial nerve |
| Mandible | Superficial subcutaneous fat above marginal mandibular branch of facial nerve |
| Ear | Above perichondrium |
| Lip | Above orbicularis oris |
| Nose | Above perichondrium/periosteum |
| Rest of face | Superficial subcutaneous fat, above the parotid duct |
| Terminal hair bearing area | Deep to hair papillae |
| Lateral neck | Superficial subcutaneous fat above spinal accessory nerve |
| Trunk/extremities | Above muscular fascia |
| Hands and feet | Subdermal |

# Repair Options: STAIRS

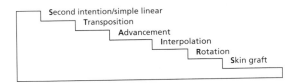

Second intention/simple linear
Transposition
Advancement
Interpolation
Rotation
Skin graft

## Second intention
### Cosmetic result of wound healing by secondary intention according to anatomical site

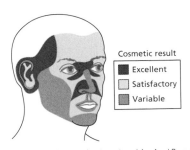

Cosmetic result
- ■ Excellent
- □ Satisfactory
- ▨ Variable

From Zitelli JA. Wound healing by secondary intention. *J Am Acad Dermatol.* 1983; 9:407–415, with permission from Elsevier.

- Ideal for
  - Concave areas: Periorbital (medial canthus), temple, conchal bowl, alar crease
  - Shallow defects (i.e. shins)
  - Fair skinned patient (wound tends to heal with whiten scar)
  - Poor operative candidates
- May take weeks/months to heal, so patient must be able to perform wound care
- May heal with atrophic, hypertrophic, white scar
- Can perform delayed repair/graft at 2–4 weeks.

## Simple linear closure
- 3–4:1 Length:width ratio
- Orient along relaxed skin tension lines at junction of cosmetic subunits.

### Relaxed skin tension line (RSTL) on the face showing orientation of simple linear closure

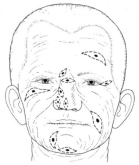

From Burge S and Rayment R. *Simple Skin Surgery.* Blackwell Scientific, 1986, with permission from Blackwell Publishing.

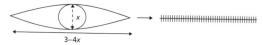

### M-plasty
- Modification of the linear closure
- GOAL: Shortens the length of a scar

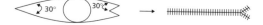

## Transposition flap

- GOAL: Redistribute tension vectors
- Flap rotates about a pivotal point at the base of the pedicle and is transposed over an island of normal skin
- Pivotal restraints may limit its movement
- Wide undermining necessary to prevent pincushioning
- Common flaps: Rhombic, bilobe, z-plasty, banner, nasolabial (melolabial).

### Rhombic

- Used for small defects where adjacent tissue is available to rotate onto defect
- Changes the tension vector along the secondary defect (perpendicular to tension across primary defect)
- Classic rhombic (Limberg) consists of parallelogram with 60° and 120°
- Common locations: Medial canthus, upper 2/3 of nose, lower eyelid, temple, peripheral cheek.

SURGERY

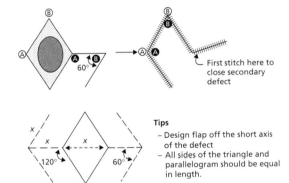

First stitch here to close secondary defect

**Tips**
- Design flap off the short axis of the defect
- All sides of the triangle and parallelogram should be equal in length.

*Modifications of rhombic flaps*
<u>Webster 30°</u>
Narrower flap, easier to close secondary defect
Less reorientation of tension vectors

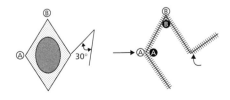

<u>Dufourmental</u>
Compromise between Limberg and Webster flap
Extend dotted lines then bisect them
Second incision parallel to defect midline

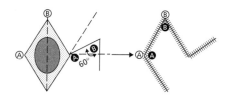

<u>Bi-rhombic flap</u>

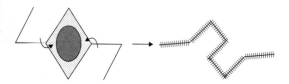

## Bilobe

- Used for small defects 1–1.5 cm in size. Common location: lower 1/3 of nose
- Tension is shared between the secondary and tertiary defects.

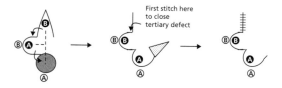

First stitch here to close tertiary defect

*Zitelli-modified bilobe flap*

- Determine location of standing cone, then draw ~90° (Zitelli modification) line
- First lobe is at 45° – equal or slightly smaller than defect
- Second lobe is at 90° to the standing cone
- Wide undermining in the submuscular plane to prevent trapdoor effect.

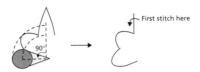

Z-plasty

- GOAL: Changing the direction of a scar or to elongate a scar
- Limbs of the Z should be of equal lengths

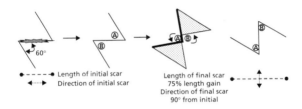

- The degree of the limbs determines both the direction and the length of final scar.

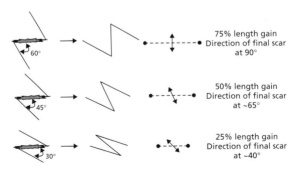

## Advancement flap

- GOAL: Modification of the linear closure, with standing cones (Burow triangle) displaced to a more desirable position (i.e. away from free margin)
- Tension vector remains parallel to the motion of the flap
- Types of advancement flaps: U-plasty, H-plasty, Burow advancement, modified crescentic advancement, O → T, island pedicle.

### U-plasty/O → U: unilateral advancement

- Burow triangles created away from defect in one direction
- Useful along eyebrow and helical rim.

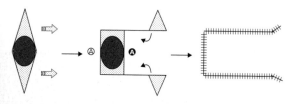

### H-plasty/O → H: bilateral advancement

- Burow triangles created away from defect bilaterally
- Useful if tissue reservoir is available bilaterally.

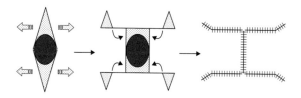

### Burow's advancement flap: unilateral advancement

- Displaces one of the standing cone to a more desirable location
- Useful if defect is along lateral upper cutaneous lip → may displace one of the standing cone to the nasolabial folds.

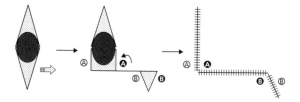

## Modified crescentic advancement flap: unilateral advancement

- Modification of the Burow triangle
- Crescentic standing cone removed along the flap to lengthen it
- Eliminates the need for excision of a standing cone.

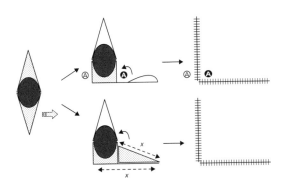

## 0 → T/T-Plasty/A → T: bilateral advancement

- Displaces one of the standing cone bilaterally
- Useful adjacent to a free margin or along the junction between two cosmetic units (brow, eyelid, forehead, lip).

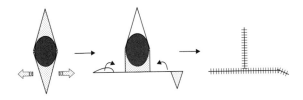

## Island pedical flap/kite/V → Y advancement

- Island of tissue detached from periphery but with underlying subcutaneous and muscular pedicle
- Caution: no undermining to base of island – must keep flap attached to underlying pedicle to ensure good blood supply.

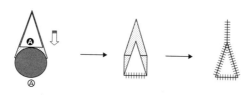

## Interpolation flap

- GOAL: Coverage of large defects requiring flap with robust blood supply
- Commonly axial pattern flap-based on named direct cutaneous artery
- Robust blood supply allow greater ratio of length to width
- Two-staged procedure
- Base is usually located at some distance from defect. Pedicle must pass over or under an intervening bridge of intact skin
- Types of flaps: Paramedian, nasolabial, abbe.

| Flap | Arterial supply | Defect location | Pedicle division |
|------|-----------------|-----------------|------------------|
| Paramedian forehead | Supratrochlear artery | Large distal nasal defect | 2–3 weeks |
| Retroauricular helical | Random flap: rich vascular supply from posterior auricular, superficial temporal, and occipital branches | Large helical rim defect | 3 weeks |
| Nasolabial | Angular artery | Large ala defect | 2–3 weeks |
| Abbe | Superior or inferior labial artery | Large lip defect | 3 weeks |

## Rotation flap
- GOAL: Covering a defect when there is an abundant surrounding tissue reservoir
- Pivotal flap with a curvilinear incision—the flap and defect form a semicircle
- Rotates in an arc about a pivotal point near the defect
- Distributes the tension vector along the curvilinear line
- Common locations: Scalp, lateral cheek, infraorbital, temple
- Types of rotation flaps: Unilateral rotation, bilateral rotation (O → Z), pinwheel, dorsal nasal flap, Tenzel/Mustarde flaps.

## Unilateral rotation flap
- Usually flap is inferiorly/laterally based to improve lymphatic drainage and decrease flap edema
- Consider backcut to improve mobility.

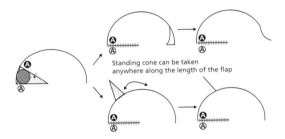

Standing cone can be taken anywhere along the length of the flap

## O → Z Plasty/bilateral rotation flap
- Useful when there is insufficient tissue reservoir for unilateral flap
- Common location: scalp.

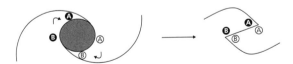

## Dorsal nasal rotation/Reiger/hatchet flap
- Useful for nasal defect <2.5 cm on the lower 2/3 of the nose, best if midline
- Flap along the entire nasal dorsal
- Undermine at the level of the perichondrium/periosteum
- Backcut in the glabella.

SURGERY

## Mustarde/Tenzel rotation flap
- Laterally based cheek rotation flap
- Useful for defect along supramedial cheek/lower eyelid
- Mustarde flap mobilizes entire cheek for defect >½ of eyelid
- Tenzel flaps mobilizes partial cheek for defect <½ eyelid.

# Skin graft
- GOAL: Surgical defect which cannot be closed with adjacent local skin or allowed to heal by second intention; useful for larger wounds, especially in areas that require tumor surveillance
- Stages of skin graft

| Stage | Events | Graft | Timeline |
|---|---|---|---|
| Imbibition | "Ischemic period" – nutrient through osmosis (bolster improves osmosis) | Dark color, edematous | 24–48 h |
| Inosculation | Anastomosis of existing blood vessels | Pink | 48–72 h (up to 10 days) |
| Neovascularization | New capillary ingrowth to graft from wound bed | Hypopigment, less edema | 6–7 days |

- Three major types:
  - (1) Full thickness skin graft (FTSG) = epidermis + full dermis
  - (2) Split thickness skin graft (STSG) = epidermis + partial dermis
  - (3) Composite graft = skin (epidermis and dermis) + additional component (cartilage or fat).

# FTSG
- Minimal contraction ~15%
- Better cosmesis than STSG – good color, texture, and thickness match
- Must have intact perichondrium/periosteum for survival – higher metabolic demand than STSG = higher rates of graft failure
- Most useful for defects less than 3 cm
- Common sites: Eyelids, medial canthus, helical rim, conchal bowl, nasal tip, digits
- Good donor sites: Preauricular/postauricular area, supraclavicular, standing cones (Burow graft), conchal bowl, upper eyelid, forehead.

# STSG
- Higher risk for contraction, poor cosmesis
- Useful for very large defects: Can use fenestration/meshing to enlarge size

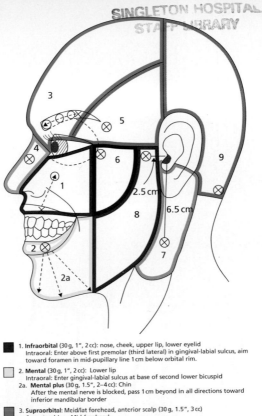

1. **Infraorbital** (30 g, 1", 2 cc): nose, cheek, upper lip, lower eyelid
   Intraoral: Enter above first premolar (third lateral) in gingival-labial sulcus, aim toward foramen in mid-pupillary line 1 cm below orbital rim.

2. **Mental** (30 g, 1", 2 cc): Lower lip
   Intraoral: Enter gingival-labial sulcus at base of second lower bicuspid
   2a. **Mental plus** (30 g, 1.5", 2–4 cc): Chin
   After the mental nerve is blocked, pass 1 cm beyond in all directions toward inferior mandibular border

3. **Supraorbital**: Meid/lat forehead, anterior scalp (30 g, 1.5", 3 cc)
   Supratrochlear: Mid-forehead
   Infratrochlear: Medial upper eyelids, upper side of nose
   Enter along the orbital rim at the lateral 1/3 of the eyebrow aiming toward the supraorbital notch. Inject 1 cc lateral to the notch, 1 cc medial to the notch, and 1 cc when the needle advances to the nasal bone.

4. **Dorsal nasal** (30 g, 1", 1–2 cc): Cartilaginous nasal dorsum and tip.
   Inject ~1 cc lateral to the distal tip of the nasal bone.

5. **Zygomaticotemporal** (30 g, 1.5", 1–2 cc): Lateral orbital rim/temple.
   Inject inferior to the zygomaticofrontal suture, 1 cm lateral to the orbital rim.
   Inject 1 cc over the lacrimal gland for upper lateral eyelid (lacrimal nerve).

6. **Zygomaticofacial** (30 g, 1.5", 1–2 cc): Superior/lateral cheek.
   Inject just lateral to the lateral/inferior border of the orbital rim.

7. **Great auricular** (30 g, 1", 1–2 cc): Lower 1/3 ear, lower postauricular
   Inject over mid-SCM, 6.5 cm below the external auditory meatus.

8. **V3-mandib** (22–23 g spinal needle, 3–4 cc): Most of cheek, upper preauric.
   Insert 90° at the sigmoid notch (b/n condyle and coranoid process)
   2.5 cm anterior to the tragus. Advance to the ptygoid plate, mark needle, retract to skin, redirect 1 cm posterior, insert to mark, then aspirate and inject.

9. **Occipital** (30 g, 1", 5 cc): Posterior scalp
   Inject medial to the occipital artery (palpate at the superior nuchal line)
   OR inject along superior medial line b/n occipital protuberance and mastoid.

**Plate 1.** Facial nerve blocks. (Courtesy of Dr. Stacey Tull.)

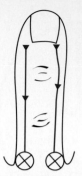

- 2 dorsal and 2 volar nerves
- Inject 1–2 cc of 2% plain lido on each side of digit distal to the MCP (or MTP) joint
- Maximum of 6–8 cc to avoid circulatory compromise

**Plate 2.** Digital nerve block. (Courtesy of Dr. Stacey Tull.)

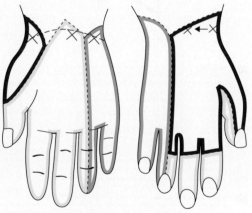

**Wrist**

■ **Radial:** Inject lateral to the radial artery at the proximal wrist crease to the midpoint of the dorsal wrist

■ **Ulnar:** Inject at the proximal wrist crease medial to the flexor carpi ulnaris (ring finger)

□ **Median:** Inject at the proximal wrist crease b/n palmaris longus and flexor carpi radialis (long finger)

**Plate 3.** Nerve block of the hand. (Courtesy of Dr. Stacey Tull.)

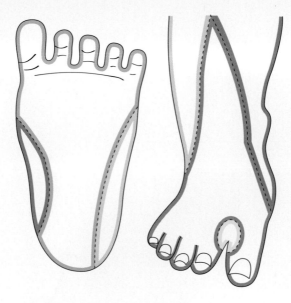

**Ankle**

- ▢ **Sural:** Inject 5 cc midway between Achilles and lateral malleolus
- ▢ **Post tibial:** Inject 3–5 cc posterior to PT artery below the medial malleolus
- ▢ **Saphenous:** Inject 5 cc along the long saphenous vein 1 cm above the medial malleolus
- ▢ **Supra peroneal:** Inject 5 cc from 5 cm above lateral malleolus to the anterior tib
- ▢ **Deep peroneal:** Skip it (mostly for deep structures)–use local for skin here.

**Plate 4.** Nerve block of the foot. (Courtesy of Dr. Stacey Tull.)

- Donor site heal by second intention can be painful
- Large grafts need to be harvested with special equipment
- Better survival than FTSG due to low nutritional requirements
  - Thin: 0.005–0.012 in.
  - Medium: 0.012–0.018 in.
  - Thick: 0.018–0.028 in.

## Composite graft

- Less likely to contract, better cosmesis
- Highest risks for necrosis due to avascular tissue (cartilage) and thicker graft
- Useful when bulk and structural support is needed (i.e. nasal alar defects).

| Types of graft | Nutritional needs | Risk of graft failure | Cosmesis and tissue match | Contraction risk | Durability/ Strength | Sensation |
|---|---|---|---|---|---|---|
| FTSG | High | Higher | Good | Low | Good | Good |
| STSG | Low | Lower | Poor | High | Poor | Fair |
| Composite | High | Highest | Good | Low | Excellent | Fair |

*Causes of graft failure*
- Poor blood and nutritional supply: Nicotine use, nutritional deficiency, collagen vascular disease
- Poor graft bed contact: Graft movement (activity, trauma, poor immobilization), hematoma, seroma
- Infection: Immunosuppression, diabetes, systemic disease, poor wound care
- Physician technique: Incomplete defatting, high tension due to inadequate size, rough tissue handling, excessive cautery.

SURGERY

# Sutures

## Absorbable

| Material | Origin | Filament | Tensile strength 50% | Absorption | Reactivity | Degradation |
|---|---|---|---|---|---|---|
| Plain gut | Animal collagen* | Twisted | 1 week | 14–80 days | High | Proteolysis |
| Fast absorbing gut | Animal collagen* | Twisted | 3–7 days | 21–42 days | High | Proteolysis |
| Vicryl rapide | Polyglactin | Braided | 5 days | 42 days | Moderate | Hydrolysis |
| Monocryl | Poliglecaprone | Monofil | 1 week | 90–120 days | Low | Hydrolysis |
| Chromic gut | Plain gut tanned with chromium salts | Twisted | 2–3 weeks | 30–80 days | High, less than plain gut | Proteolysis |
| Dexon | Polyglycolic acid | Braided | 2–3 weeks | 90 days | Low | Hydrolysis |
| Vicryl | Polyglactin | Braided | 3 weeks | 80–90 days | Moderate | Hydrolysis |
| PDS | Polydioxanone | Monofil | 4 weeks | 180 days | Low | Hydrolysis |
| Maxon | Polyglyconate | Monofil | 4 weeks | 180 days | Very low | Hydrolysis |

*Gut made from mucosal/submucosa of sheep or beef intestine.

## Non-absorbable

| Material | Origin | Filament | Tensile strength | Reactivity | Elasticity | Handling |
|---|---|---|---|---|---|---|
| Silk | Silk | Braided or twisted | Low, 3–6 months | High | Inelastic Soft suture | Best |
| Prolene/ Surgilene | Polypropylene | Monofil | High, 2 years | Least | Very elastic Stiff suture | Fair–good |
| Ethilon/Monosol/ Dermalon | Nylon | Monofil | High, losing 10–20%/year | Low | Mild elasticity Stiff suture | Fair |
| Surgilon/Nurolon/ Mersilene | Nylon Polyester | Braded Monofil or braided | High, losing 10–20%/year High, permanent | Moderate Low | Mild elasticity Mild elasticity | Good Very good |
| Ethibond/Dacron Novafil | Polybutester | Monofil | High | Low | Very elastic | Very good |

## Suture removal time

| Area | Removal time (days) |
|---|---|
| Face | 4–5 |
| Neck | 5–7 |
| Scalp | 7 |
| Trunk | 7–12 |
| Extremities | 10–14 |

## Electrosurgery*

| Modality | Terminals | Gap output | Voltage | Amperage | Capability |
|---|---|---|---|---|---|
| Electrodessi-cation | 1 | Markedly damped | High | Low | Superficial destruction |
| Electrofulgu-ration | 1 | Markedly damped | High | Low | Superficial destruction (spark gap) |
| Electrocoagu-lation | 2 | Moderately damped | Mod | Mod | Deep penetration and destruction, Good hemostasis |
| Electrosection | 2 | Undamped | Low | High | Cutting |

*Electrocautery: not electrosurgery, no electric current, uses heat conduction.

## Wound Healing

| Time | Tensile strength vs. baseline |
|---|---|
| 1 week | 5% |
| 1 month | 40% |
| 1 year | 80% |

- Three phases of wound healing: Inflammatory (days) → Proliferation/ Granulation (weeks) → Remodeling (months)
- Platelets are the first cells to appear
- Collagen: Early in wound healing, Collagen III predominates, then later replaced by Collagen I.

SURGERY

# Wound dressing

|  | Brand name | Composition | Absorptive | Others | Indications |
|---|---|---|---|---|---|
| **Adhesive dressing** | | | | | |
| Hydrocolloids | Duoderm | Hydrophilic base and adhesive with polyurethane | Good, forms gel with exudates | May leave in place × 1 week | Pressure ulcers, second intention wounds |
| Film dressing | Tegederm Op-site Bioocclusive | Polyurethane file | None (may cause fluid collection) Gas permeable | Impermeable to bacteria | Best used in conjunction with alginate/hydrogen. Good for monitoring wounds. Lacerations/abrasions/STSG donor site |
| **Non-adhesive dressing** | | | | | |
| Alginates | Sorbsan algiderm | Alginic acid | Highly | Hemostatic agent: releases $Ca^{++}$ | Highly exudative wounds |
| Hydrogels | Vigilon tegagel | 1% water, cross-linked polymers Semitransparent gel | Highly | Cooling/pain relief | Abrasion wounds (post laser, peels) |
| Foam dressing | Flexzan Allevyn Vigifoam | Hydrophilic foam, polyurethane, silicone | Moderate, gas and water permeable | Compresses chronic leg wounds, conforms to body contours | Pressure ulcer, exudative wound |
| Gauze dressing | Telfa pad Vaseline gauze, Xeroform | | Excellent | Cheap, readily available | Use to cover nonocclusive, nonadherent dressing |

SURGERY

# Antiseptic Scrubs

| Agent | Mechanism of action | Gram+ | Gram− | Mycobacteria | Viruses | Fungi | Spores | Speed of action | Residual activity | Other |
|---|---|---|---|---|---|---|---|---|---|---|
| Alcohol 60–95% | Denature proteins (bacterial cell wall) | +++ | +++ | +++ | +++ | +++ | − | Fast | None | Flammable with laser/cautery. Allow to dry on surface |
| Chlorhexidine 2–4% (Hibiclens) | Impairs cell membrane | +++ | ++ | + | +++ | + | − | Intermed | Excellent | Ototoxicity, keratitis, skin irritant |
| Iodine 3% (Lugol) | Oxidation | +++ | +++ | +++ | +++ | ++ | + | Intermed | Minimal | Skin irritant inactivated by blood/sputum |
| Iodophors-(Betadine) Povidone-iodine 7.5–10% | Oxidation/ substitution by free iodine: disrupts S–H and N–H bonds, C=C bonds in fatty acids | +++ | +++ | + | ++ | ++ | − | Intermed (needs to dry) | Minimal | Skin irritant (less than iodine). Inactivated by blood/sputum. May cross-react with radiopaque iodine. Surfactant + iodine = iodophor |

| | Mechanism of action | | | | | | Speed | | Comments |
|---|---|---|---|---|---|---|---|---|---|
| TechniCare PCMX Chloroxylenol | Disrupt cell membrane | +++ | + | + | + | Unknown | Slow | Good | Addition of EDTA increases its activity against Pseudomonas |
| Triclosan 0.2–2% | Disrupts cell wall, inhibits fatty acid synthesis, binds bacterial enoyl-acyl carrier protein reductase (ENR, *fabl*) | +++ | ++ | + | +++ | − | Unknown | Intermed | Good | Forms chloroform and dioxins when combined with chlorine in tap water |
| Benzalkonium (Quaternary ammonium) | Dissociation of cell membranes; disrupts intermolecular interactions | ++ | + | +/− | + Lipophilic +/− | Unknown | Slow | Good | Use only in combination with alcohols. Eyedrop preservative. Easily inactivated by cotton gauze/organic materials |

Adapted from *CDC. MMWR Recomm Rep.* 2002; 25:51(RR-ˈ6):1–48

SURGERY

# Lasers

| Laser | Wavelength (nm) | Type | Depth (µm) | Target | Usage |
|---|---|---|---|---|---|
| $CO_2$ | 10,600 | IR | 20 | Water | Resurface, destruction, coagulation, cut |
| Erbium:YAG | 2940 | IR | 1 | Water | Superficial resurface, destruction |
| Holmium:YAG | 2100 | IR | 200 | Water | Superficial resurface, destruction |
| Nd:YAG | 1064 | IR | 1600 | Mel, Hb | Deep dermal pigment, black/ blue tattoo, epilation, non-ablative resurface, leg veins, telangiectasia |
| Diode | 800, 810, 930 | R | 1400 | Mel | Dermal pigment, epilation, leg veins, vascular |
| Q-switched alexandrite | 755 | R | 1300 | Mel | Tattoo (black, blue, green), epilation, pigmentation |
| Q-switched ruby | 694 | R | 1200 | Mel | Epidermal/Dermal pigment, tattoo (black, blue, green), epilation |
| Argon-pumped dye | 630, 514, 488 | O, G, B | 600 | Hb, mel | Vascular, epidermal pigment |
| PDL | 585–595 | Y | 600 | Hb, mel | Vascular, hypertrophic scar |
| Copper (bromide) vapor | 578, 511 | Y, G | 400, 300 | Hb, mel | Vascular, epidermal pigment |
| Krypton | 568, 531 | Y, G | 400 | Hb, mel | Vascular, epidermal pigment |
| Frequency doubled Q-switched Nd:YAG/ KTP | 532 | G | 400 | Mel, Hb | Vascular, epidermal pigment, red tattoo |
| Flash lamp pumped PDL | 510 | G | 300 | Mel, Hb | Vascular, hypertrophic scar |
| Argon | 488, 514 | B | 200, 300 | Mel, Hb | Vascular, epidermal pigment |
| Pulse excimer | 351, 308, 193 | UV | 0.5 | Protein | Psoriasis, vitiligo, LASIK |

IR: infrared; R: red; O: orange; Y: yellow; G: green; B:blue; UV: ultraviolet; Mel: melanin; Hb: hemoglobin.

| | Unit | Definition |
|---|---|---|
| Energy | J | |
| Power | W | Rate of energy delivery, laser output |
| Fluence | $J/cm^2$ | Amount of energy delivered per area |
| Pulse width | sec | Duration of laser exposure |
| Spot size | mm | Diameter of laser beam |
| Thermal relaxation time | sec | Time needed for the heated target to cool by 50% of its peak temperature through diffusion |
| Chromophore | | Target of laser |

**Laser principles** (LASER = Light Amplification by Stimulated Emission of Radiation)

1. monochromatic (single wavelength)
2. coherent (in phase with time and space)
3. collimated (parallel waves)

**Selective photothermolysis:** Selective heating of a target chromophore occurs when

1. selected wavelength is preferentially absorbed by the target chromophore
2. energy is high enough to damage the chromophores
3. pulse duration of the laser is shorter than the thermal relaxation of the target

$$\text{Laser output} = \text{Power (W)} = \frac{\text{Fluence } (J/cm^2) \times \text{Spot size (mm)}}{\text{Pulse width (sec)}}$$

To increase laser output → Increase fluence
→ Increase spot size
→ Decrease pulse width

## Thermal relaxation time

| Chromophore target | Size ($\mu$m) | Thermal relaxation time |
|---|---|---|
| Melanosome | 0.5–1.0 | 20–40 ns |
| Tattoo pigment particles | 0.5–100 | 20 ns – 3 ms |
| Epidermis | 50 | 1 ms |
| Telangiectasias | 30–50 | 1 ms |
| Blood vessel | 100–300 | 5–30 ms |
| Melanin in hair follicle | 200 | 20–100 ms |

## Laser treatment of tattoo pigment

| Tattoo | Pigment | Wavelength absorbed (nm) | Laser |
|---|---|---|---|
| Black | Carbon (India ink), iron oxide, logwood | 1064 | Nd:YAG |
| | | 755 | Q-switched alexandrite |
| | | 694 | Q-switched ruby |
| Blue | Cobalt aluminate | 1064 | Nd:YAG |
| | | 755 | Q-switched alexandrite |
| | | 694 | Q-switched ruby |
| Green | Chromic oxide, lead chromate, malachite, ferro- and ferricyanides, phthalocyanine dyes, Curcuma | 755 | Q-switched alexandrite |
| | | 694 | Q-switched ruby |
| Yellow | Cadmium sulfide | No good laser | |
| Red | Mercury sulfide (cinnabar), cadmium selenide, iron oxide (may turn black with laser tx) | 532 | Q-switched Nd:YAG |
| | | 510 | PDL |

## Photoinduced eye injury

| | Wavelength (nm) | Exposure risk | Ocular target | Eye effect |
|---|---|---|---|---|
| UVB/UVC | 200–320 | Sunburn | Cornea | Photokeratitis (Snow blindness) |
| UVA | 320–400 | PUVA, Excimer | Lens | Photochemical UV cataract, delayed (years) |
| Visible | 400–760 | Ruby, PDL, Argon | Retina (melanin, photoreceptors) | Photochemical and thermal retinal injury (Flash blindness) |
| Infrared A | 760–1400 | Nd:YAG | Retina | Same as above |
| Infrared B | >1400 | $CO_2$, Erb:YAG | Cornea (water) | Corneal burn |

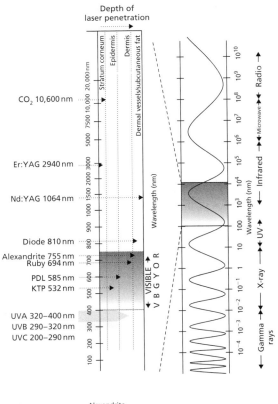

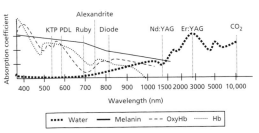

# Photodynamic Therapy

## Basic principles

- Components: (1) Photosensitizer, (2) light source, and (3) tissue oxygenation
- Two steps: (1) Administration of photosensitizer (topical or systemic), and (2) irradiation with visible light
- Effects:
  - Through Type 2 photo-oxidative reactions, PDT produces cytotoxic reactive oxygen species (singlet oxygen, superoxide anion, hydroxyl radical, hydrogen peroxide) → oxidation of amino acids, proteins, lipids → necrosis, apoptosis
  - Modifies immune responses (i.e. cytokine expression)
  - For acne, targets sebaceous glands and decreases P. acnes (P. acnes accumulates porphyrins).

## Applications

AKs, acne, BCC, Bowen, photoaging, verruca vulgaris, hidradenitis suppurativa, sebaceous hyperplasia.

## Photosensitizer properties and options

| Methyl aminolevulinic acid (MAL) | Aminolevulinic acid (ALA) |
| --- | --- |
| METVIX® cream 160 mg/g | Levulan® Kerastick® topical solution 20% |
| More lipophilic (some passive) transmembrane diffuse | More hydrophilic (needs active transport) |
| Deeper penetration | Poorer penetration* |
| Intracellularly, MAL is demethylated to ALA | Not a photosensitizer but converted to protoporphyrin IX (through heme biosynthesis pathway) |
| Red light (Aktilite) | Blue light (Blu-U) |
| FDA approved for treatment of AK. Approved in Europe for treatment of BCC | FDA approved for treatment of AK |

\* Can increase ALA penetration by increasing the application time, occluding, scrubbing with acetone, or using iontophoresis or electroporation.

- Selectivity: MAL and ALA (1) concentrate in tumor cells and newly formed endothelium and (2) require specific wavelengths to become activated
- Heme pathway:
  - In the cytoplasm, ALA → porphobilinogen → uroporphyrinogen III → coproporphyrinogen III
  - In the mitochondria, coproporphyrinogen III → protoporphyrinogen IX → protoporphyrin IX → iron incorporated by ferrochelatase

- Systemic photosensitizers have tetrapyrrolic structure and are given intravenously due to their low cutaneous penetration; examples: HpD and porfimer sodium (Photofrin®).

### Light source
- ALA and MAL converts to protoporphyrin IX, which has an absorption peak at the Soret band (~405 nm, within blue light) as well as peaks at higher wavelengths (Q-bands – at 510, 545, 580, and 630 nm)
- Q-band peaks are ~15× smaller than the Soret band peak
- Red light (Aktilite 630 nm) penetrates deeper into skin than blue light (Blu-U – 405–420 nm).

### Adverse effects
- Topical: Mild, transient burning pain, pruritus, erythema, edema, crusting, scaling
- Systemic: Longer-lasting generalized phototoxicity and sensitivity (sometimes months), photophobia, ocular pain, pigmentary changes, N/V, liver toxicity, metallic taste, SLE exacerbation.

### Precautions/contraindications
- Contraindicated in patients with porphyria, cutaneous sensitivity to the light source's wavelength(s), allergies to porphyrins or any part of the ALA solution/MAL cream (MAL cream contains peanut/almond oils)
- Contraindicated in patients who are pregnant or breast-feeding
- Patients should review all medications (OTC, herbal, rx – TCNs, thiazides, griseofulvin, sulfonamides, sulfonylureas, phenothiazines) which may impact (1) photosensitivity and (2) ALA/MAL penetration (retinoids)
- Deep recurrence can occur with partial (superficial only) tx of malignancies.

### Protocol

*ALA PDT*
- Wash treatment area with non-soap cleanser. Consider acetone scrub prior to applying ALA
- Per package instructions: Crush Levulan Kerastick at two points, then sequentially down the stick. Shake stick vertically for 2 min. Must be used within 2 h of resuspension
- Avoid applying ALA to ocular/mucosal surfaces
- For large areas, wait 30 min to 2 h after applying ALA (~15 h ok for small isolated lesion)
- For anesthetic effect, may apply topical lidocaine immediately following ALA application
- Avoid bright artificial light and sunlight during incubation period

- Use protective glasses
- If situated 2–4 in. from Blu-U light, tx time ~ 16 min, 40 s (10 J/cm²).
- After tx, avoid sunlight (or intense light) for 2 days (sunscreen will not block visible light)
- Re-tx in 2 months prn.

*MAL PDT*

- Curette treatment area to remove scale
- Apply MAL cream (nitrile gloves and spatula) under occlusion
- Avoid sunlight, bright artificial lights, or cold during 3-h incubation period
- Use protective glasses
- Tx time: 8–10 min. at 5–8 cm from red light (37 J/cm²)
- Re-tx in 1 week prn.

## UV Spectrum

| | | |
|---|---|---|
| Infrared | >760 nm | |
| Visible | 400–760 nm | |
| UV | <400 nm | |
| UVAI | 340–400 nm | Soret band (400–410 nm) |
| UVAII | 320–340 nm | Wood lamp (320–400 nm, peak at 365 nm) |
| UVB | 290–320 nm | NBUVB (311 nm) |
| UVC | 200–290 nm | |

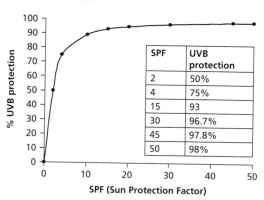

| SPF | UVB protection |
|---|---|
| 2 | 50% |
| 4 | 75% |
| 15 | 93 |
| 30 | 96.7% |
| 45 | 97.8% |
| 50 | 98% |

## UV Protection Measurements

- SPF = Sun Protection Factor = sunscreen protected:unprotected ratio of duration of UVB exposure to produce 1 MED
- Water-resistant product maintains SPF level after 40 min of water immersion
- Waterproof (very water-resistant) maintains SPF level after 80 min of water immersion
- Measures of UVA protection: persistent pigment darkening, immediate pigment darkening, protection factor UVA
- Critical Wavelength (CW) = wavelength at which the integral of the spectral absorbance curves equals 90% of the integral from 290–400 nm (CW of at least 370 nm for broad-spectrum sunscreen).

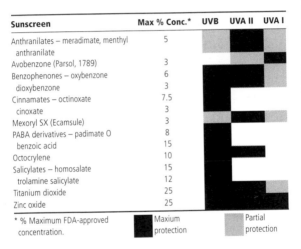

| Sunscreen | Max % Conc.* | UVB | UVA II | UVA I |
|---|---|---|---|---|
| Anthranilates – meradimate, menthyl anthranilate | 5 | | | |
| Avobenzone (Parsol, 1789) | 3 | | | |
| Benzophenones – oxybenzone | 6 | | | |
| dioxybenzone | 3 | | | |
| Cinnamates – octinoxate | 7.5 | | | |
| cinoxate | 3 | | | |
| Mexoryl SX (Ecamsule) | 3 | | | |
| PABA derivatives – padimate O | 8 | | | |
| benzoic acid | 15 | | | |
| Octocrylene | 10 | | | |
| Salicylates – homosalate | 15 | | | |
| trolamine salicylate | 12 | | | |
| Titanium dioxide | 25 | | | |
| Zinc oxide | 25 | | | |

\* % Maximum FDA-approved concentration.  ■ Maxium protection   ▨ Partial protection

## UV Associations/Specificities

| UVA | UVB | UVA and UVB |
|---|---|---|
| Immediate tanning | Delayed tanning | AKs |
| Photoaging (UVA > UVB) | Photocarcinogenesis (UVB>UVA) | Fine wrinkles |
| Hydroa vacciniforme | Persistent light reaction | Solar urticaria |
| Phytophotodermatitis | Sunburn | (or visible light) |
| Photoallergic drug reaction | Xeroderma pigmentosa | |
| PMLE (UVA>UVB, UVC, or visible) | Cockayne syndrome | |
| | Lupus erythematosus photosensitivity (UVB>UVA) | |

# Glogau Wrinkle Scale

| Glogau type | 1 | 2 | 3 | 4 |
|---|---|---|---|---|
| | **No wrinkles** | **Wrinkles in motion** | **Wrinkles at rest** | **Only wrinkles** |
| **Age (years)** | ~20–30 s | ~30–40 s | ~50–60 s | ~60–70 s and older |
| **Photoaging** | Early photoaging | Early-moderate photoaging | Advanced photoaging | Severe photoaging |
| **Pigmentary changes** | Mild/early pigmentary changes | Early lentigines | Dyschromia, telangiectasia | Yellow-gray discoloration |
| **Keratoses/ skin cancers** | No keratoses | Palpable keratoses | Visible keratoses | Skin cancers |
| **Wrinkles** | Minimal wrinkles | Dynamic wrinkles– parallel smile lines | Wrinkles without motion | Wrinkles throughout |

# Fitzpatrick Skin Type

| Skin type | Color | Tanning response |
|---|---|---|
| Type I | White | Always burns, never tans |
| Type II | White | Usually burns, sometimes tans |
| Type III | White | Sometimes burns mildly, always tans |
| Type IV | Olive | Rarely burns, always tans |
| Type V | Dark brown | Never burns, tans very easily |
| Type VI | Black | Never burns, tans very easily |

# Peeling Agents

| Depth of peel | Layer | Peel | Amount | Component |
|---|---|---|---|---|
| **Very superficial** | Strateum corneum/ ganulosum | Retinoids | | Retinoic acid |
| | | TCA 10–25% | 1 coat | Trichloroacetic acid (TCA) |
| | | Resorcin 20–30% | 5–10 min | Resorcinol |
| | | Gycolic 30–50% | 1–2 min | Alpha hydroxy acid |
| | | Salicylic acid | | Beta hydroxy acid |
| | | Jessner | 1–3 coats | Resorcinol/ Salicylic acid/ Lactic acid/ETOH |

continued p. 224

SURGERY

| Depth of peel | Layer | Peel | Amount | Component |
|---|---|---|---|---|
| **Superficial** | Basal layer/ Papillary dermis | TCA 35% | 1 coat | Trichloroacetic acid |
| | | Gycolic 50–70% | 5–20 min | Alpha hydroxy acid |
| | | Resorcin 50% | 30–60 min | Resorcinol |
| **Medium** | Upper reticular dermis | Combination Peels | | Jessner + 35% TCA |
| | | | | $CO_2$ + 35% TCA Glycolic 70% + 35% TCA 50% TCA |
| **Deep** | Mid-reticular dermis | Baker-Gordon | | Phenol/ septisol/ croton oil |
| | | Phenol 88% | | Carbolic acid |

## TCA peel

- End point is frosting (self-neutralizing).
- Depth based on number/amount of application (wait 3–4 min after each application to assess amount of frost).
- May use cold compress after appearance of light frost to reduce discomfort.

## TCA peel frost level

| Level | Frosting | Depth of peel | Healing time |
|---|---|---|---|
| 0 | No frost, minimal erythema | Removes stratum corneum | |
| 1 | Partial light frost, some erythema | Superficial peel | 2–4 days |
| 2 | White frost with erythema show through | Full thickness epidermal peel | 5 days |
| 3 | Solid white frost, no pink | Papillary dermis | 5–7 days |

## Jessner solution

Resorcinol (14 g); salicyclic acid (14 g); lactic acid (14 g); ethanol 95% (100 ml)

- Salicylate toxicity: Tinnitus, headache, nausea
- Recorcinol toxicity: Methemoglobinemia, syncope, thyroid suppression.

## Baker-Gordon phenol

88% Phenol (3 cc); Distilled water (2 cc); Septisol (8 drops); Croton oil (3 drops)
- Rapidly absorbed through skin, metabolized by the liver, excreted by renal system
- Risk of renal failure, hepatotoxicity, and cardiac arrhythmias.

## Cook total body peel

70% glycolic acid gel followed immediately by 35–40% TCA
- Neutralize with 10% sodium bicarbonate solution once scattered frosting is noted.

## Pre-peel prep

- Cleanse with Septisol to remove oils. Rinse thoroughly.
- Wipe area with alcohol.
- Degrease area with 100% acetone to further debride oil and streateum corneum.
- Apply white petrolatum to corners of eyes, mouth and nose to protect areas.

## Post-peel wound care

- Vinegar soak 3–4× per day with 0.25% acetic acid compress (1 tbs white vinegar in 1 pint warm water).
- White petrolatum or emollient to face and neck. May cover neck with saran wrap.

# Botulinum Toxin

- Produced by *Clostridium botulinum* (Gram-negative anaerobic bacterium)
- FDA approved 4/2002 for glabella region. Off label use for other areas.
- Mechanism of action
  - Block Ach release from presynaptic nerve terminal by cleaving SNARE complex
    - BTX-A: cleaves SNAP-25
    - BTX-B: cleaves synaptobrevin/VAMP.
- Reconstitution
  - Potency can be maintained for up to 6 weeks
  - Reconstitution with sterile saline with preservative (0.9% benzyl alcohol) provides local anesthetic effect.
- Response
  - Clinical effect 1–3 days following injection with maximal effect by 2 weeks

| Diluent added (0.9% NaCl) | 1.0 ml | 2.0 ml | 2.5 ml | 4.0 ml | 8.0 ml |
|---|---|---|---|---|---|
| Resulting dose/units per 0.1 ml | 10.0 U | 5.0 U | 4.0 U | 2.5 U | 1.25 U |

- Benefits last 3–4 months
- Adverse effects/complications
  - *Common*: redness, ecchymosis, headache, bruising, edema, inflammation, erythema
  - *Ptosis*: minimize by careful selection of injection site (1–1.5 cm away from the orbital rim).
- If ptosis, use Iopidine (apraclonidine) drops. α2-adrenergic agonist which stimulates Muller's muscles to provide an elevation of 1–3 mm.
- Contraindications: infection at site of injection, known hypersensitivity to formulation.
- Caution:
  - Peripheral motor neuropathic disease, neuromuscular disorder (myasthenia gravis, Eaton-Lambert have increased risk of systemic side effects)
  - Aminoglycosides, penicillamine, and Ca$^+$ channel blockers may potentiate BOTOX
  - Pregnancy category C
  - Lactation: not known whether toxin is excreted in human milk.

## Botox injection sites

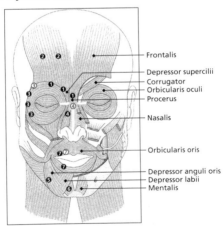

Frontalis
Depressor supercilii
Corrugator
Orbicularis oculi
Procerus
Nasalis
Orbicularis oris
Depressor anguli oris
Depressor labii
Mentalis

Recommended sites are denoted as dark numbered circles. Optional sites are denoted as white numbered circles.

Modified from Sommer B and Sattler G (eds). Botulinum toxin in aesthetic medicine. Boston: Blackwell Science, Ltd.: 2001, with permission from Blackwell Publishing.

SURGERY

## Botox injection sites

| Location | Muscles | Recommended units | Comments |
|---|---|---|---|
| ❶ Glabella frown lines | Corrugator, procerus, orbicularis oculi, depressor supercilii | 20–30 U women 30–40 U men | Keep >1 cm superior to orbital rim |
| ❷ Horizontal forehead lines | Frontalis | 10–2 U women 20–3 U men ~ 2–8 sites at 1 cm apart | Avoid treating lower 1/3 of lateral forehead to avoid brow ptosis |
| ❸ Crow's feet | Lateral fibers of orbicularis oculi | 6–15 U per side subdermal plane | keep >1–1.5 cm lateral to orbital rim |
| ❹ Bunny lines | Upper nasalis Procerus | 2–4 U per side | 1 U midline if needed to procerus |
| ❺ Marionette lines and mouth frown | Depressor anguli oris | 5–10 U | Inject 1 cm lateral and 1–2 cm inferior to angle of mouth |
| ❻ Mental crease | Mentalis | 5–10 U | Deep injection |
| ❼ Perioral rhytides | Orbicularis oris | 1–2 U per quadrant | Superficially over vermillion |
| ❽ Platysmal bands | Platysma | 10–3C U women 10–4C U men | Grasp band and inject into belly of muscle |

# Fillers

| Brand name (Company) | Composition | How supplied | Approx x. Cost (US$) | Duration of effect | FDA approval/CE mark | Location of injection | Side effects/ adverse effects |
|---|---|---|---|---|---|---|---|
| **COLLAGEN** | | | | | | | |
| Zyderm I (Inamed, division of Allergan) | Bovine collagen 35 mg/ml. Contains 0.3% lidocaine | 0.5, 1.0, 1.5 ml | 145 (1 ml) | 3–4 months | FDA 1981 CE mark 1995 | Superficial dermis – superficial rhytids, scars | Hypersensitivity to bovine collagen. Need two skin testing (2–4 weeks apart). Wait 4 weeks before treatment Lidocaine sensitivity |
| Zyderm II (Inamed) | Bovine collagen 65 mg/ml. Contains 0.3% lidocaine | 0.5, 1.0 ml | 150 (1 ml) | 3–4 months | FDA 1983 CE mark 1995 | Mid-dermis – moderate rhytids | |
| Zyplast (Inamed) | Bovine collagen 35 mg/ml cross-linked with glutaraldehyde. Contains 0.3% lidocaine | 1.0, 1.5, 2.0, 2.5 ml | 165 (1 ml) | 3–5 months | FDA 1985 CE mark 1995 | Deep dermis – deep rhytids, lip augmentation | |
| Cosmoderm I (Inamed) | Human collagen 35 mg/ml. Contains 0.3% lidocaine | 1.0 ml | 175–205 (1 ml) | 3–4 months | FDA 2003 | Superficial dermis – superficial rhytids, scars | Lidocaine sensitivity |
| Cosmoderm II (Inamed) | Human collagen 65 mg/ml. Contains 0.3% lidocaine | 1.0 ml | 200 (1 ml) | 3–4 months | FDA 2003 | Mid-dermis – moderate rhytids | |

continued p. 230

SURGERY

229

| Brand name (Company) | Composition | How supplied | Approx. Cost (US$) | Duration of effect | FDA approval/CE mark | Location of injection | Side effects/ adverse effects |
|---|---|---|---|---|---|---|---|
| Cosmoplast (Inamed) | Human collagen 35 mg/ml crosslinked with glutaraldehyde. Contains 0.3% lidocaine | 1.0, 1.5 ml | 235 (1 ml) | 3–4 months | FDA 2003 | Deep dermis – deep rhytids, lip augmentation | |
| Evolence (ColBar LifeScience/ OrthoNeutrogena) | Porcine collagen 35 mg/ml. Glymatrix technology crosslink type I collagen to ribose – mimic human collagen. Dispersed in phosphate buffered saline | 1.0 ml | 250+ (1 ml) | Up to 12 months | FDA 2008. CE 2004. | Upper to mid-dermis | Non-human collagen with potential for allergic reaction, though pre-testing is not required |
| **HYALURONIC ACID** | | | | | | | |
| Restylane fine line (Medicis) | Hyaluronic acid 20 mg/ml. Gel bead size 100μ. By bacterial fermentation from streptococci bacteria | 0.4 ml | 250–500 (0.4 ml) | 3–6 months | Not FDA approved. CE mark | Superficial dermis – superficial rhytids, scars | |
| Restylane (Medicis) | Hyaluronic acid 20 mg/ml. Gel bead size 250μ. By bacterial fermentation from streptococci bacteria | 0.4, 1.0 ml | 200 (1 ml) | 4–6 months | FDA 2003. CE mark | Mid-dermis – moderate/ severe rhytids, folds, lip | Rare allergic/ hypersensitivity reactions, granulomas |

| Product | Composition | | | | | Adverse reactions |
|---|---|---|---|---|---|---|
| Perlane (Medicis) | Hyaluronic acid 20 mg/ml Gel bead size 1000μ. By bacterial fermentation from streptococci bacteria | 1.0 ml | 250 (1 ml) | 3–9 months | FDA 2007 | Deep dermis – severe rhytids, folds | Rare allergic/hypersensitivity reactions, granulomas |
| Hylaform (Inamed) | Hyaluronic acid 5.5 mg/ml 20% cross-linking. Derived from rooster comb | 0.4, 0.75 ml | 175 (0.7 ml) | 3–6 months | FDA 2004 CE 1995 | Mid/deep dermis – moderate/severe rhytids, lips | Contraindicated if allergic to avian product. Rare allergic/hypersensitivity reactions, granulomas |
| Hylaform plus (Inamed) | Hyaluronic acid 5.5 mg/ml 20% cross-linking. Larger particle size. Derived from rooster comb | 0.4, 0.75 ml | 200 (0.7 ml) | 3–6 months | FDA 2004 CE 1995 | Deep dermis – severe rhytids | |
| Juvederm ultra (Allergan) | Hyaluronic acid 24 mg/m produced by Streptococcus equi | 0.8 ml | 200 (0.8 ml) | 6–12 months | FDA 2006 | Mid/deep dermis – mod/severe rhytids, folds, lip | |
| Juvederm ultra plus (Allergan) | Hyaluronic acid 30 mg/ml produced by Streptococcus equi | 0.8 ml | 250 (0.8 ml) | 6–12 months | FDA 2006 | Deep dermis – severe rhytids, folds | |
| Captique (Allergan) | Hyaluronic acid 5.5 mg/ml | 0.75 ml | 200 (0.75 ml) | 3–5 months | FDA 2004 | Mid/deep dermis – mod/severe rhytids, folds, lip | |

Adapted from Injectables at Glance. The American Society for Aesthetic Plastic Surgery, http://www.surgery.org/download/injectablechart.pdf, 11/25/07. Sengelmann RD et al. Soft-tissue augmentation. In Robinson JK et al. (eds). Surgery of the Skin. Philadelphia: Mosby, 2005.

SURGERY

| Brand name (Company) | Composition | How supplied | Approx x. Cost (US$) | Duration of effect | FDA approval/CE mark | Location of injection | Side effects/ adverse effects |
|---|---|---|---|---|---|---|---|
| **SYNTHETIC FILLERS** | | | | | | | |
| Radiesse formerly Radiance (Bioform Medical) | 55.7% calcium hydroxylapatite (25–45μ) microspheres | 0.3, 1.3 ml | 500 (1.3 ml) | 12 months + | FDA 2006 | Subdermis – deep rhytids and folds, lipatrophy | Rare allergic reactions. Reports of granulomas, lumps |
| Artefill (Artes Medical) | 20% polymethylmethacrylate microspheres (32–40μ) suspended in 3.5% bovine collagen with 0.3% lidocaine | 0.4, 0.8 ml | 700–800 | Permanent filler up to 5 years + | FDA 2006 CE 1994 | Deep dermis – deep rhytids, folds | Lidocaine sensitivity. Potential for sensitivity to bovine collagen, need skin test 4 weeks prior. Reports of allergic reactions, foreign body granulomas 0.01% |
| Sculptra Or New-Fill (Dermik Laboratories) | Poly-l-lactic acid Mix 5 cc sterile water + 1 cc 1%. Lidocaine for total 6 cc product | 1 vial (150μg) reconstituted to 6 ml | 480 | Up to 2 years after 1st tx. Need 3–6 tx spaced 2–4 weeks apart | FDA 2004 | Deep dermis/subcutaneous plane – restoration and correction of facial fat loss (HIV lipoatrophy) | Potential for lumpiness – need to massage area post treatment |
| Silikon (Alcon) AdatoSil (Bausch & Lomb) | Silicone, pure polymers from siloxane | 1 vial 8.5 ml (2 ml max per tx) | | Permanent | Off-label use. FDA approved for retinal tamponade | Subcutaneous plane – deep rhytids, folds | Granuloma formation, migration, inflammatory reactions |

## HOMOLOGOUS MATERIAL

| | | | | | | | |
|---|---|---|---|---|---|---|---|
| Autologen (Collagenesis) | Autologous human collagen, elastin, glycosaminoglycans, and fibronectic. Prepared from patient tissue | No longer available | – | 4 months–2 years | No longer available | Mid-dermis – mod/severe rhytids, lip, folds | |
| Dermalogen (Collagenesis) | Pooled human cadaveric proteins, primarily type I and III collagens | No longer available | – | 3–6 months | No longer available | Mid and deep dermal filler for rhytids and folds | |
| Fascian (Fascia Biosystems) | Freeze-dried irradiated cadaveric fascia lata reconstituted with saline and 0.5% lidocaine | 3 ml various particle size | 125 | 3–8 months | FDA approved not required. Tissue bank regulations | Superficial, mid, deep dermis based on particle size | Potential for hypersensitivity to polymyxin B sulfate, bacitracin, gentamicin |
| Isolagen (Isolagen Technologies) | Autologous fibroblasts culture from 3 mm punch biopsy from patient | 3 ml | 1000–1500 | Unclear | Phase III trials | Mid-/deep dermis | Need test dose 2 + weeks before tx |

# Sclerotherapy

| Mechanism of action | Brand name | Sclerosing agent | FDA approval | Maximum dosage | Pain | Necrosis | Pigmentation | Other |
|---|---|---|---|---|---|---|---|---|
| Detergent/ emulsifier | Sotradecol Fibro-vein | Sodium tetradecyl sulfate | Yes, 1946 | 10 cc of 3% solution | Mild/Minimal | Occasional, at conc. >1% | +++ | 0.1–0.3% anaphylaxis |
| | Sclero-vein Aethoxysklerol | Polidocanol | Approved in Europe only | 20 cc of 3% solution | Minimal | Rare | ++ at high concentrations | 0.2% anaphylaxis |
| | Scleromate | Sodium morrhuate | Yes, 1930 | 10 cc | Moderate | Frequent | +++ | 3–10% cases of anaphylaxis (highest risk) |
| | Etholamin | Ethanolamine oleate | Off-label use; for esophageal varices only | 10 cc | Mild | Occasional | +++ | Risk of RBC hemolysis and renal failure allergic rxn |

| | | Hypertonic saline 23.4% (NaCl) | Off-label use | 10–20 cc | Painful, muscle cramps | Significant if extravasated | ++ | No allergic rxn |
|---|---|---|---|---|---|---|---|---|
| Hyperosmotic agent | Hypertonic saline | | | | | | | |
| | Sclerodex | 10% Saline + No 5% dextrose | No | 10–20 cc | Painful | Significant if extravasated | + | Low risk of allergic rxn |
| Chemical irritant | Chromex Scleremo | Glycerin 72% | No | 5–10 cc | Moderate | Rare | Least likely | Viscous solution, rare allergic rxn |
| | Varigloban, Variglobin, Sclerodine | Polyiodine iodine | No | 3 cc of 6% | Painful | Occasional | ++ | Viscous solution, rare allergic rxn- to iodine. Renal insufficiency |

Adapted from Sadick N, Li C. Small Vessel Sclerotherapy. *Dermatol Clin.* 2001; 19:475–81; Duffy DM. Cutaneous necrosis following sclerotherapy. *J Aesthetic Dermatol Cosmetic Surgery.* 1999; 1:157–68.

# Determine vessel size using needle gauge

| Use needle gauge to determine vessel size | |
| --- | --- |
| **Needle Gauge** | **Vessel Size** |
| 30 gauge | 0.32 mm |
| 25 gauge | 0.50 mm |
| 18 gauge | 1.25 mm |

# Recommended maximum effective concentration of sclerosant to minimize side effects

| Vessel size (mm) | Recommended maximum effective concentration (%) | | | |
| --- | --- | --- | --- | --- |
| | Sotradecol | Polidocanol | Hypertonic saline | Glycerin |
| 0.1–0.5 | 0.1–0.2 | 0.25–0.5 | 11.7 | 50–72 |
| 0.6–0.9 | 0.2–0.3 | 0.25–0.75 | 11.7–23.4 | – |
| 1.0–3.0 | 0.2–0.5 | 0.5–2.0 | 23.4 | – |
| > 4 mm | 0.5–1.0 | 2.0–5.0 | – | – |

# Part 3
# Drugs and Therapies

*Handbook of Dermatology: A Practical Manual.* By Margaret W. Mann,
David R. Berk, Daniel L. Popkin, and Susan J. Bayliss. Published 2009 by Blackwell Publishing,
ISBN: 978-1-4051-8110-5.

# Medication Quick Reference

## Topical steroids

### CLASS 1 – SUPERPOTENT

| | | | | |
|---|---|---|---|---|
| Betamethasone dipropionate | Diprolene | O/G | 0.05% | 15, 50 g |
| Clobetasol propionate | Temovate | O/Cr | 0.05% | 15, 30, 45 g |
| | Temovate | S | 0.05% | 25, 50 ml |
| | Cormax | S | 0.05% | 25, 50 ml |
| | Olux | F | 0.05% | 100 g |
| Diflorasone diacetate | Psorcon | O | 0.05% | 15, 30, 60 g |
| Halobetasol propionate | Ultravate | O/Cr | 0.05% | 15, 50 g |

### CLASS 2 – POTENT

| | | | | |
|---|---|---|---|---|
| Amcinonide | Cyclocort | O | 0.1% | 15, 30, 60 g |
| Betamethasone dipropionate | Diprosone | O | 0.05% | 15, 50 g |
| Desoximetasone | Topicort | O/Cr | 0.25% | 15, 60 g |
| | Topicort | G | 0.05% | 15, 60 g |
| Diflorasone diacetate | Florone | G | 0.05% | 15, 60 g |
| | Maxiflor | O | 0.05% | 15 g |
| Fluocinonide | Lidex | O/Cr G | 0.05% | 15, 30, 60, 120 g |
| Halcinonide | Halog | O/Cr | 0.1% | 15, 30, 60, 240 g |

### CLASS 3 – UPPER MID-STRENGTH

| | | | | |
|---|---|---|---|---|
| Betamethasone dipropionate | Diprosone | Cr | 0.05% | 15, 50 g |
| Betamethasone valerate | Valisone | O | 0.1% | 15, 45 g |
| Diflorasone diacetate | Florone, Maxiflor | Cr | 0.05% | 15 g |
| Fluticasone propionate | Cutivate | O | 0.005% | 15, 30, 60 g |
| Mometasone furoate | Elocon | O | 0.1% | 15, 45 g |
| Triamcinolone acetonide | Aristocort | Cr | 0.5% | 15 g |

### CLASS 4 – MID-STRENGTH

| | | | | |
|---|---|---|---|---|
| Betamethasone valerate | Luxiq | F | 0.12% | 100 g |
| Desoximetasone | Topicort LP | Cr | 0.05% | 15, 60 g |
| Fluocinolone acetonide | Synalar-HP | Cr | 0.2% | 15, 60 g |
| | Synalar | O | 0.025% | 60 g |
| Flurandrenolide | Cordran | O | 0.05% | 15, 30, 60 g |
| Triamcinolone acetonide | Aristocort, Kenalog | O | 0.1% | 15, 60, 240 g, 1 lb |

### CLASS 5 – LOWER MID-STRENGTH

| | | | | |
|---|---|---|---|---|
| Betamethasone dipropionate | Diprosone | L | 0.05% | 20, 60 g |
| Betamethasone valerate | Valisone | Cr/L | 0.1% | 15, 45 g |
| Clocortolone | Cloderm | Cr | 0.1% | 15, 45, 90 g |

continued p. 240

DRUGS AND THERAPIES

| Fluocinolone acetonide | Synalar | Cr | 0.025% | 15, 60 g |
| Fluocinolone acetonide | Dermasmooth/ FS | Oil | 0.01% | 4 oz |
| Flurandrenolide | Cordran | Cr | 0.05% | 15, 30, 60 g |
| Fluticasone propionate | Cutivate | Cr | 0.05% | 15, 30, 60 g |
| Hydrocortisone butyrate | Locoid | Cr | 0.1% | 15, 45 g |
| Hydrocortisone valerate | Westcort | Cr | 0.2% | 15, 45, 60 g |
| Prednicarbate | Dermatop | Cr | 0.1% | 15, 60 g |
| Triamcinolone acetonide | Kenalog | Cr/L | 0.25% | 15, 60, 80 g |

## CLASS 6 – LOW

| Alclometasone dipropionate | Aclovate | O/Cr | 0.05% | 15, 45, 60 g |
| Betamethasone valerate | Valisone | L | 0.1% | 60 g |
| Desonide | DesOwen | Cr | 0.05% | 15, 60, 90 g |
| | Tridesilon | Cr | 0.05% | 5, 15, 60 g |
| | Desonate | G | 0.05% | 60 g |
| | Verdeso | F | 0.05% | 50, 100 g |
| Fluocinolone acetonide | Synalar | Cr/S | 0.01% | 15, 60 g |
| Triamcinolone acetonide | Aristocort | Cr/L | 0.1% | 15, 60, 240 g |

## CLASS 7 – LEAST POTENT

Topicals with hydrocortisone 0.5%, 1.0%, 2.5% (Cortisporin, Hytone, U-cort, Vytone), dexamethasone, flumethasone, methylprednisolone and prednisolone

Cr: Cream; F: Foam; G: Gel; L: Lotion; O: Ointment; S: Solution.

## Non-steroidals

| Tacrolimus | Protopic | O | 0.03, 0.1% | 30, 60 g |
| Pimecrolimus | Elidel | Cr | 0.1% | 15, 30, 100 g |

## Commonly used drugs in dermatology
### Acne Vulgaris/Rosacea
Accutane 0.5 – 1 mg/kg/day divided qd-bid (Goal = 120–150 mg/kg). 10,20,30,40 mg

Azelex 20% Cr – 30, 50 g

BP LQ 2.5,5,10%; bar 5, 10%; L &Cr 5, 10%; G 2.4,4,5,6,10,20%

Cleocin T 1% S, L – 60 ml, 1% G – 30, 60 g, 1% pledgets – 60/box

Differin 0.1% Cr, G – 15, 45 g

Erythromycin 2% O – 25 g; 2% G – 27, 50 g

Evoclin 1% F – 50, 100 g

Finacea 15% G – 30 g

Klaron L – 59 ml

Metronidazole 1% Cr – 30 g; 0.75% Cr – 30,45 g; 0.75% G – 29 g; 0.75% L – 59 ml

Retin-A Micro 0.04%, 0.1% G – 20, 45 g; Generic 0.025%, 0.05%, 0.1% Cr –20, 45 g; Generic 0.025%, 0.1% G – 15, 45 g

Sulfacet R L – 25 ml

Tazorac 0.05%, 0.1% Cr – 15, 30, 60 g

### Antibiotics – topical
Mupirocin/Bactroban bid/tid 2% Cr, O – 15, 30 g
Polysporin – (bacitracin + polymyxin) – OTC
Silvadene 1% Cr – 20, 50, 400, 1000 g

### Antibiotics – systemic
Bactrim DS bid
Keflex 500 mg bid-qid; 250, 500 mg tab
Tetracycline 500 mg bid; 250, 500 mg tab
Doxycycline 100 mg bid; 50, 100 mg tab
Minocycline 100 mg bid; 50, 100 mg tab

### Antibiotic preoperative prophylaxis
1 h prior to surgery
Amoxicillin: 2 g; 500 mg tab
Cephalexin: 2 g; 500 mg tab
### If allergic to penicillin
Clindamycin: 600 mg; 300 mg tab
Azithromycin/Clarithromycin: 500 mg; 500 mg tab

### Antifungal
Ciclopirox (Penlac) 8% nail S – 6.6 ml
Diflucan/Fluconazole 150–300 mg Qwk; 150 mg
Griseofulvin 20 mg/kg/d; 250, 500 mg, 125 mg/5 ml
Lamisil/Terbinafine 250 mg po qd, 250 tab; OTC 1% C, S, spray
Loprox/Ciclopirox 1% Cr, L – 15, 30, 90 g
Mentax/Butenafine 1% Cr – 15, 30 g
Micatin/Miconazole 2% Cr – 15, 30, 90 g
Nizoral/Ketoconazole 400 mg then sweat, 200 mg tab; 2% Cr – 15, 30,
   60 g; 2% wash – 120 ml
Specatazole/Econazole 1% Cr – 15, 30, 85 g
Sporanox/Itraconazole 200 mg qd or pulse dose 200 mg bid × 7 days q month
Thymol 4% in alcohol: 30 cc disp. c dropper.
Naftin 1% G, Cr – 15, 30, 60 g
Zeasorb – AF powder/miconazole 2%

### Antiparasitics
Elimite/Permethrin – Cr 5% – 60 g
Ivermectin 0.2 mg/kg × 1; 6 mg tab

### Antivirals
Aldara/Imiquimod 3×/week qhs; Cr 5% – 1 box = 12 pks
Abreva/Docosanol 5×/day OTC Cr 10% – 2 g
Denavir/Penciclovir Q2 h × 4 days; Cr 1% – 2 g
Valtrex 2 g bid × 1 day; 500, 1000 mg tab
Zovirax/Acyclovir Q3 h × 5 – 7 days; O 5% – 2, 10 g

## Antihistamines

Allegra/Fexofenadine 60 mg bid or 180 mg qd; 60, 180 mg tab
Atarax/Hydroxyzine 10–50 mg q4–6 h; 10, 25 mg, 10 mg/5 ml
Clarinex/Desloratadine 5 mg qd; 5 mg tab
Claritin/Loratadine 10 mg qd; OTC 10, 5/5 ml
Doxepin 10–75 qhs; 10, 25, 50 mg tab
Zyrtec/Cetirizine 5–10 mg; 5, 10, 5/5 ml

## Bleaching agents

Azelex 20% Cr – 30, 50 g
Hydroquinone (Epiqquin Micro, Lustra, Triluma, others) bid. 4%
   Cr – 30, 60 g

## Chemotherapy

Aldara/Imiquimod. For AK, BCC qhs $\times$ 8–12 weeks. Cr 5% – 1 box = 12
   single use 250 mg packets
Efudex/Fluorouracil. For AK qd-bid $\times$ 2–6 weeks. 5% Cr – 25 g; 2%,
   5% S – 10 ml
Solaraze/diclofenac bid $\times$ 3 months; Cr 5% – 30, 45 g

## CTCL

Bexarotene tabs 200–300 mg/m$^2$ qd; 75 tab
Nitrogen mustard bid.10 mg% in Aquaphor 2 lb
Targretin/Bexarotene Gel qd-bid. 1% G – 60 g

## Psoriasis

Dovonex/Calcipotriene bid. 0.005% O, Cr – 30, 60, 100 g; scalp S – 60 ml
Dermazinc with clobetasol spray. Write Dermazinc 4 oz. compound with
   50 mcg micronized clobetasol, disp. 4 oz.
Liquor Carbonis Detergens (LCD): Must be compounded: TMC 0.1% oint
   compounded with 10% LCD, disp.1 lb.
Oxsoralen ultra 0.4–0.6 mg/kg 1–2 h prior to PUVA. 10 mg tab
Tazorac/Tazarotene qd. Cr 0.05%, 0.1% – 15, 30, 60 g, G 0.05%,
   0.1% – 30, 100 g

## Miscellaneous

Biotin 2.5 mg qd
Colchicine 0.3 mg, titrate to diarrhea; 0.6 mg tab
Drysol 20% solution; QHS until effective then spaced out; S – 35, 37.5, 60 ml
Elidel/Pimecrolimus bid; Cr 1% – 15, 30, 100 g
Folic acid 1 mg qd; 1 mg tab
Lac-hydrin (lactic acid) bid; Cr 12% – 140, 385 g; L 12% – 150, 360 ml
Niacinamide 500 mg Tid; 500 mg tab
Propecia/Finesteride 1 mg qd; 1 mg tab
Protopic/Tacrolimus bid; Cr 0.03, 0.1% – 30 g
Robinul 1 mg qd, titrate to effect; 1 mg tab
Trental 400 mg Tid; 400 mg tab
Vaniqa/Eflornithine bid. Cr 13.9% – 30 g

# Systemic Medications

## Anti-malarials

| Drug (Brand name) Trade size | Dose | Labs to follow | Mechanism | Side effects | Interactions | ♀ |
|---|---|---|---|---|---|---|
| **Diaminodiphenyl sulfone** (Dapsone) 25/100 mg | 50 mg/day then increase to 100–200 mg/day (take with food) | Baseline: CBC, **G6PD**, CMP, UA, neuro exam (check reflex). F/U: CBC qwk × 4, qmos × 6, then q6mos; CMP, neuro exam q3–4 mos | *Antimicrobial* (antagonist of dihydropteroate synthetase → prevents formation of folic acid) and *anti-inflamm* (inhibits PMN chemotaxis, Ig binding; inhibits myeloperoxidase) | **Hemolysis** (dose-related), **methemoglobinemia** (dose-related; decreased incidence with cimetidine), **agranulocytosis** (idiosyncratic), hypersensitivity syndrome – mono-like, **neuropathy** (motor), hepatitis | Rifampin, antimalarials, sulfonamides, probenecid, folate antagonists, TMP | C |
| **Hydroxychloroquine** (Plaquenil) 200 mg | 200–400 mg/day (6.5 mg/kg/day) | Baseline: eye exam, **G6PD**, CBC; F/U: **eye exam:** q1–5 years; **Amsler grid** qmos, CBC qmo (→ q6mos) | ALL anti-malarials: Intercalate into DNA preventing transcription; disrupt UV $O_2$ radical formation; inhibit IL-2 synthesis; inhibit chemotaxis; reduce platelet aggregation; Inhibit endosome acidification | Blue pigment, GI upset (brand name medication with decreased GI upset), corneal deposition, hemolysis, **retinopathy** (peripheral fields), **psoriasis/ PCT flares**, cardiac toxicity with overdose (2–6g), CNS stimulant | Cimetidine, digoxin, kaolin, magnesium trisilicate; Avoid combination of chloroquine/ hydroxychloroquine | C |
| **Chloroquine** (Aralen) 250/500 mg | 250 mg/day (4.0 mg/kg/day) | Same as Plaquenil | | SAME as Plaquenil PLUS bleaches hair, increased ocular risk | *Smoking decreases effectiveness and worsens underlying lupus | C |
| **Quinacrine** (Atabrine) 100 mg | 100 mg/day | Same as Plaquenil EXCEPT no eye exam, no G6PD | | SIMILAR to Plaquenil BUT **no ocular toxicity, yellow hyperpigment**, no hemolysis | SAME as above BUT safe to use with chloroquine or hydroxychloroquine | C |

*continued p. 244*

**DRUGS AND THERAPIES**

243

# Immunosuppressive agents

| Drug | Dose | Labs to follow | Mechanism | Side effects | Interactions | ♀ |
|---|---|---|---|---|---|---|
| Prednisone (1,2.5,5, 10,20,50 mg) | Variable | If long-term therapy (>3 months of >20 mg/day): BP, PPD, DEXA-scan; supplement Ca$^{++}$ (1000 mg)/Vit D (800IU) and bisphosphonate | Decreases AP-1, cyclooxygenase, NF-kB. Decreases proinflammatory cytokines (esp. IL-2) | Hyperglycemia, insomnia, HTN, infection, osteoporosis, avascular necrosis, poor wound healing, peptic ulcer, water retention, adrenal insufficiency, cushingoid, glaucoma, myopathy, electrolyte imbalance (hypoK, hyperNa) | Metabolized by CYP3A4 | C |
| Methotrexate (Rheumatrex) 2.5 mg | Begin at 5 mg up to 25 mg qwk PO/IM **dose with folate 1 mg qd | Baseline CBC, CMP, Hep panel F/U: CBC/LFTs qwk x 4 → q3mo; LIVER BX: q1–1.5gm; Grade I/II = continue; IIIA (mild fibrosis) = continue, rebx in 6 months; IIIB (severe)/ IV (cirrhosis) = stop | Inhibits dihydrofolate reductase; Cell-cycle specific (S phase); inhibits thymidylate synthetase, methionine synthetase, and AICAR; increases local adenosine (anti-inflammatory effects related to adenosine) | Hepatotoxic, cancer, BM depression, HA, pulm fibrosis/pneumonitis, alopecia, photosensitivity, UV burn recall; GI; increases homocysteine (↑ CV risk); anaphylactoid rxn reported (test dose at 5 mg); Leucovorin rescue | EtOH, NSAIDs, TCNs, retinoids, TMP/SMX, dapsone cyclosporin, probenecid, phenytoin, dipyridamole, chloramphenicol, phenothiazines | X |
| Azathioprine (Imuran) 50 mg | 1–3 mg/kg/day, increase by 0.5 mg/kg/day q4wks | Baseline: CBC, LFT, TPMT; F/U: CBC, LFT qmo × 3 → q2mo Consider PPD | 6-Thioguanine (active metabolite via HGPRT) incorporates into DNA; inhibits de novo purine synthesis (lymphocytes) | N/V, BM suppression, oral ulcers, hepatotoxicity, cancer (lymphoma, SCC), infxn, curly hair, hypersensitivity syndrome at 14 days (fever/shock) | Allopurinol (↓ dose by 75%), warfarin, ACE-I, TMP/SMX, sulfasalazine, IUDs | D |

**DRUGS AND THERAPIES**

| Drug | Dose | Baseline/Follow-up | Mechanism | Side Effects | Interactions | ♀ |
|---|---|---|---|---|---|---|
| **Mycophenolate mofetil** (Cellcept 500 mg; Myfortic 180/360 mg) | 0.5–2 g bid (cellcept 1000 = myfortic 720) | Baseline: CBC, LFTs; F/U: CBC: qwk × 4 → qmo, LFTs qmo | Inhibits **inosine monophosphate dehydrogenase → de novo** purine biosynthesis (lymphs) | GI symptoms (Myfortic = enteric coated, less GI effects), BM depression, hepatotoxicity | Cholestyramine, iron, magnesium/aluminum hydroxide, acyclovir | D |
| **Thalidomide** (Thalidomid) 50 mg | 50–300 mg qh | Baseline: hCG, neuro exam, **SNAP;** F/U: hCG qwk × 4 then q2–4 wks; neuro q3mos; SNAP prn | Decreases TNF-α; inhibits angiogenesis; inhibits PMN phagocytosis; inhibits monocyte chemotaxis | Birth defects, sedation, constipation, peripheral **neuropathy** (sensory), leukopenia | Sedatives, histamine, serotonin, prostaglandin | X |
| **Cyclosporine** (Neoral) 25/100 mg | Start at 2.5 mg/kg/day 5 mg/kg/day (without food) | Baseline, q2wks (→ qmo): CBC, BMP, LFTs, FLP, Mg, Uric Acid, BP; F/U: **Creatinine Cl** q6mo; Trough levels if > 5 mg/kg/day | Binds cyclophilin → inhibits calcineurin activation of NF-AT; inhibits IL-2, IFN-γ synthesis | **Nephrotoxic, HTN** (use CCB, no ACE/diuretic), hyperlipidemia, infxn, cancer, HA, acne, hyperK/uricemia, hirsutism, hypoMg, paresthesias, gingival hyperplasia | Metabolized by CYP3A4 (liver), P-gp (intestine) – Azoles, Macrole, CCB, **grapefruit juice**, MTX, SSR, ticlopidine; additive toxicity with nephrotoxic drugs | C |
| **Cyclophosphamide** (Cytoxan) 25/50 mg | 1–3 mg/kg/day or IV pulse 1 g/m² qmo; increase fluid intake (>3 l/day) | Baseline: CBC, CMP, UA; F/U: CBC qwk x 8 then qmo; CMP qmo; **UA** qwk × 12 then q2–4 wks **forever;** cystoscopy: yearly or if microscopic hematuria; **urine cytology** @ >50 gm | Cell cycle-independent; Covalent DNA binding; B-cell suppression | BM depression, **hemorrhagic cystitis** (acrolein metabolite), **carcinogenesis** (esp. TCC of bladder), hepatotoxicity, reproductive toxicity, anagen effluvium, mucositis, SIADH, pneumonitis/fibrosis, infections, nail ridging, pigmented bands on teeth, diffuse hyperpigmentation | Allopurinol, chloramphenicol, succinylcholine, digoxin, doxorubicin, barbiturates, cimetidine, halothane, nitrous oxide | D |

♀: Pregnancy Category

continued p. 246

## Systemic retinoids

| Drug | Dose | Labs to follow | Mechanism | Side effects | Interactions | ♀ |
|------|------|----------------|-----------|--------------|--------------|---|
| **Isotretinoin** (Accutane) 10/20/30/40 mg | 0.5–1 mg/kg/day with food. Total dose based on body weight = 120–150 mg/kg | Baseline: hCG, LFT, FLP; F/U: hCG, LFT, FLP qmo. *Half Life:* 10–20 h Pregnancy Avoidance = 30 days | *All Retinoids:* Affect cell growth/differentiation, morphogenesis, inhibit malignant cell growth, alter cellular cohesiveness, inhibit AP-1, NF-kB, ornithine decarboxylase, TLR-2; Increase dermal collagen I, hyaluronic acid, elastic fibers, fibronectin, transglutaminase and Th1 skewing | **Dryness,** myalgia/arthralgia, tendinitis, hyperostosis (long term), pseudotumor cerebri, HA, depression, transaminase elevation, alopecia (telogen effluvium), decreased night vision, PGs, photosensitivity, staph infxns, IBD association | Tetracyclines (risk of pseudotumor cerebri), MTX (hepatotoxicity) Vitamin A, macrolides, azoles, rifampicin, alcohol, phenytoin, mini-pill contraceptive, photosensitizers, carbamazepine | X |
| **Acitretin** (Soriatane) 10/25 mg | 25–50 mg/day with food | Baseline: CBC, LFT, FLP, hCG, BUN/Cr; F/U: hCG, CBC qmo; LFT, FLP q2wks → qmo → q3mo *Half life:* 50 h Pregnancy Avoidance = 3 years | *Isotretinoin:* no specific receptor; *Acitretin:* all RAR receptor subtypes; *Bexarotene:* all RXR receptor subtypes | SAME as Accutane but difference is duration of tx; **longer pregnancy avoidance** (3 years), more alopecia, more hyperostosis. Alcohol can convert acitretin to etretinate (accumulates in fat) | | X |
| **Bexarotene** (Targretin) 10/75 mg | 300 mg/m²/day with food (fatty foods improve bioavailability for retinoids) | Baseline: FLP, CBC, LFT, **TSH/T4,** hCG; F/U: FLP qwk until stable then q1–2 mo; CBC, LFT, hCG qmo × 3–6 months; TSH/T4 q8wks *Half life:* 7 h Pregnancy Avoidance = 30 days | | SAME as other retinoids PLUS more marked **hypertriglyceridemia, central hypothyroidism, leukopenia,** cataracts, hypoglycemia | Same as above; gemfibrozil | X |

# Biologics

| Drug | Dose | Labs to follow | Mechanism | Side effects | Interactions | ♀ |
|---|---|---|---|---|---|---|
| **Alefacept** (Amevive) 15 mg | 15 mg IM qw × 12 wks (in office) | Baseline: WBC CD4, PPD; F/U: CD4 qwk (hold dose if <250 cells/μl) | Recombinant fusion protein Fc IgG1 binds to **CD2** on T cells (CD45RO+); causes activated T-cell apoptosis | **Leukopenia**, infection, cancer, chills, hepatic injury (transaminitis) | None | B |
| **Efalizumab** (Raptiva) | 1 mg/kg SQ weekly | Baseline: PPD, CBC (platelets); F/U: CBC qmo x 3, then q3mos | Humanized murine antibody (anti-CD11a); inhibits **LFA1 – ICAM 1** interaction by binding CD11a subunit of LFA1 on T cells; prevents T cell activation & diapedesis | Rebound with discontinuation, flare on therapy, infection, cancer, injection site reaction, **thrombocytopenia** | None | C |
| **Etanercept** (Enbrel) 25/50 mg | 25–50 mg SQ 2 × per wk × 3 mos then 50 mg qwk | Baseline: PPD and/or CXR Consider CMP, HepB, HepC, CBC, HIV | Recombinant fusion protein Fc IgG1 to TNF receptor; binds **soluble TNF-α** | Injection site rxn, infection (**TB** reactivation), cancer, CHF, **demyelinating disease**, lupus-like syndrome, paradoxical pustular psoriasis | None | B |
| **Infliximab** (Remicade) | 3–10 mg/kg IV; Week 0, 2, 6 then q8wks | Baseline: PPD and/or CXR. Consider CMP, HepB, HepC, CBC, HIV | Murine chimeric monoclonal antibody to TNF-α; binds **soluble and transmembrane TNF-α** | SAME as Enbrel but slightly increased risk; infusion reactions | None | B |

♀: Pregnancy Category

continued p. 248

**DRUGS AND THERAPIES**

247

| Drug | Dose | Labs to follow | Mechanism | Side effects | Interactions | ♀ |
|------|------|---------------|-----------|--------------|--------------|---|
| **Adalimumab** (Humira) | 40 mg SQ q other week | Baseline: PPD and/or CXR. Consider CMP, HepB, HepC, CBC, HIV | Humanized monoclonal antibody to TNF-α; binds **soluble and transmembrane TNF-**α | SAME as Enbrel | None | B |
| **Rituximab** (Rituxan) | Chemo: 375 mg/m2 × 4, q week RA: 1g × 2, qo week | Baseline: CBC Follow CD19 q6–12 mos | Anti-CD20 monoclonal antibody | Infusion rxn (worst with first infusion), JC virus infx resulting in PML, severe mucocutaneous reactions | None | C |
| **Kineret** (Anakinra) | RA dosing: 100 mg SQ daily Indicated for Periodic Fever Syndromes | Baseline: PPD and/or CXR. Consider CMP, HepB, HepC, CBC, HIV | IL-1 receptor antagonist | SAME as Enbrel | None | C |
| **IVIg** | 2 g/kg over 2–5 days. Also see TEN protocol p. 285 | Baseline: IgA levels (use Gammagard in IgA deficiency). BMP; evaluate for heart failure | Immunomodulatory | Fluid overload, anaphylactic shock (in IgA deficiency), rare reports of hemolytic anemia, ARF, and aseptic meningitis | None | C |

Nomenclature of biologics: mab (monoclonal antibody); ximab (chimeric); zumab (humanized); umab 'human'; cept (receptor-antibody fusion protein).
♀: Pregnancy Category

# General Reference

## Metric measurements
15 ml = 15 cc = 1 tablespoon
5 ml = 5 cc = 1 teaspoon
250 ml = 8 oz
454 g = 16 oz
30 g = 1 oz

## Dose calculations
1% = 1 g/100 ml = 10 mg/cc
0.1% = 0.1 g/100 ml = 1 mg/cc

## Drug dispensing and absorption
1 g Cream (or ~0.95 g Ointment) → covers 100 cm$^2$
1 Fingertip Unit (FTU) = 2 cm of cream on fingertip = 0.5 g

|  | 1 Application(G) | bid × 1 week(G) |
|---|---|---|
| Adult full body | 10–30 | 170 |
| Head and neck | 2 | 10 |
| Hands and feet | 2 | 10 |
| Single arm | 3 | 15 |
| Single leg | 4 | 30 |
| Trunk | 8 | 60 |

Percutaneous absorption by anatomic site: scrotum > cheeks > abdomen and chest > scalp and axillae > back > forearms > palms > ankles > soles.

# Corticosteroid

|  | Equivalent dose (mg) | Glucocorticoid potency | Mineralo-corticoid potency | Duration (h) (half life) |
|---|---|---|---|---|
| Hydrocortisone | 4 | 1 | 1 | 8–12 |
| Cortisone acetate | 5 | 0.8 | 0.8 | 8–12 |
| Prednisone | 1 | 3.5–5 | 0.8 | 18–36 |
| Prednisolone | 1 | 4 | 0.8 | 18–36 |
| Triamcinolone | 0.8 | 5 | 0 | 18–36 |
| Methylprednisolone | 0.8 | 5–7.5 | 0.5 | 18–36 |
| Dexamethasone | 0.15 | 25–80 | 0 | 36–54 |
| Betamethasone | 0.12–0.15 | 25–30 | 0 | 36–54 |

| Drug name (Trade Name)*<br>–Formulation, dosage | Trade size | ♀ |
|---|---|---|
| *Available in Generic | ♀: Pregnancy Category | |

## Acne – Topical

### Antibiotics

| | | |
|---|---|---|
| **Benzoyl peroxide 5%/clindamycin 1%** | | |
| Duac gel | 45 g | C |
| Benzaclin gel | 25, 50 g | C |
| **Benzoyl peroxide 5%/erythromycin 3%\*** | | |
| Generic gel | 23, 46 g | C |
| Benzamycin | 46 g, 60/box | C |
| **Clindamycin\*** | | |
| Cleocin T 1% solution, lotion | 60 ml | B |
| 1% gel | 30, 60 g | B |
| 1% pledgets | 60/box | B |
| Evoclin 1% foam | 50, 100 g | B |
| **Erythromycin\*** | | |
| Akne-Mycin 2% ointment | 25 g | B |
| Emgel 2% gel | 27, 50 g | B |
| **Metronidazole** | | |
| Noritate 1% cream | 30 g | B |
| MetroCream 0.75% | 30, 45 g | B |
| MetroGel 0.75% gel | 29 g | B |
| MetroLotion 0.75% lotion | 59 ml | B |
| **Sodium sulfacetamide 10%** | | |
| Klaron lotion | 59 ml | C |
| **Sulfa 5%/sodium sulfacetamide\* 10%** | | |
| Generic lotion | 25 ml | C |
| Novacet lotion | 30, 60 ml | C |
| Plexion TS cream | 30, 90 g | C |
| Avar Gel; Avar Green gel | 45 g | C |
| Clenia emollient cream | 28 g | C |
| Sulfacet R lotion | 25 ml | C |
| Rosula gel | 45 ml | C |

### Keratolytics

| | | |
|---|---|---|
| **Azelaic acid** | | |
| Azelex 20% cream | 30, 50 g | B |
| Finacea 15% gel | 30 g | B |

*Available in Generic

**Benzoyl peroxide\*** (BP) — Antibacterial/keratolytic for comedonal acne; may bleach clothing

| Rx | Benzac AC 2.5%, 5%, 10% emollient gel | 60, 90 g | C |
|----|----|----|----|
| | Benzagel 5%, 10% gel | 45 g | C |
| | Brevoxyl 4%, 8% gel, lotion/cleanser | 42.5, 90 g | C |
| | Generic BP 2.5%, 5%, 10% gel, wash | | C |
| | Triaz 3%, 6%, 10% gel | 42.5 g | C |
| OTC | Clearasil 10% cream, lotion | | C |
| | Oxy balance 10% gel | | C |

## Retinoids:

**Adapalene** *(specific for RAR-beta and gamma)*

| Differin 0.1% cream, gel | 15, 45 g | C |
|----|----|----|
| Differin 0.3% gel | 45 g | C |

**Tretinoin\*** *(binds all RAR, no RXR)*

| Avita 0.025% cream, gel | 20, 45 g | C |
|----|----|----|
| Retin-A Micro 0.04%, 0.1% gel | 20, 45 g | C |
| Generic 0.025%, 0.05%, 0.1% cream | 20, 45 g | C |
| Generic 0.025%, 0.1% gel | 15, 45 g | C |
| Renova 0.02%, 0.05% cream | 40, 60 g | C |
| Ziana 0.025% (+ clindamycin 1.2%) gel | 30, 60 g | C |

**Tazarotene** *(specific for RAR-beta and gamma)*

| Avage 0.1% cream | 15, 30 g | X |
|----|----|----|
| Tazorac 0.05%, 0.1% cream | 15, 30, 60 g | X |
| Tazorac 0.05%, 0.1% gel | 30, 100 g | X |

# Acne – Systemic

## Antibiotics

| **Tetracycline\*** (Sumycin)<br>250–500 mg bid-qid<br>Do not use in age < 8 years | 250, 500 mg<br>Susp 125/5 ml | D |
|----|----|----|
| **Doxycycline\*** (Adoxa, Doryx,<br>Vibramycin) po qd-bid<br>(Periostat) po bid<br>(Oracea) po qd<br>SE: photosensitivity, dizziness, esophagitis:<br>take w/8 oz water. Do not take w. calcium.<br>Not for age <8 years | 50, 100 mg<br><br>20 mg<br>40 mg | D |
| **Minocycline\*** (Dynacin, Minocin)<br>50–100 mg po qd-bid<br>SE: gray discoloration of skin/teeth,<br>lupus-like syndrome, pseudotumor cerebri.<br>Not for age <8 years | 50, 75, 100<br>50 mg/5 ml | D |
| **Erythromycin\*** (E-mycin, Erytab)<br>250–500 mg po qid or 333 mg po tid,<br>or 500 mg po bid<br>PEDs: 50 mg/kg/day divided qid<br>SE: nausea, diarrhea | 250,333,500 mg<br>Susp 200/5, 400/5 ml | B |

\*Available in Generic

## Retinoids

**Isotretinoin\*** (Accutane,                        10, 20, 40 mg     X
Amnesteem, Sotret, Claravis) 13-cis RA – unclear receptor affinity)
0.5–1 mg/kg/day divided qd-bid
☑LABS: Baseline – 2 neg βhcg, lipids, LFTs (for Medicaid + CBC, glucose).
Monthly – βhcg, lipids, LFTs.
SE: dryness, teratogen, HA, arthralgias/myalgias, ↓ night vision, depression, lipid
abnormalities.

## Others

**Spironolactone\*** (Aldactone)                     25, 50, 100 mg     X
25–200 mg qd, start 25–50 mg
Weakly antiandrogenic effects for PCOS patients
SE: hyperkalemia, gynecomastia, hypotension

# Alopecia

**Finasteride** (Propecia)                             1 mg     X
Androgenetic alopecia in men: 1 mg po qd
**Minoxidil\*** (Rogaine)                         2% women; 5% men     C
For men or women: usually use 5% solution.    60 ml
1 ml bid to dry scalp

# Analgesics

Dose: 1–2 tabs po q4–6 h PRN pain (in increasing strength)

| | | | |
|---|---|---|---|
| Darvocet | Propoxyphene + Acetaminophen<br>N-50 (50/325); N-100 (100/325) | 50/325 mg<br>100/325 mg | C |
| Tylenol #3 | Codeine + Acetaminophen<br>*Can cause constipation-Rx w<br>Colace 100bid | 15/300 mg (#2)<br>30/300 mg (#3)<br>60/300 mg (#4) | C |
| Vicodin | Hydrocodone + Acetaminophen | 5/500 mg<br>7.5/500 mg | C |
| Percocet | Oxycodone + Acetaminophen<br>* Very strong, almost never<br>prescribed in Derm. Use for 5/325 mg<br>major abd surgeries, etc. | 2.5/325 mg<br>5/325 mg<br>7.5/325 mg | C |

*Available in Generic

## Anesthetics – Topical

| **EMLA** Lidocaine 2.5% + prilocaine 2.5% | | | | 5, 30 g | B |
|---|---|---|---|---|---|
| Age area | Weight (kg) | Max dose (g) | Max area (cm²) | | |
| 1–3 months | <5 | 1 | 10 | | |
| 4–12 months | 5–10 | 2 | 20 | | |
| 1–6 years | 10–20 | 10 | 100 | | |
| 7–12 years | >20 | 20 | 200 | | |

May cause methemoglobinemia in children.

| | | |
|---|---|---|
| **LMX 4** Lidocaine 4% cream | 30 g | B |
| **LMX 5** Lidocaine 5% cream | 15, 30 g | B |
| **Lida-Mantle** Lidocaine 3% cream | 28, 85 g | B |
| **Lida-Mantle HC** Lidocaine 3% + 0.5% HC | 28, 85 g | C |
| **Pramosone** Pramoxine + 1% or 2.5% | 60, 120 ml solution | C |
| hydrocortisone – topical for itching | 30, 60 g cream | |
| | 30 g ointment | |

## Antibiotics

### Topical/Antiseptic

| | | |
|---|---|---|
| **Mupirocin\*** (Bactroban/Centany) 2% cream, ointment apply bid-tid for impetigo, wound infections; for nasal MRSA eradication, use 0.5 g in each nostril bid × 5 days | 15, 30 g | B |
| **Bacitracin** + **Polymyxin\*** (Polysporin) | OTC | C |
| **Silver sulfadiazine\*** (Silvadene) 1% cream | 20, 50, 400 1000 g | B |
| **Retapamulin** (Altabax) 1% ointment bid × 5 days for methicillin sensitive s. aureus or s. pyogenes | 5, 10, 15 g | B |
| **Chlorhexidine\*** (Hibiclens 4% cleanser) Good antimicrobial agent for bacteria, fungus, and yeast. For MRSA eradication | 120, 240, 480, 960, 3840 ml | B |
| **Gentamicin\*** (Garamycin cream/ointment 0.1%) For pseudomonas coverage (i.e. nails, wound) | 15 g | D |

\*Available in Generic

**DRUGS AND THERAPIES**

## Systemic

| | | |
|---|---|---|
| **Amoxicillin\*** (Amoxil)<br>250–500 mg po tid<br>Child: 20–40 mg/kg/day po divided tid | 250, 500 mg<br>Susp 125/5<br>250 mg/5 ml | B |
| **Augmentin\*** (Amoxicillin + Clavulanic acid)<br>500–875 mg po bid/250–500 mg po tid<br>Peds: 20–40 mg/kg/day divided tid | 250, 500, 875 mg<br>Susp 200/5<br>400 mg/5 ml | B |
| **Azithromycin\*** (Zithromax) macrolide.<br>500 mg po × 1; then 250 mg qd 5 days<br>500 mg po qd for 3 days | Zpak: 250 mg<br>TriPak: 500 mg | B |
| **Cefaclor** (Ceclor) second gen. cephalosporin.<br>250–500 mg po tid. 250 mg/5 ml<br>Peds: 20–40 mg/kg/day po divided tid | 250, 500 mg<br>Susp 125/5,<br>250 mg/5ml | B |
| **Cephalexin\*** (Keflex) first gen cephalosporin<br>250–500 mg po qid<br>Peds: 40 mg/kg/day po divided bid | 250, 500 mg<br>Susp<br>250 mg/5 ml | B |
| **Ciprofloxacin\*** (Cipro) second gen. quinolone.<br>250–750 mg po bid<br>Interactions: antacids, sucralfate, Fe, Zn,<br>theophylline, warfarin, cyclosporine | 250, 500,<br>750 mg | C |
| **Clarithromycin\*** (Biaxin)<br>250–500 mg po bid<br>Peds: 7.5–mg/kg po bid | 250, 500 mg<br>Susp 125/5,<br>250 mg/5 ml | C |
| **Clindamycin\*** (Cleocin)<br>150–450 mg po qid<br>Peds: 8–25 mg/kg/day divided tid-qid<br>May cause C. difficile colitis | 75, 150, 300 mg<br>Susp<br>75 mg/5 ml | B |
| **Doxycycline\*** (Adoxa, Doryx, Vibramycin)<br>50–100 mg po qd-bid<br>SE: photosensitivity, dizziness, esophagitis:<br>take w/8 oz water. Do not take with calcium.<br>Not for age <8 years | 50, 100 mg | D |
| **Erythromycin\***<br>SE: nausea, diarrhea | | B |
| E-mycin, Erytab<br>250–500 mg po qid or 333 mg po tid, or<br>500 mg po bid | 250, 333, 500 mg | B |
| Erythromycin ethyl<br>succinate – EES,Eryped 400 mg po qid<br>Peds: 50 mg/kg/day divided qid | 400 mg | B |
| | 200 mg/5 ml<br>400 mg/5 ml | B |
| **Minocycline\*** (Dynacin, Minocin)<br>50–100 mg po qd-bid.<br>SE: blue-gray discoloration of skin/teeth, lupus-like<br>syndrome, pseudotumor cerebri.<br>Not for age <8 years | 50 mg/5 ml<br>50, 75<br>100 mg | D |

\*Available in Generic

**Rifampin\*** 10–20 mg/kg/day, max 600 mg qd        150, 300 mg        C
   P450 drug interactions: antacids, calcium channel
    blockers, steroids, cyclosporine, digoxin, dapsone,
    quinolones, warfarin, L-thyroxine.

**Tetracycline\*** (Sumycin)        250, 500 mg        D
   250–500 mg bid-qid
   Not for age < 8 years

**Trimethoprim-sulfamethoxazole\*** (Septra, Bactrim)     Sulfa (mg)/TMP (mg)  C
   1 tab (double-strength) po bid        400/80
   Peds: 0.5 kg/kg po bid;        800/160 (DS)
    10 kg – 1 tsp bid        Sus 200/40 per 5 ml
    20 kg – 2 tsp bid
    30 kg – 3 tsp bid
    >40 kg –4 tsp bid or 1 DS tab bid

## Antibiotic preoperative prophylaxis

See p. 184 for use of antibiotic prophylaxis for endocarditis indicated for surgical procedure on infected tissue in patients with high-risk cardiac lesion.

## Antibiotic regimens

|  | **First line** | **Second line** |
|---|---|---|
| Acne, perioral dermatitis | MCN 50–100 mg qd-bid<br>DCN 50–100 mg qd-bid<br>TCN 500 mg bid | Erythromycin<br>TMP-SMZ |
| Anthrax | Cipro 500 mg bid × 60 days<br>Peds: 20–30 mg/kg/d<br>  divided q12 × 60 days | DCN 100 mg bid × 60 day<br>Peds > 8 years 2.2 mg/kg<br>  bid × 60 days |
| Bacillary angiomatosis | Clarithro 500 mg bid<br>Azithromycin 250 mg qd<br>Cipro 500–750 mg bid | Erythromycin 500 mg Qid<br>DCN 100 mg bid |
| Bite: Cat<br>*Pasteurella multocida* | Augmentin 875/125 mg bid<br>Or 500/125 mg tid | Cefuroxime 0.5 g q12 h<br>DCN 100 mg bid |
| Bite: Dog<br>*Pasteurella multocida* | Augmentin 875/125 mg bid<br>Or 500/125 mg tid | Clinda 300 Qid<br>+TMP-SMX Cinda +<br>Floroquinone |
| Bite: Human | Augmentin 875/125 mg bid<br>× 5 days | If infxn: Clinda + Cipro |

*continued p. 256*

\*Available in Generic

| | First line | Second line |
|---|---|---|
| Bite: Spider – (Brown Recluse) | Dapsone 50 mg qd may help | |
| *Borrelia recurrentis* | Doxycycline | Erythromycin |
| *Campylobacter jejuni* | Floroquinone | Erythromycin |
| Cellulitis (extremity) | Nafcillin 2 g Q4h IV | Erythromycin, Z-Pak |
| | Dicloxacillin 500 Q6 h | Augmentin |
| | Cefazolin 1 g Q8h IV | 875/125 mg bid |
| Cellulitis (Face) | Vanco 1 g IV Q12h | Amoxicillin/Penicillin |
| *Clostridium perfringens* | Clindamycin + PCN G | Doxycyline |
| Erythrasma (*Corynebact. minutissimum*) | Erythro 250 mg Qid × 14 days | Topical agents |
| Kawasaki syndrome | IVIG 2 g/kg over 12 h + ASA 80–100 mg/kg/day divided in 4 doses then 3–5 mg/kg/day qd × 6–8 weeks | |
| Impetigo | Dicloxicillin 125–500 mg Qid | Azithromycin, Clarithromycin |
| | Bactroban topically | Erythromycin |
| Lyme disease (*Borrelia burgdorferi*) | Exposure: DCN 200 mg ×1 Tx: for 14–21 days DCN 100 bid Amoxicillin 500 Tid Cefuroxime 500 bid | Erythro 250 Qid |
| Meningococcus (*N. meningitides*) | PCN G | Cefuroxime |
| Mycoplasma | Azithromycin Clarithromycin Erythromycin Fluoroquinone | Doxycyline |
| Pseudomonas aeruginosa | Cipro 500–750 mg bid | Third generation Cephalo Imipenem, Aztreonam |
| Rickettsia: RMSF | DCN 100 mg bid × 7 days | Chloramphenicol 500 mg Qid × 7 days |
| Staphylococcus | Clindamycin TMP-SMX | Erythromycin |
| Staph scalded skin | Nafcillin or Oxacillin 2 g IV Q4h × 5–7 days Ped: 150 mg/kg divided Q6h | |
| Streptococcus | PCN G | Erythromycin Azithromycin Clarithromycin |

Bites: need tetanus prophylaxis.
Modified from the Sanford Guide 2006

## STDs

| Disease | Symptoms | First line therapy | Second line therapy |
|---------|----------|--------------------|--------------------|
| Gonorrhea (and treat for Chlamydia) | Male: urethritis with discharge | Cefixime 400 mg | Gatifloxacin 400 mg |
| | Female: endocervicits with discharge | Cipro 500 mg Ofloxacin 400 mg and Azithromycin 1 g DCN 100 mg bid × 7 days | Enoxacin 400 mg Lomefloxacin 400 mg and Azithromycin 1 g DCN 100 mg bid × 7 days |
| Chancroid (*Haemophilus ducreyi*) | Deep ulcer, Pain, 50% adenopathy | Azithromycin 1 g × 1 Ceftriazone 250 mg IM ×1 | Erythromycin 500 mg Qid×7 days Cipro 500 mg bid × 3 days |
| Lymphogranuloma Venereum (*Chlamydia trachomatis*) | Herpetiform vesicle, NO PAIN, +LAD/ Groove sign | DCN 100 mg bid × 21 days | Erythromycin 500 mg Qid × 21 days |
| Granuloma Inguinale (*Klebsiella granulomatis*, formerly *Calymmato-bacterium granulomatis*) | Ulcer with beefy granulation tissue, NO PAIN, NO LAD + Donovan bodies | DCN 100 bid × 21 days TMP-SMX DS bid × 21 days | Erythromycin Cipro |
| Syphilis (*Treponema pallidum*) | Indurated chancre, NO PAIN, +LAD | Benzathine PCN G 2.4 million units IM x 1, repeat in 1 week | DCN 100 mg bid × 14 days TCN 500 mg Qid × 14 days |

*Pregnant mothers who are PCN allergic should get desensitization then treat with PCN.

## Antifungals

### Topical
*Classes:* polyenes bind ergosterol; azoles inhibit 14-alpha demethylase; allylamines inhibit squalene epoxidase.

| Rx | | | |
|----|--|--|--|
| | **Butenafine*** (Mentax) 1% cream | 15, 30 g | B |
| | **Ciclopirox** (Loprox) 1% cream, lotion | 15, 30, 90 g | B |
| | **Ciclopirox** (Penlac) 8% nail solution | 6.6 ml | B |
| | **Econazole*** (Spectazole) 1% cream | 15, 30, 85 g | C |
| | **Ketoconazole*** (Nizoral) 2% cream | 15, 30, 60 g | C |
| | **Ketoconazole** (Nizoral) 2% shampoo | 120 ml | C |

continued p. 258

*Available in Generic

| | | |
|---|---|---|
| **Ketoconazole** (Xolegel) 2% gel | 15 g | C |
| **Miconazole\*** (Micatin) 2% cream, powder, spray | 15, 30, 90 g | C |
| **Naftifine\*** (Naftin) 1% gel, cream | 15, 30, 60 g | B |
| **Oxiconazole** (Oxistat) 1% cream | 15, 30, 60 g | B |
| **Sertaconazole** (Ertazco) 2% cream | 30 g | C |
| **Thymol** 4% in alcohol | 30 ml with dropper | |

| | | | |
|---|---|---|---|
| OTC | **Clotrimazole** (Lotrimin, Mycelex) 1% cream, solution, lotion | | B |
| | **Ketoconazole** (Nizoral) 1% cream, shampoo | | C |
| | **Miconazole** (Zeasorb-AF Powder) 2% powder | | C |
| | **Miconazole** (Monistat) 2% cream | | C |
| | **Terbinafine** (Lamisil) 1% cream, solution, spray | | B |
| | **Selenium sulfide** (Selsun, Head and Shoulder) 1%, 2.5% shampoo | | C |

## Systemic

| | | |
|---|---|---|
| **Griseofulvin\*** (Grifulvin, Grisactin, Fulvicin) | | C |
| *Microsize:* 500–1000 mg po qd. | 250, 500 mg | |
| *Peds:* 20 mg/kg/day divided bid, | | |
| max 1 g/days × 6–8 weeks | 125 mg/5 ml | |
| Take with food (fatty meals increase absorption) | | |
| Do not take if pregnant, h/o hepatic failure, porphyria, lupus | | |
| May cause agranulocytosis, OCP failure, lupus, photosensitivity, disulfiram-like reaction | | |
| CYP3A4 inducer: decreases levels of warfarin, CSA, OCPs | | |
| *Mechanism:* inhibits microtubules | | |
| **Fluconazole\*** (Diflucan) | 50,100,150, | |
| *Onychomycosis:* 150–300 mg | 200 mg | C |
| 1 dose q wk, for 3–12 months | 10 or 40 mg/ml | |
| Peds: 3–6 mg/kg/day | | |
| *Do not take:* cisapride – fatal arrhythmia | | |
| *Increases effects of:* warfarin, CSA, phenytoin, zidovudine, theophylline, terfenadine (CYP2C9 and 3A4 inhibitor) | | |
| Rifampin decreases Fluconazole levels & cimetidine/HCTZ increase Fluconazole levels | | |
| *Mechanism:* inhibits lanosterol 14-α demethylase | | |
| **Itraconazole\*** (Sporanox) | 100 mg | C |
| *Onychomycosis:* 200 mg qd or pulse dose 200 mg bid × 1 week/month | 10 mg/ml | |
| Peds: pulse dose 1 week/month (10–20 kg = 50 mg qd; 20–30 mg = 100 mg qd; 30–40 mg = | | |

*continued p. 259*

\*Available in Generic

DRUGS AND THERAPIES

100/200 alternate; 40–50 kg = 200 mg qd;
>50 kg = 200 mg bid)
☑ Check LFTs after 4 weeks.
Treat 6 weeks-fingernails, 12 weeks-toenails
*Tinea versicolor*: 200 mg ×1, repeat in 1 week
*Tinea capitis*: 3–5 mg/kg/day divided qd-bid
for 1 month
Take with orange juice/ carbonated beverage
*Do not take*: cisapride (arrhythmia)
Contraindication: ventricular dysfunction
CYP3A4 inhibitor: increases effects of: felodipine, CSA, digoxin, warfarin,
statins, oral hypoglycemics
*Mechanism*: inhibits lanosterol 14-α demethylase

**Ketoconazole\*** (Nizoral) 200 mg po qd.    200 mg    C
*Tinea versicolor*: 400 mg ×1, repeat in 1 week
*Peds >2 years*: 3.3–6.6 mg/kg/day po given qd.
☑ Check LFTs if long-term use, Q2wks × 2 mos
Take with orange juice/ carbonated beverage
CYP3A4 inhibitor
*Do not take*: cisapride, pimozide, quinidine (arrhythmia)
*Increases effects of*: warfarin, CSA, phenytoin, theophylline
Rifampin, PPI decrease Ketoconazole levels
*Mechanism*: inhibits lanosterol 14-α demethylase

**Nystatin\*** Swish and swallow 4–6 ml Qid    100,000    C
For oral candidiasis    units/ml
*Mechanism*: associates with ergosterol
to produce pores

**Terbinafine\*** (Lamisil)    250 mg    B
*Onychomycosis*: 250 mg po qd × 12 weeks, or
pulse dose 250 mg bid for 1 wk/mo × 3 months
*Tinea capitis*: Peds 3–6 mg/kg/day for 1 month.
<20 kg – ¼ tab po qd; 20–40 kg – ½ tab po qd;
>40 kg – 1 tab po qd.
☑ Check LFTs baseline and q6wks.
May cause SCLE, taste or visual disturbance, headache, diarrhea
Lowers CSA level. CYP2D6 inhibitor: increases theophylline, TCA, narc levels.
Rifampin decreases and cimetidine/terfinadine increases
terbinafine levels. Caution with hepatic or renal insufficiency.
*Mechanism*: inhibits squalene epoxidase

**Amphotericin** B (Amphocin)    B
*For Systemic Fungal Infection* dose varies
0.3–1 mg/kg/day IV, start 0.25 mg/kg/day and increase by
5–10 mg/day. Max 1.5 mg/kg/day
☑ Check renal function, Mg, K+, LFT, CBC.
*Mechanism*: associates with ergosterol to produce pores

\*Available in Generic

## Antifungal regimens

### Candidal infection
*Perleche:* Ketoconazole cream, Miconazole cream bid until resolve
*Intertrigo:* Clotrimazole cream, Miconazole cream bid until resolve
  then use Miconazole or Zeasorb AF powder to keep area dry
*Oral Candidiasis/ Thrush:* Nystatin swish and swallow qid
  Clotriamazole troche 5×per/day
*Chronic Paronychia:* Thymol solution bid

### Pityrosporum folliculitis: (P. ovale or P. orbiculare)
*Topical:* Loprox cream, lotion; Nizoral cream, shampoo; Selenium sulfide
*Oral:* Nizoral 200–400 mg qd

### Onychomycosis
Also need to use topical antifungal cream bid indefinitely

| | | | |
|---|---|---|---|
| Topical | **Ciclopirox (Penlac):** Apply lacquer to affected nails qd; apply new coats on top of previous coats. | 6.6 ml | B |
| | **Thymol** 4% in alcohol Drip onto & around affected nails bid | 30 ml with dropper | |
| Oral | Treat fingernails for 6 weeks, toenails for 12 weeks. | | |
| | **Itraconazole** (Sporanox) 200 mg po qd; pulse dose 200 mg po bid for 7 days, off for 21 days. ☑Labs: +/ − LFTs after 4 weeks | 100 mg | C |
| | **Terbinafine** (Lamisil) 250 mg po qd ☑Labs: LFTs baseline, Q6wks | 250 mg | B |
| | **Fluconazole** (Diflucan) 150–300 qwk No need to check labs | 50, 100, 150, 200 mg | C |

### Tinea versicolor
*Mild:* Topical treatment with Nizoral shampoo, Nizoral cream
*Severe:* Oral agents

Ketoconazole (Nizoral) [200 mg]
    200 mg po qd × 5 days
    Or 400 mg po × 1, 1–2 h before exercise. Let sweat dry, leave on
    as long as possible. Repeat in 1 week

Itraconazole (Sporanox) [100 mg]
    200 mg po × 1, repeat in 1 week

Maintenance treatment with Nizoral shampoo, Nizoral cream

**Tinea capitis** (almost exclusively in children)
  Griseofulvin: 20 mg/kg/d divided bid × 6–8 weeks [250, 500 mg or 125/5 ml]
  Itraconazole (Sporanox): 3–5 mg/kg/d × 4–6 weeks [100 mg or 10 mg/ml]

**Tinea corporis**
  Rx: Spectazole, Naftin bid to area until resolve
  OTC: Lamisil, Lotrimin bid to area until resolve

# Antiparasitics

| | | |
|---|---|---|
| **Permethrin\*** (Elimite) For scabies:<br>Apply from neck to soles of feet, leave on overnight for 8–12 h, wash off in am; repeat in 1 week | 5% cream<br>60 g | B |
| **Permethrin\*** (Nix) For lice:<br>Apply cream rinse to hair/scalp, leave on 10 min, shampoo hair. Repeat in 1 week. Use nit comb | 1% soln.<br>60 ml | B |
| **Ivermectin** (Stromectol) For scabies | 6 mg | C |

| Single dose of 0.2 mg/kg | |
|---|---|
| Weight:(kg) | Dose |
| 15–24 | ½ tab (3 mg) |
| 25–35 | 1 tab (6 mg) |
| 36–50 | 1 ½ tab (9 mg) |
| 51–65 | 2 tab (12 mg) |
| 66–79 | 2 ½ tab (15 mg) |
| ≥ 80 | 0.2 mg/kg |

*Mechanism:* blocks invertebrate glutamate-gated Cl channels, leading to paralysis and death

| | | |
|---|---|---|
| **Precipitated sulfur** For scabies<br>Apply to entire body below head on three successive nights; bather 24 h after each application | 6% in petrolatum | C |
| **Lindane** (Kwell) For scabies<br><br>Adults: apply thin layer from chin to toes; use on dry skin and shower off 10 h later; repeat in 1 week<br>*Second-line secondary to neurotoxicity (not for use in neonates or infants)* | 1% lotion or cream | C |
| **Malathion** (Ovide) For lice<br>Apply to dry hair/scalp. Wash out after 8–12 h. Repeat in 1 week. Use nit comb. *(Best efficacy among chemical pediculicides)* | 0.5% lotion | B |

\*Available in Generic

# Antivirals

## For HSV labialis – topical agents

| | | | |
|---|---|---|---|
| **Penciclovir** (Denavir) | Apply cream to lesions q2 while awake x 4 days | 1% cream 2 g | B |
| **Acyclovir** (Zovirax) | Apply ointment 5×per/day for 5 days | 5% ointment 2, 10 g | B |
| **Docosanol** (Abreva) | Apply cream 5×per/day for 5–10 days (efficacy same as placebo) | OTC 2 g | B |

## For HSV 1 or 2 – oral agents

| | Primary | Recurrent | Suppression | Dosage | |
|---|---|---|---|---|---|
| **Valacyclovir** (Valtrex) | Labialis: 2 g q12 h × 1 day, OR 500 mg bid × 5 days Genital: 1 g bid × 10 days | 500 mg bid × 5 days | <10×/year: 500 mg qd >10×/year 1 g qd | 500 mg, 1 g | B B |
| **Famciclovir** (Famvir) | Labialis: 500 mg tid×5 days Genital: 250 mg tid × 7–10 days | 125 mg bid × 5 days | 250 mg bid | 120, 250, 500 mg | B B |
| **Acyclovir*** (Zovirax) | 400 mg tid ×10 days 200 mg 5×per/day × 10 days 5 mg/kg/d IV q8 h | 400 mg tid × 5 days, OR 800 mg bid× 5 days | 400 mg bid | 200, 400, 800 mg 200 mg/5 ml 250, 500 mg IV | B |

## For HSV disseminated disease

| | | | |
|---|---|---|---|
| **Acyclovir*** (Zovirax) | 5–10 mg/kg IV q8 h for 7 days if > 12 years | 200, 400, 800 mg | B |
| | Neonatal: 400 mg tid during third trimester | 250, 500 mg IV | |

## For herpes zoster/VZV

| | | | |
|---|---|---|---|
| **Valacyclovir** (Valtrex) | 1 g po tid × 7 days | 500 mg, 1 g | B |
| **Famciclovir** (Famvir) | 500 mg po qid × 7 days | 125, 250, 500 mg | B |
| **Acyclovir*** (Zovirax) | 800 mg 5×/day × 7–10 days | 200, 400, 800 mg | B |

Mechanism: These nucleoside analogs are phosphorylated by viral thymidine kinase to form a nucleoside triphosphate which then inhibits HSV DNA polymerase action.

*Available in Generic

## For genital warts

| | | | |
|---|---|---|---|
| **Imiquimod** (Aldara) | Apply to genital warts 3× weekly at night | 5% cream 1 box = 12 or 24 pks of 250 mg each | C |
| **Podofilox** (Condylox) | Apply to genital warts bid 3 days/week consecutive | 0.5% gel, soln 3.5 g | C |
| **Podophyllin/Benzoin** (Podocon-25) | MD applies. Pt leave on for 1–6 h then wash off | 15 ml | X |

## For verruca vulgaris

| | | | |
|---|---|---|---|
| Compound W pad | 40% Salicylic Acid | OTC | / |
| Compound W gel | 17% SA with colloidion | | |
| Canthacur-PS | 30% SA, 5% podophyllin, 1% cantharidin | MD applies | |
| Cidofovir | 3% topical solution bid until resolve | Compound by pharm | C |
| Bleomycin | Place 0.5–1 mg/ml solution onto wart then prick it into wart with needle | | |
| Candida Antigen | Inject intradermally into wart by MD. Dilute 1:1 with 1% Lidocaine. Inject 0.1–0.2 cc per wart. Limit total to 0.3–0.5 cc. Repeat q 3 weeks x 3 visit to see if respond. | | |

## For molluscum

| | |
|---|---|
| Canthacur | 0.7% cantharidin. Apply by MD with toothpick |

# Antihistamines

### Sedating (usually use at night)

| | | | |
|---|---|---|---|
| **Diphenhydramine\*** (Benadryl) | 25–50 mg q6–8 h. Peds: 5 mg/kg/d divided q4–6 h | OTC 25, 50 mg 12.5 mg/5 ml | B |
| **Hydroxyzine\*** (Atarax, Vistaril) | 10–50 mg po q4–6 h. Peds (<6 years): 2 mg/kg/d divided q6 h | 10, 25, 50 mg Susp 10 mg/5 ml | C |
| **Cyproheptadine\*** (Periactin) | 4 mg tid; max 32 mg/d Peds (2–5 years): 2 mg bid-tid Peds (6–12 years): 4 mg bid-tid | 4 mg Susp 2 mg/5 ml | B |

\*Available in Generic

## Non-sedating

| | | | |
|---|---|---|---|
| **Loratadine*** (Claritin) | 10 mg po qd<br>Peds (2–5 years): 5 mg qd | OTC 10 mg<br>Susp 5 mg/5 ml | B |
| **Desloratadine** (Clarinex) | 5 mg po qd | 5 mg | C |
| **Fexofenadine** (Allegra) | 60 mg po bid<br>or 180 mg po qd<br>Peds (6–12 years):<br>30 mg bid | 30, 60, 180 mg | C |
| **Cetirizine** (Zyrtec) | 5–10 mg qh<br>Peds (2–6 years):<br>2.5 mg qh<br>max 5 mg qd.<br>*(may be sedating)* | 5, 10 mg<br>Susp 5 mg/5 ml | B |

## H2-blockers for angioedema, systemic mastocystosis

| | | | |
|---|---|---|---|
| **Famotidine**<br>(Pepcid) | 20 mg qd-bid | 20, 40 mg<br>40 mg/5 ml | B |
| **Cimetidine**<br>(Tagamet) | 400 mg qd-qid | 300, 400, 800 mg | B |
| **Ranitidine**<br>(Zantac) | 150 mg qd-bid | 150, 300 mg<br>15 mg/ml | B |

# Antipruritic

## Topical

| | | |
|---|---|---|
| **Pramoxine** (Pramosone) – topical anesthetic<br>+1% or 2.5% hydrocortisone | 30 g O<br>30, 60 g C<br>60, 120 ml L | C |
| **Doxepin** (Zonalon) 5% Cream – Apply q 3–4 h × 1 week<br>max; may cause systemic effect if applied to >10% BSA | 30, 45 g C | B |
| Sarna lotion (Menthol 0.5%, Camphor 0.5%) | OTC | / |
| Aveeno anti-itch cream (calamine 3%,<br>Camphor 0.47%, Pramoxine 1%) | OTC | / |
| Calamine lotion | OTC | / |
| Gold bond cream (Menthol 1%, Pramoxine 1%) | OTC | / |

## Oral

| | | | |
|---|---|---|---|
| **Doxepin**<br>(Sinequan) | 10–75 mg qh<br>Tricyclic antidepressant<br>with high affinity for H1 receptor.<br>Do NOT use with MAOI | 10, 25, 50 mg | B |

*Available in Generic

| Promethazine hydrochloride (Phenergan) | 12.5 mg Qid, 25 mg qh CNS depressant, antiemetic, anticholinergic, sedative antihistamine (H1) | 12.5, 25, 50 mg | C |
|---|---|---|---|
| Amitriptyline (Elavil) | 10–25 mg to 150 mg qd For anxiety, neuropathic pain. TCA | 10, 25, 50 mg | D |
| Naltrexone (RevVia, Depade) | 25–50 mg qd Opioid antagonist | 25, 50 mg | C |
| Ondansetron (Zofran) | 8 mg bid Blocks serotonin 5HT3 & opioid receptors | 4, 8, 24 mg | B |
| Cholestyramine (Questran) | 4–16 mg qd For cholestastic pruritus. Bile acid resin. Do not take other meds for 4 h | 4, 378 g | B |
| Rifampin | 300–600 mg qd (10 mg/kg/d) For pruritus from primary bilary cirrhosis. Increases metabolism/ excretion of bile acid | 150, 300 mg | C |
| Pimozide (Orap) | Start 1 mg qd to 0.2 mg/kg/d For delusions of parasitosis Increases toxicity of MAOI, CNS depressant May cause extrapyramidal effects ☑ Check ECG-may cause long QT | 1, 2 mg | C |

DRUGS AND THERAPIES

## Bleaching Agents/Depigmenting Agents

All contain hydroquinone which inhibits enzymatic oxidation of tyrosine to 3-(3,4-dihydroxyphenyl-alanine [dopa]). Some agents also contain topical steroids, retinoids, sunscreen (SS); glycolic acid (G).

| Hydroquinone* 4% cream | | | | |
|---|---|---|---|---|
| EpiQuin Micro | | $30, 60 | 30, 60 g | C |
| | | $80–100 | 30 g | C |
| Lustra 4% cream | G | $80, 140 | 28.4, 56.8 g | C |
| Lustra AF 4% cream | G, SS | $80,140 | 28.4, 56.8 g | C |
| Claripel 4% cream | SS | $100–150 | 28, 45 g | C |
| Glyquin 4% cream | 10% G, SS | $80–100 | 30 g | C |
| Triluma 4% cream | 0.01% Fluocinolone 0.05% Tretinoin | $120 | 30 g | C |

continued p. 266

*Available in Generic

| Benoquin 20% cream – final depigmentation | Monobenzone 20% Apply bid until effect (2–4 months) | $ 50–70 | 35.4 g | C |
|---|---|---|---|---|

**Others**

| Azelex cream 20% | bid to affected area | | 30, 50 g | B |
|---|---|---|---|---|

# Topical Chemotherapy

## Actinic keratoses (AK)

| **Fluorouracil** (Efudex) | Apply qd-bid × 2–6 weeks or until irritated | 5% Cream 25 g | X |
|---|---|---|---|
| **Fluorouracil** (Carac) | Apply qd-bid × 2–6 weeks or until irritated | 0.5% Solution 10 ml | X |
| **Diclofenac** (Solaraze) | Apply bid × 8–12 weeks NSAID | 3% Gel 50, 100 g | B |
| **Imiquimod** (Aldara) | Apply qh × 8–12 weeks | 5% Cream 1 box = 12 pks of 250 mg each | C |

## Basal cell carcinoma (BCC) – superficial BCC

| **Imiquimod** (Aldara) | Apply qh × 8–12 weeks | 5% Cream 1 Box = 12 pks of 250 mg each | C |
|---|---|---|---|

# CTCL

**Topical agents** (see also Class I topical steroids and CTCL in General Dermatology section for systemic treatments)

| **Bexarotene** (Targretin Gel) | Apply to area qd-bid as tolerated | 1% gel 60 g tube | X |
|---|---|---|---|
| **Nitrogen mustard Mechlorethamine** (Mustargen) | Apply to plaques of CTCL bid | 10 mg% in Aquaphor. 2 lb | D |

## Oral agent

| **Bexarotene** (Targretin) | 200–300 mg/m$^2$ qd with meal | 75 mg | X |
|---|---|---|---|

## Other agent

| Interferon α 2a<br>(Roferon A) | 6–9 million IU SC 3×per/wk<br>Use in combination with PUVA | 3, 6, 9 million<br>IU prefilled syringes | C |
|---|---|---|---|

# Psoriasis

## Topical agents (see also topical steroids)

| Dermazinc with<br>Clobetasol Spray | DermaZinc 4 oz compound<br>with 50 mcg micronized<br>clobetasol | 4 oz | C |
|---|---|---|---|
| Calcipotriene (Dovonex) | 0.005% Ointment<br>0.005% Cream<br>Scalp solution | 30, 60, 100 g<br>30, 60, 100 g<br>60 ml | C |
| Tazorotene (Tazorac) | 0.05%, 0.1% Cream<br>0.05%, 0.1% Gel | 15, 30, 60 g<br>30, 100 g | X |
| Betamethasone/<br>calcipotriene (Taclonex) | 0.064%/0.005%<br>ointment | 60, 100 g | C |

## Tar (apply in direction of hair growth)

| Crude coal tar (CCT) | 1–10% Compound in<br>petrolatum base | | C |
|---|---|---|---|
| Tar Gel (Estar 5%,<br>Psorigel 7.5%) | Cover with<br>vaseline to<br>prevent drying | 90, 120 ml | C |
| Liquor Carbonis<br>Detergens (LCD) | Triamcinolone 0.1%<br>ointment compound<br>with 10% LCD | 1 lb | C |
| Tar Shampoo<br>Neutrogena T-Gel | Apply to scalp, leave<br>for 5–10 min<br>then rinse | OTC | C |

## Systemic agents

| Methoxypsoralen<br>(Oxsoralen Ultra) | 0.4–0.6 mg/kg po 1–2h<br>prior to PUVA | 10 mg | C |
|---|---|---|---|

| Weight (kg) | Dose (mg) |
|---|---|
| <30 | 10 |
| 30–65 | 20 |
| 65–90 | 30 |
| >90 | 40 |

**See toxic drug chart**
Retinoids: **acitretin** (Soriatane); Biologics: **alefacept** (Amevive), **efalizumab**
(Raptiva), **etanercept** (Enbrel), **infliximab** (Remicade).

DRUGS AND THERAPIES

# Seborrheic Dermatitis

(see Topical Steroids, Keratolytics)

| Carmol scalp treatment | Sodium sulfacetamide 10% lotion | 90 ml Lotion | B |
|---|---|---|---|
| Derma-Smoothe/FS | Fluocinolone acetonide 0.1%, peanut oil, mineral oil | 120 ml Oil | C |
| Ovace | Sodium sulfacetamide 10% wash | 180, 360 ml wash | B |
| Nizoral | Ketoconazole 2% cream | 15,30,60 g | C |
| | Ketoconazole 2% shampoo | 120 ml | C |
| | Ketoconazole 1% shampoo | OTC | C |
| Selsun, Head and Shoulders | Selenium sulfide 1%, 2.5% shampoo | OTC | C |

# Hypertrichosis

| **Eflornithine** 13.9% (Vaniqa) | Apply to affected area bid | 30 g | C |
|---|---|---|---|

# Hyperhidrosis

| **Aluminum Cl** (Drysol 20% CertainDry 12.5% Xerac-AC 6.25%) | Apply to underarms qh until desired effects, then space out. Combines with intraductal keratin to produce a functional closure. | 35, 37.5, 60 ml | / |
|---|---|---|---|
| **Glycopyrrolate** (Robinul) | Start 1 mg, titrate to effect Antimuscarinic anticholinergic – inhibits ACh at autonomic cholinergic nerves. SE: anhidrosis/hyperthermia, blurred vision, urinary retention, constipation, tachycardia | 1 mg | B |
| **Botulinum Toxin A** (Botox) | 50 units per axilla q4–6 mos Blocks release of ACh via inhibiting SNAP-25 | | C |

Other treatment modalities include iontophoresis and liposuction.

## Wound Care

| | | | |
|---|---|---|---|
| **Acetic acid** | | 35, 37.5, 60 ml | C |
| **Burow's solution/ Domeboro** Aluminum acetate | Dissolve one pack into 1 pint of water | 12, 100, 1000 tabs/box | / |
| **Dakin's solution** Sodium hypochlorite | 0.25% Solution 0.5% Solution | 480, 3840 ml 480 ml | C |

## Vitamins/Nutritional Supplements

| | | | |
|---|---|---|---|
| **Biotin** (Appearex 2.5 mg) | 1 tab qd – for nails/ biotin deficiency | 30 tabs | / |
| **Folic Acid** (Vitamin B9) | 1 mg qd For MTX toxicity prophylaxis | 100 tabs | A |
| **Niacinamide** (Niacin, Vitamin B3) | 500 mg tid Suppression of antigen/ mitogen-induced lymphoblast transformation. For BP | 500 mg | C |
| **Nicomide** (NOT niacin) | Contains nicotinamide 750 mg + copper 1.5 mg, folic acid 0.5 mg, zinc 25 mg for acne rosacea | 60 tabs | A |

## Miscellaneous Meds

| | | | |
|---|---|---|---|
| **Colchicine** | Start 0.3 mg qd- titrate to diarrhea 0.6 mg po bid-tid Prevents assembly of microtubules ☑ Check CBC, U/A, BMP q3mos | 0.6 mg | C |
| **Pentoxyfyline** (Trental) | 400 mg Tid For treatment of peripheral vascular disease, painful diabetic neuropathy ☑ Check serum creatinine/BUN baseline | 400 mg | C |
| **SSKI/Potassium Iodide** 1 drop = 47 mg KI | 5–15 drops Tid Alters host immune/non-immune response, for use in EM, E. nodosum, Sporothrichosis ☑ Check TSH, T4. Monitor for Wolff-Chaikoff effect – excess iodide can inhibit binding of iodine in the thyroid gland resulting in cessation of thyroid hormone synthesis | 30, 240 ml | D |

# Cytochrome P-450 Interactions

| CYP2D6 | Substrates | Amiodarone, Antipsychotics, Beta Blockers, Antidepressants (TCA's, SSRIs, Venlafaxine) |
|---|---|---|
| | | Narcotics (Codeine, Tramadol) |
| | **Inducers** | **Rifampin, Dexamethasone** |
| | Inhibitors | Potent: Amiodarone, SSRIs, Ritonavir |
| | | Antipsychotics, Celecoxib, |
| | | H1-Antagonists: Cimetidine, Hydroxyzine |
| CYP3A4 | Substrates | Antiarrhythmic (Amiodarone, Digoxin, Quinidine) |
| | | Anticonvulsant (Carbamazepine, Verapamil) |
| | | Antidepressant (Amitriptyline, SSRI) |
| | | Immunosuppressive (Steroids, Dapsone, Tacrolimus, Cyclophosphamide, Cyclosporine) |
| | | Others: Antihistamines, Benzodiazepine, CCBs, Estrogens, Erythromycin, Omeprazole, Statins, Protease Inhibitors, Theophylline, |
| | **Inducers** | **Anticonvulsants (Phenobarbital, Phenytoin, Carbamazepine)** |
| | | **Anti-TB (INH, Rifampin), Glucocorticoids, St. John's Wort, Efavirenz, Nevirapine, Glitazones, Griseofulvin** |
| | Inhibitors | Antibiotics (Erythromycin, Clarithromycin Fluoroquirolone) |
| | | Azoles, CCBs, Cimetidine, Protease Inhibitors, SSRI, Grapefruit Juice |
| CYP1A2 | Substrates | TCA's, Theophylline, Haloperidol, |
| | | Propranolol, Verapamil, R-Warfarin |
| | | Estradiol, Tacrine, Clozapine, |
| | | Naproxen, Zileuton, Zolmitriptan |
| | **Inducers** | **Omeprazole, Rifampin, Ritonavir** |

| | |
|---|---|
| Inhibitors | **Nafcillin, Phenobarbital, Phenytoin** |
| | **Smoking, Charbroiled meats** |
| | **Broccoli, Brussel Sprouts, Cabbage** |
| | Fluoroquinolones, Fluvoxamine, Paroxetine, |
| | Amiodarone, Cimetidine, Ticlopidine |
| | Grapefruit Juice |
| **CYP2C9** | |
| Substrates | Phenytoin, S-Warfarin, NSAIDs, |
| | Sartans (Losartan), Sulfonylureas |
| | Tricyclic antidepressants, Valproic acid |
| **Inducers** | **Rifampin, Secobarbital, Ethanol** |
| Inhibitors | Azoles, Ritonavir, INH, TMP-SMX |
| | Statins, Fluvoxamine |
| | Zafirlukast, Amiodarone |

# Pregnancy Categories of Commonly Used Dermatologic Agents

| Class B | Class C |
|---|---|
| Acyclovir | Adapalene (Differin) |
| Alefacept (Amevive) | Bacitracin preps (Polysporin) |
| Amoxicillin | Benzaclin & Benzamycin |
| Amphotericin topical | Benzoyl peroxide |
| Augmentin | Calcipotriene (Dovonex) |
| Azithromycin (Zithromax) | Carmol |
| Azelaic acid (Azelex, Finevin) | Ciprofloxacin |
| Butenafine (Mentax) | Clarithromycin |
| Cephalexin (Keflex) | Cyclosporine |
| Cetirizine (Zyrtec) | Desloratadine (Clarinex) |
| Chlorhexidine (Hibiclens) | Econazole (Spectazole) |
| Ciclopirox (Loprox, Penlac) | Eflornithine (Vaniqa) |
| Clindamycin | Fexofenadine (Allegra) |
| Clotrimazole topical | Fluconazole (Diflucan) |
| Cimetidine | Griseofulvin – po |
| Cyproheptadine | Hydroquinones – topical |
| Diclofenac (Solaraze) | Hydroxychloroquine (Plaquenil) |
| Diphenhydramine | Hydroxyzine |
| Docosanol (Abreva) | Imiquimod |
| Doxepin | Itraconazole (Sporanox) |
| Erythromycin po/ topical | Ivermectin |
| Etanercept (Enbrel) | Ketoconazole (Nizoral) |
| Famciclovir | Levofloxin |
| Famotidine (Pepcid) | Methoxypsoralen |
| Glycopyrrolate (Robinul) | Miconazole (Micatin, Zeasorb) |
| Imiquimod | Minoxidil |
| Infliximab (Remicade) | Neomycin preps (Neosporin) |
| Lidocaine cream (LMX) | Nystatin |
| Loratadine (Claritin) | Pimecrolimus |
| Metronidazole topical | Rifampin |
| Mupirocin (Bactroban) | Sertazconazole (Ertaczo) |
| Naftifine (Naftin) | Sirolimus (Rapamune) |
| Oxiconazole (Oxistat) | Sodium sulfacet/sulfur (Avar, Plexion, Rosula) |
| Penciclovir topical | Sodium sulfacetamide (Klaron) |
| Penicillin | Steroids – systemic & topical |
| Permethrin (Elimite, Nix) | Sulfonamides |
| Silvadene | Tacrolimus – systemic & topical |
| Solaraze | Tretinoin (Renova) |
| Terbinafine – po & topical | Trimethoprim-sulfamethoxazole |
| Valacyclovir | |
| Zithromax | |

| | Class D | Class X |
|---|---|---|
| | Azathioprine (Imuran) | Acitretin |
| | Doxycycline | Finasteride (Propecia) |
| | Gentamicin topical | Fluorouracil (Efudex, Carac) |
| | Minocycline | Isotretinoin (Accutane, Amnesteem) |
| | Mycophenolate mofetil (Cellcept) | Methotrexate |
| | Nitrogen mustard | Tazarotene (Tazorac) |
| | Tetracycline | Thalidomide |

B: Generally considered safe to use.
C: No evidence of harm to fetus.
D: Some significant risks. Use only if benefits outweigh risks.
X: Evidence of fetal abnormalities. Should not be used in pregnancy.

## Common Dermatologic Drugs and Teratogenic Effects

| | Medication | Teratogenic effects |
|---|---|---|
| Analgesics | Acetaminophen | Analgesic of choice, low dose not linked with identifiable risk throughout pregnancy |
| | NSAIDs | Caution in final trimester: fetal/neonatal hemorrhage and premature closure of ductus arteriosus |
| | Opioids | Respiratory depression and withdrawal symptoms |
| Antimicrobial | Tetracyclines | Dental staining and enamel hypoplasia (limited data for minocycline and doxycycline) |
| | Voriconazole | Known teratogen |
| | Lindane, malathion, permethrin | Although FDA category B, low risk and historically well tolerated, precipitated sulfur is often preferred given theoretical toxicity |
| Miscellaneous | Prednisone | Small risk of orofacial clefts |
| | Lidocaine with epinephrine | No appreciable risk for small excisional biopsies |

From Leachman and Reed. The use of dermatologic drugs in pregnancy and lactation. *Dermatol Clin.* 2006 24: 167–97.

## Dermatologic Drugs Reportedly Associated with Contraceptive Failure

| Medication | Contraceptive agent | Proposed mechanism |
|---|---|---|
| Azathioprine | Intrauterine devices | Unknown |
| NSAIDs | Intrauterine devices | Unknown |
| Griseofulvin | Oral contraceptives | Increased estrogen metabolism by hepatic microsomal enzyme induction |

*continued p. 274*

DRUGS AND THERAPIES

| Medication | Contraceptive agent | Proposed mechanism |
|---|---|---|
| Rifampin | Oral contraceptives | Increased estrogen metabolism by hepatic microsomal enzyme induction or reduced enterohepatic circulation of estrogens |
| Tetracycline | Oral contraceptives (unlikely to play causal role in contraceptive failure) | Reduced enterohepatic circulation of estrogens |
| Sulfonamides | Oral contraceptives (unlikely to play causal role in contraceptive failure) | Reduced enterohepatic circulation of estrogens |

# Drug Eruptions

Common medications that can cause cutaneous eruptions. When these diseases start abruptly, flare, or are not controlled by conventional therapies, re-evaluate diagnosis and consider complicating factors such as medication list.

| Disease | Medications |
|---|---|
| Acne | Corticosteroids, oral contraceptives, androgens, ACTH, lithium, phenytoin, halogens, isoniazid, haloperidol, radiation, sirolimus |
| AGEP | Beta-lactam antibiotics (most common), macrolides, mercury (association with loxocelism), diltiazem, hydroxychloroquine, terbinafine, imatinib |
| Alopecia | ACE inhibitors, allopurinol, anticoagulants, antidepressants, antiepileptics, azathioprine, bromocriptine, beta-blockers, cyclophosphamide, didanosine, ECMO, hormones, indinavir, interferons, NSAIDs, oral contraceptives, methotrexate, retinoids, tacrolimus |
| Beau lines/ onychomadesis | Carbamazepine, cefaloridine, chemotherapy (taxanes), cloxacillin, dapsone, fluorine, itraconazole, lithium, metoprolol, phenophtaleine, psoralens, retinoids, radiation, sulfonamides, tetracyclines |
| Bullous pemphigoid | Ampicillin, captopril, chloroquine, ciprofloxacin, enalapril, furosemide, neuroleptics, penicillamine, penicillins, phenacetin, PUVA, salicylazosulfapyridine, sulfasalazine, terbinafine |
| Dermatomyositis-like | Hydroxyurea (most common), lovastatin, simvastatin, omeprazole, BCG vaccine, penicillamine, tegafur, tamoxifen |
| Hypersensitivity/ DRESS | Phenobarbital, phenytoin, carbamazepine, minocycline, sulfonamides, dapsone, allopurinol, gold, nevirapine, abacavir, lamotrigine |
| Erythema nodosum | Oral contraceptives (most common), echinacea, halogens, penicillin, sulfonamides, tetracycline |

| | |
|---|---|
| Fixed drug eruptions | Trimethoprim-sulfamethoxazole, phenolphthalein, NSAIDs, anticonvulsants, tetracyclines |
| GA-like | Gold therapy, diclofenac, allopurinol, quinidine, intranasal calcitonin, amlodipine |
| Hair curling/kinking | Retinoids, indinavir, antineoplastics, valproate, azathioprine |
| Hair straightening | Interferon, lithium |
| Hypertrichosis | Acetazolamide, cyclosporin, minoxidil, phenytoin, psoralens, steroids, streptomycin, zidovudine |
| Interstitial granulomatous drug reaction | Anti-hypertensives (ACE inhibitors, calcium channel blockers, beta-blockers), antidepressants, anticonvulsants, antihistamines, lipid lowering agents |
| Leukocytoclastic vasculitis | Allopurinol, penicillins, sulfonamides, anti-TNF agents, quinolones, hydantoins, insulin, tamoxifen, thiazides, retinoids, anti-influenza vaccines, interferons, sympatomimetic illicit drugs (ANCA+ vasculitis: hydralazine, propylthiouracil, MCN, leukotriene inhibitors; Necrotizing – bortezomib) |
| Lichenoid eruptions (usually sun-exposed areas, may be confluent) | Antimalarials, thiazides, demethylchlortetracycline, fenofibrate, enalapril, quinine, quinidine |
| Linear IgA dermatosis | Vancomycin, atorvastatin, captopril, carbamazepine, diclofenac, glibenclamide, lithium, phenytoin, amoidarone, piroxicam |
| Lupus erythematosus, definite association | Minocycline, methyldopa, chlorpromazine, procainamide, hydralazine, quinidine, isoniazide |
| Lupus erythematosus, possible association | Beta-blockers, methimazole, captopril, nitrofurantoin, carbamazepine, penicillamine, cimetidine, phenytoin, ethosuximide, propylthiouracil, sulfasalazine, levodopa, sulfonamides, lithium, trimethadione |
| Lupus erythematosus, unlikely association | Allopurinol, penicillin, chlorthalidone, phenylbutazone, gold, salts, reserpine, griseofulvin, streptomycin, methysergide, oral contraceptives |
| Lupus erythematosus, subacute cutaneous | Thiazides>terbinafine, verapamil, diltiazem, buproprion, enalapril, nifedipine, infliximab, etanercept, statins, interferon-alfa, leflunomide, acebutolol |
| Melanonychia | Chemotherapy, hydroxyurea, psoralens, zidovudine |
| Nail brittleness | Antiretrovirals, chemotherapy, retinoids |
| Nail, decreased growth | Cyclosporin, heparin, lithium, methotrexate, zidovudine |
| Nail, increased growth | Azoles, levodopa, oral contraceptives |
| Nail pigmentation | Antimalarials (blue-brown), anthraline (brown-black), clofazamine (dark brown), gold (yellow), minocycline (blue-gray), tar (brown-black), tetracyclines (yellow) |
| Paronychia | Antiretrovirals, cyclophosphamide, EGF receptor antagonists, fluorouracil, methotrexate, retinoids |
| Pemphigus | *Thiols*: ACE inhibitors, penicillamine, gold sodium thiomalate, mercaptopropionylglycine, pyritinol, thiamazole, thiopronine |

continued p. 276

**DRUGS AND THERAPIES**

| Disease | Medications |
|---|---|
| | *Nonthiols*: aminophenazone, aminopyrine, azapropazone, cephalosporins, heroin, hydantoin, imiquimod, indapamide, levodopa, lysine acetylsalicylate, montelukast, oxyphenbutazone, penicillins, phenobarbital, phenylbutazone, piroxicam, progesterone, propranolol, rifampicin |
| Photoonycholysis | Quinolones, tetracyclines, psoralens, quinine, captopril, chlorpromazine, thiazides, taxanes |
| Photosensitivity | ACE inhibitors, amiodarone, amlodipine, celecoxib, chlorpromazine, diltiazem, furosemide, griseofulvin, lovastatin, nifedipine, phenothiazine, piroxicam, quinolones, sulfonamides, tetracycline, thiazides |
| Pseudolymphoma | Phenytoin, ACE inhibitors, penicillamine |
| Pseudoporphyria | Amiodarone, bumetanide, chlorthalidone, cyclosporine, dapsone, etretinate, fluorouracil, flutamide, furosemide, hydrochlorothiazide/triamterene, isotretinoin, NSAIDs, oral contraceptives, tetracycline |
| Pseudotumor cerebri | Minocycline, tetracycline, doxycycline (most frequently reported tetracyclines in descending order), vitamin A analogs, corticosteroids (especially in withdrawal), nalidixic acid, sulfonamides, lithium, thyroxine, growth hormone, amiodarone, tamoxifen |
| Psoriasis | Antimalarials, beta-blockers, NSAIDs, penicillin, tetracycline, ACE inhibitors, G-CSF, interferons, lithium, corticosteroid withdrawal, anti-TNF agents |
| Pyogenic granulomas | Cyclosporin, EGF receptor antagonists, indinavir, retinoids, |
| Raynaud phenomenon | Ergot compounds (methysergide), OCPs containing estrogen and progesterone, non-selective beta-blockers (propranolol), chemotherapy, polyvinyl chloride |
| Serum sickness | Antithymocyte globulin, penicillin, vaccines (pneumococcal, rabies, horse serum derivatives) |
| Serum sickness–like | Cefaclor (most common), other beta-lactams, minocycline, propranol, streptokinase, sulfonamides, NSAIDs, rituximab, buproprion, infliximab |
| SJS/TEN | Sulfonamides, antiepileptics, allopurinol, NSAIDs, antiretrovirals |
| Sweet syndrome | All-*trans*-retinoic acid, celecoxib, GCSF, nitrofurantoin, oral contraceptives, tetracyclines, trimethoprim-sulfamethoxazole |
| Thrombotic microangiopathy | CSA, mitomycin C, tacrolimus |
| Urticaria | Opiates, ibuprofen, aspirin, polymyxin B, tartrazine, beta-lactams (immunologic), dextran |

Adapted from Knowles and Shear. Recognition and management of severe cutaneous drug reactions. *Dermatol Clin.* 2007; 25:245–53; Callen JP. Newly recognized cutaneous drug eruptions. *Dermatol Clin.* 2007; 25:255–61; Piraccini and Iorizzo, Drug reactions affecting the nail unit: diagnosis and management. *Dermatol Clin.* 2007; 25:215–21; Bolognia, Jorizzo and Rapini. *Dermatology.* St. Louis: Mosby, 2003.

DRUGS AND THERAPIES

# Chemotherapeutic Agents and Skin Changes

| Cutaneous manifestation | Chemotherapeutics |
|---|---|
| **Alopecia (most common reaction to chemotherapy, usually anagen effluvium)** | |
| Irreversible alopecia | Cyclophosphamide, busulfan |
| Hair texture change upon regrowth (dry and dull) | Doxorubicin |
| **Hyperpigmentation** | |
| Serpentine supravenous hyperpigmentation | Fluorouracil, fotemustine, vinorelbine, docetaxel, sometimes with combination chemotherapy |
| Hair color change from light to black | Cyclophosphamide |
| Flag sign | Methotrexate |
| Flagellate streaks with pruritus | Bleomycin |
| Dusky pigmentation, similar to Addison's except no mucous membrane involvement | Busulfan – "busulfan tan" |
| Areas of pressure | Cisplatin |
| Acral | Tegafur |
| Occluded areas | Thiotepa, BCNU |
| Banded hyperpigmentation of nails | Bleomycin, cyclophosphamide, daunorubicin, doxorubicin, fluorouracil, melphalan, vincristine |
| Oral hyperpigmentation: mucous membrane | Doxorubicin, fluorouracil |
| Oral hyperpigmentation: gingival | Cisplatin (transient lead line) |
| Oral hyperpigmentation: teeth | Cyclophosphamide |
| Yellowish discoloration | Sunitinib |
| **Interaction with ultraviolet light** | |
| Most phototoxic | Fluorouracil, dacarbazine, methotrexate |
| Photoallergy | Flutamide, tegafur |
| Photo-onycholysis | Mercaptopurine, taxanes |
| Ultraviolet recall | Methotrexate, suranim |
| Reverse UV recall (reactivation of healed extravasation ulcer) | Mitomycin |
| Squamous cell carcinoma | Fludarabine |
| **Inflammation of keratoses** | |
| Actinic keratosis | Fluorouracil, doxorubicin, sorafenib, capecitabine |
| Seborrheic keratosis | Cytarabine |
| **Hypersensitivity reactions** | |
| Type I hypersensitivity (i.e. urticaria, anaphylaxis) most common | L-asparaginase, paclitaxel, docetaxel, mitomycin-C |
| Type I hypersensitivity (i.e. urticaria, anaphylaxis) severe | Methotrexate |

continued p. 278

DRUGS AND THERAPIES

| Cutaneous manifestation | Chemotherapeutics |
|---|---|
| Type IV hypersensitivity (i.e. contact dermatitis) | Mitomycin-C (groin), mechlorethamine, carmustine |
| Fixed drug in patients with SLE on cyclophosphamide | Mesna |
| Flushing (results in skin thickening and hyperpigmentation, stop treatment) | Mithramycin, mitomycin, plicamycin |

## Nail dystrophies

| | |
|---|---|
| Subungal abscess | Docetaxel (subungual hemorrhage – docetaxel, sunitinib) |
| Nail bed changes | EGFR inhibitors (splinter hemorrhages – sunitinib, sorafenib) |
| Onycholysis | Bleomycin, cyclophosphamide, fluorouracil, methotrexate, mitoxantrone, doxorubicin, paclitaxel |
| Leukonychia | Anthracyclines, cisplatinum, cyclophosphamide, vincristine |

## Miscellaneous

| | |
|---|---|
| Raynaud's phenomenon (vasoconstriction) | Bleomycin, vinblastine, cisplatin, gemcitabine, rituximab |
| Flushing (vasodilation) | Anthracyclines, asparaginase, bleomycin, cisplatin, dacarbazine, taxanes |
| Capillary leak syndrome – edema (skin and lungs), erythema, pruritus, vascular collapse | Taxanes, gemcitabine, IL-2, sirolimus, docetaxel, G-CSF |
| Scleroderma-like reaction | Bleomycin, docetaxel, paclitaxel, melphalan, gemcitabine |
| Ulcers | Hydroxyurea (leg), methotrexate, interferon, bleomycin |
| Acanthosis nigricans | Diethylstilbestrol |
| Furunculosis | Fluoxymesterone, methotrexate |
| Pustular psoriasis | Aminoglutethimide |
| Sticky skin (acquired cutaneous adherence) | Doxorubicin, ketoconazole |
| Acute intermittent porphyria | Chlorambucil, cyclophosphamide |
| Dermatomyositis-like reaction | Hydroxyurea, tamoxifen, tegafur |
| Discoid lupus | Fluorouracil, tegafur (SCLE-taxanes) |
| Bullous pemphigoid | Dactinomycin, methotrexate |
| Exacerbation of psoriasis and autoimmune disorders (also injection site reactions) | Interferons, IL-2 |
| Sweet's syndrome | GCSF |
| Erythema nodosum | Azathioprine |
| Increased skin neoplasms | Hydroxyurea, suranim |
| Folliculitis | Dactinomycin |
| Lichen planus | Hydroxyurea, tegafur |
| Leukoderma | Topical thiotepa |
| Acneiform eruption | EGF receptor inhibitors (i.e. cetuximab), actinomycin D, docetaxel |

| Cutaneous manifestation | Chemotherapeutics |
|---|---|
| Edema (>eyes & ankles), pigmentation changes | Imatinib (edema is thru PDGFR) |
| Conjuctivitis | Cytarabine |
| Excessive lacrimation | Docetaxel |
| Blue sclera | Mitoxantrone |
| Pseudolymphoma | Gemcitabine (also erysipelas-like reaction) |
| Baboon syndrome | Hydroxyurea (also amoxicillin, ampicillin, nickel, heparin, mercury) |
| Neutrophilic eccrine hidradenitis | Cytarabine, bleomycin, GCSF |
| Acral erythema = hand-foot; Syndrome = Burgdorf's; Syndrome = "Palmar-plantar erythrodysesthesia" | Cytarabine, doxorubicin, fluorouracil, sorafenib (bullous variant: cytarabine, methotrexate, tegafur (PPK)) |
| Radiation recall | Dactinomycin, doxorubicin, docetaxel, etoposide gemcitabine, methotrexate |
| Radiation enhancement | Doxorubicin, dactinomycin, 5-bromodeoxyuridine |
| **Extravasation** | |
| Necrosis (vesicant) | Doxorubicin, daunorubicin (large ulcerations), bleomycin, doxorubicin, vinblastine, vincristine |
| Rx: aspiration, cold packs, except vinca alkaloids require heat. Otherwise specific antidotes as below | |

## Antidote to extravasation of chemotherapeutic agents

| **Antidote** | **Specific drug** |
|---|---|
| Sodium thiosulfate (neutralizes vesicant) | Mechlorethamine cisplatin |
| Dimethlysulfoxide (free radical scavenger), dexrazoxane | Anthracyclines, mitomycin C |
| Vinca alkaloids | Hyaluronidase |

Adapted from Sanborn and Sauer. Cutaneous reaction to chemotherapy: commonly seen, less described, little understood. *Dermatol Clin.* 2008; 26:103–19; Guillot et al. Mucocutaneous side effects of antineoplastic therapy. *Expert Opin Drug Saf.* 2004; 579–87; Bolognia, Jorizzo, and Rapini. *Dermatology.* St. Louis: 2003.

# UV Light Treatment

## UVA/UVB dosing

| Skin type | UVA | | | UVB | |
|---|---|---|---|---|---|
| | Initial dose (J/cm²) | Increment (J/cm²) | Max | Initial dose (mJ/cm²) | Increment (mJ/cm²) |
| I | 0.5 | 0.5 | 5 | 20 | 5 |
| II | 1.0 | 0.5 | 8 | 25 | 10 |

continued p. 280

| III | 2.0 | 0.5–1.0 | 12 | 30 | 15 |
| IV | 3.0 | 0.5–1.0 | 14 | 40 | 20 |
| V | 4.0 | 1.0–1.5 | 16 | 50 | 25 |
| VI | 5.0 | 1.0–1.5 | 20 | 60 | 30 |

Classify patient with erythroderma as Type I skin.

## NBUVB dosing

| Skin type | Initial dose (mJ) | Increase (mJ) | Estimated goal ~4× initial dose |
| --- | --- | --- | --- |
| I | 130 | 15 | 520 |
| II | 220 | 25 | 880 |
| III | 260 | 40 | 1040 |
| IV | 330 | 45 | 1320 |
| V | 350 | 60 | 1400 |
| VI | 400 | 65 | 1600 |
| Vitiligo | 170 | 30 | Unknown |

## PUVA

- *Absolute contraindication*: Photosensitivity (lupus, albinism, XP), porphyria, pregnancy, lactation.
- *Relative contraindication*: Melanoma or family history of melanoma, personal history of non-melanoma skin ca, prior radiation, arsenic, photosensitizing meds (simply note use then "start slow and go slow"), severe cardiac/liver/renal disease, pemphigus/pemphigoid, immunosuppression, inability to understand details of tx.
- *Photosensitizing meds*: Griseofulvin, phenothiazine, nalidixic acid, salicylanilides, sulfonamides, TCN, thiazides, MTX, retinoids.

### Choosing appropriate patients

- Usually reserved for severe disease or patients unresponsive to UVB
- Good choice for patients whose disease will likely require maintenance (i.e. long history of severe psoriasis or CTCL).
- Good choice for thicker plaques, palmar/plantar disease, or erythematous/pustular disease due to deeper penetration.
- Better in darker skin (Type III or above).

### General precautions

- *Eye protection*: It is absolutely necessary on day of treatment
- *General sun protection*: Patients need to be more cautious with sun exposure to avoid risk of burning, worsening photoaging, and

"hardening" their skin with natural sunlight which makes them less responsive to phototherapy
• *Genital coverage for men*: Wear athletic support or sock over genitals. No full coverage underwear as most psoriasis and CTCL patients have involvement of their buttocks

**8-METHOXYPSORALEN** = Oxsoralen Ultra 10 mg caps
**Dose 0.6 mg/kg**
Take 1.5–2 h before treatment with food/milk.
**Side effects:** Nausea, anorexia, dizziness, HA, malaise, phototoxic reaction

> *Nausea*: decrease dose by 10 mg, take with food, rarely anti-emetics. *Treatment for nausea*: Divide dose, take with food.
> *PUVA Burns*: UVB burns present within 12–24 h, PUVA burns are delayed 48 h but can be as late as 96 h. Prevent repeat burns by careful questioning of patients by phototherapy nurses, patient education, and always skipping a day between tx (i.e. MWF) to give a burn time to present itself.
> *PUVA Itch*: It can be intractable and can last for weeks. Make sure patient's skin is hydrated and then back off on light as soon as patients complain (see below). This itch usually does NOT respond to anti-pruritic agents.

**Long-term side effects:** Photoaging, non-melanoma skin ca, potential for increase melanoma risk, cataracts (prevent with eye protection), genital cancer (shield)

**Clearing schedule**
• Usually takes 10 treatments to tell if responsive
• If no response, increase additional 0.5 J/tx
• If after 15 treatments and no response, increase dose by 10 mg
• Correctable causes for non-response: missed tx, inadequate oxsoralen concentration in the skin (patient not pigmenting), patient not taking med, or taking medication which increases liver enzyme (i.e. carbamazepine, phenytoin)
• Takes 25–30 treatments to achieve control (3 months)

**Maintenance schedule**
• Once clearance is achieved, maintain dose but space out visits (i.e. qwk × 4, then qow × 4, then q mo)

**Missed treatment**

| | |
|---|---|
| Missed 1 tx | Hold dose as previous |
| Missed >1 tx | Decrease by 0.5 J for each tx missed |
| Missed >3 tx | May need to return to starting dose |

**Pruritus protocol (i.e. PUVA itch)**

| | |
|---|---|
| Mild | Use moisturizer, increase UVA by 0.5 J |
| Severe | Stop UVA for a few days to see if light induced. (If yes, then decrease by 2–3 J) |
| Intractable | Localized: shield area, keep UVA constant |
| | Generalized: Stop tx until clear, then resume 2–3 J below pruritic dose |

**Erythema protocol**

| | |
|---|---|
| None | Increase per skin type |
| Minimal | (Erythema occurs but resolves by next appointment) |
| | Hold UVA dose content, do not increase until resolve |
| Marked | (Erythema occurs and does not resolve by next appointment) |
| | Stop tx until erythema resolve |
| Edema | Do not treat |

# Washington University Dermatology Toxic Epidermal Necrolysis (TEN) Protocol

Based on current published data and reviews on the treatment of TEN. Courtesy of Dr. Amy Cheng and Dr. Grace Bandow

## Diagnosis of TEN

### History

- Fever, cough, sore throat, constitutional sxs may occur 1–3 days prior to rash.
- Burning eyes, photophobia, burning/painful skin starts on torso/face.
- Drug exposure 1–3 weeks prior.

### Physical Exam

- Initial lesions are poorly defined macules with dusky centers/bullae with surrounding erythema, that is two zones of color, not a classic target with three zones.
- Full thickness necrosis leads to Nikolsky sign (lateral shearing) and wrinkled paper skin. Detachment occurs in areas of pressure (palms/soles). Denuded areas are oozing dark red.
- Mucosal involvement: urethra, GI, vulva, anus, eyes, mouth, tracheobronchial tree.

**Common culprits:** Sulfa, PCN, quinolones, cephalosporins, carbamazepine, phenobarbital, phenytoin, valproic acid, NSAIDs, allopurinol, lamotrigine, HAART.

## Workup for suspected TEN
- CBC, CMP, LFTs, albumin, lytes, baseline CXR.
- Skin biopsy for frozen section and H&E, IgA.
- Do not need to culture the skin unless you think they are septic.

## Triage algorithm for TEN patients
1. What is the total body surface area affected?
   A. <10% TBSA (including areas of erythema)    →Continue to Step 2
   B. >10% TBSA    →Continue to Step 4
2. Is the patient:
   A. <10 year old or >50 year old    →Continue to Step 4
   B. Between 11 and 49 year old    →Continue to Step 3
3. Does the patient have underlying medical problems?
   A. Yes (CHF, Renal, Pulm, Diabetes, Others)    →Continue to Step 4
   B. No → OK To: Manage on the Floor with Wound Care Consult
      Reevaluate Daily: If progresses or needs more extensive wound care,
      then transfer to ICU for care. Wound care alone justifies ICU transfer
4. ICU Care: (If no Burn Unit is readily available) Transfer to Unit based on
   underlying concerns
   A. Significant Medical Co-morbidities:
      – MICU
      – Wound Care Consult
   B. No-Significant Medical Co-morbidities:
      – SICU
      – Wound Care Consult

## Treatment for all TEN patients
1. Start IVIg immediately. Check IgA levels first, but do not wait for
   results to start treatment because it can take several days. See
   Appendix I below for starting IVIg.
2. Identify and STOP ALL non-vital medications.
3. Consider additional dialysis if needed for patients with ESRD.
4. Consultations:
   a. Ophthalmology. 40% of TEN survivors have disabling ocular
      symptoms including scarring and blindness.
   b. Nutrition. Massive protein loss may require enteral or parenteral
      feeding.
   c. Consult additional services (pulmonary, GI, urology, OB-GYN for
      mucosal involvement) prn system involvement.
5. Evaluate percentage of TBSA affected daily.
6. Evaluate mucosal involvement daily: eyes, GU, pulmonary.
7. Wound care:
   a. Swab mouth, nose, involved orifices with saline daily. Apply
      mupirocin ointment. Non-sulfa antibiotic ointments and eye drops

are usually recommended by ophtholmology. They should follow daily to break up synechiae.

b. Vaseline with vaseline gauze to denuded skin (alternatives: Exudry, Telfa or Acticoat dressings, kept wet with sterile saline). Vaseline on intact blisters. Leave necrotic intact epidermis in place. Leave normal skin alone. Do not use Silvadene! (It has a sulfa moiety.)

8. Monitor electrolytes, albumin, fluids and replace accordingly – patients lose a lot transdermally but can get overloaded with high volume of IVIg if CHF or renal failure.

9. Warming to combat massive heat loss.

10. Avoid taping, debridement, or skin trauma.

11. Prophylactic antibiotics are not recommended: may cause worsening drug reactions and increase resistance.

12. Prednisone is controversial. Questionable benefit of short course in early TEN. Most do not recommend because of increased infections and mortality in septic patients.

13. Output follow up: ophtho, GI, GYN, urology, etc. based on involvement for evaluation and tx of strictures, phimosis, synechiae, etc.

## Appendix I: American Burn Association Burn Center Referral Criteria

1. second or third degree burns >10% body surface area in patients <10 year old or >50 year old.

2. second and third degree burns >20% TBSA any age group.

3. Significant burns of face, hands, feet, genitalia.

4. Full-thickness burns that involve more than 5% of TBSA in other age groups.

5. Significant electric injury, including lightning injury.

6. Significant chemical injury.

7. Lesser burn injuries w/ associated inhalation injury, concomitant mechanical trauma or significant pre-existing medical disorders.

8. Burn injury in patients who will require special social, emotional, or long-term rehab support.

## Appendix II: SCORTEN Score (Risk factors for death in both SJS and TEN)

One point for each factor:

> Age > 40
> Malignancy
> Heart rate > 120
> BUN > 10 mmol/l
> Serum glucose > 250 mg/dl
> Bicarb < 20 mEq/l
> Initial BSA involved with epidermal detachment > 10%

Mortality rates are as follows:

$$
\begin{array}{ll}
\text{SCORTEN } 0\text{–}1 & = 3.2\% \\
\text{SCORTEN } 2 & = 12.1\% \\
\text{SCORTEN } 3 & = 35.3\% \\
\text{SCORTEN } 4 & = 58.3\% \\
\text{SCORTEN } > 5 & = 90\%
\end{array}
$$

## Appendix III: IVIg

Avoid in patients with known IgA deficiency and anaphylaxis to previous IVIg infusions.

Need monitored bed for administration (especially if IgA levels not available, frequently test not available over the weekend at many hospitals).

*Gammagard* is the IgA-deficient brand that needs to be specially ordered for IgA deficient or unknown status patients.

Dose 3 g/kg/total over 3–4 days as tolerated (slow infusion rate if necessary for ESRD or CHF patients; some cases demonstrated benefit w/2 g or 1.5 g)
Write orders to dose the infusion rate at

> 30 cc per hour × 1 h
> 60 cc per hour × 2nd h
> 120 cc per hour after that
> For example     70 kg patient would get 70 g/d
>                 × 3 days
> 70 g is about 1600 cc of Gammar P
> This would take ~12.5 h to infuse.

DRUGS AND THERAPIES

## Appendix IV: References

1. Magina S, Lisboa C, Leal V *et al.* Dermatological and ophthalmological sequels in toxic epidermal necrolysis. *Dermatology* 2003; 207:33–6.
2. Freedberg IM, Eisen A *et al. Fitzpatrick's Dermatology in General Medicine.* 2003.
3. Bologna JL, Jorizzo JL *et al. Dermatology.* 2003.
4. Townsend C, Evers MB. *Sabiston Textbook of Surgery.* 2004.
5. Lissia M, Figus A, Rubino C. Intravenous immunoglobulins and plasmapheresis combined treatment in patients with severe toxic epidermal necrolysis: preliminary report. *Br J Plast Surg.* 2005; 58:504–10.
6. Tan AW, Thong BY *et al.* High-dose immunoglobulins in the treatment to toxic epidermal necrolysis: an Asian series. *J Dermatol.* 2005; 32:1–6.
7. Nassif A, Moslehi H *et al.* Evaluation of the potential role of cytokines in toxic epidermal necrolysis. *J Invest Dermatol.* 2004; 123:850–55.
8. Chave TA, Mortimer MJ, Sladden MJ *et al.* Toxic epidermal necrolysis: current evidence, practical management and future directions. *Brit J Dermatol.* 2005; 153: 241–45.

# Index